The double burden of malnutrition
Case studies from six developing countries

84

FOOD AND AGRICULTURE ORGANIZATION OF THE UNITED NATIONS
Rome, 2006

ISBN 92-5-105489-4

CONTENTS

Foreword   v
Acroynms   vii

Assessment of the double burden of malnutrition in six case study countries   1

The double burden of malnutrition in China, 1989 to 2000   21

Assessment of dietary changes and their health implications   43
in countries facing the double burden of malnutrition: Egypt, 1980 to 2005

The double burden of malnutrition in India   99

Food consumption, food expenditure, anthropometric status and   161
nutrition-related diseases in Mexico

Dietary changes and their health implications in the Philippines   205

Dietary changes and the health transition in South Africa: 259
implications for health policy

Trends towards overweight in lower- and middle-income countries: 305
some causes and economic policy options

Workshop recommendations   327

Foreword

There is growing recognition of the emergence of a "double burden" of malnutrition with under- and overnutrition occurring simultaneously among different population groups in developing countries. This phenomenon is not limited to upper-income developing countries, but is occurring across the globe in countries with very different cultures and dietary customs. There is accumulating evidence that when economic conditions improve, obesity and diet-related non-communicable diseases may escalate in countries with high levels of undernutrition. There is also evidence to indicate that undernutrition *in utero* and early childhood may predispose individuals to greater susceptibility to some chronic diseases.

Historically the menu of programmes to address nutrition problems in developing countries has focused primarily on reducing undernutrition and has met with varying degrees of success. There are only a handful of programmes, mainly in high-income countries, which have had some success in reducing the burgeoning growth of overweight, obesity and associated non-communicable diseases. It is now being understood that more aggressive strategies are needed and that attention to both under- and overnutrition should be incorporated into nutrition action plans and programmes.

This publication is the result of a multi-country effort to assess the extent of the double burden of malnutrition in six case study countries and identify programmes currently in place or needed to prevent and manage nutritional problems. The work represents ongoing efforts by FAO to document changes in diet and monitor population-level nutritional status and the prevalence of diet-related non-communicable diseases.

The case studies presented in this publication were prepared using existing secondary data in China, Egypt, India, Mexico, the Philippines and South Africa. Collaborating institutes include the Chinese Center for Disease Control and Prevention, the National Nutrition Institute, Egypt, the Nutrition Foundation of India, the National Institute of Public Health, Mexico, the Food and Nutrition Research Institute, the Philippines and the Medical Research Council, South Africa. The project was supported financially by the FAO-Norway Partnership Programme.

For many of those involved in preparing the case studies, this was a valuable opportunity to reassess priority nutrition problems and review programmes in place to address the problems. Some of the case study countries were already systematically monitoring patterns of dietary intake, nutritional status and risk factors related to non-communicable diseases, while others acknowledged a need to improve monitoring efforts. Most recognized the need to intensify efforts to prevent and manage overweight and obesity and disease processes associated with overnutrition, while maintaining efforts to eliminate undernutrition and micronutrient deficiencies.

Kraisid Tontisirin
Director
Nutrition and Consumer Protection Division

Aknowledgements

Special thanks go to all of the authors whose papers appear in this publication. Particular acknowledgement is due to Dr Osman Galal, School of Public Health, University of California Los Angeles for his considerable assistance and contribution to the Egypt case study. We would also like to thank Terri Ballard, Ruth Charrondiere and Cristina Lopriore, Food and Agriculture Organization; Pirjo Pietinen, Department of Nutrition, National Public Health Institute, Finland; Dr David Sanders and Thandi Puoane, School of Public Health, University of the Western Cape and Dr Veronica Tuffrey, Centre for Public Health Nutrition, University of Westminster for their assistance in reviewing one or more of the papers in this publication.

24HDR	24-hour dietary recall
AE	adult equivalent
AIS	acquired immune deficiency syndrome
ARC	Agriculture Research Centre (Egypt)
ASR	age-standardized incidence rate
ASSA	Actuarial Society of South Africa
BHS	barangay health station (the Philippines)
BMD	bone mass density
BMI	body mass index
BP	blood pressure
CAPMAS	Central Agency for Public Mobilization and Statistics (Egypt)
CED	chronic energy deficiency
CHD	coronary heart diseases
CHNS	China Economic, Population, Nutrition and Health Survey
CU	consumption unit
CVD	cardiovascular disease
DALY	disability-adjusted life year
DES	dietary energy supply
DLHS	District-Level Household Survey (India)
DR-NCD	diet-related non-communicable disease
DWCD	Department of Women and Child Development (China)
EDHS	Egypt Demographic and Health Survey

EHDR	Egypt Human Development Report
EMR	East Mediterranean Region
FAO	Food and Agriculture Organization of the United Nations
FBG	fasting blood glucose
FCT	Food Composition Table (the Philippines)
FHSIS	Field Health Service Information System (the Philippines)
FNRI-DOST	Food and Nutrition Research Institute, Department of Science and Technology (the Philippines)
FTRI	Food Technology Research Institute (Egypt)
GDP	gross domestic product
GDI	gender development index
GNP	gross national product
HCV	hepatitis C virus
HDI	human development index
HES	Health Examination Survey (Egypt)
HIV/AIDS	human immunodeficiency virus/acquired immunodeficiency syndrome
HPE	Health Profile of Egypt
HSRC	Human Sciences Research Council (South Africa)
IARC	International Agency for Research on Cancer
ICCIDD	International Council for Control of Iodine Deficiency Disorders
ICD	International Classification of Diseases
ICMR	Indian Council of Medical Research
ICN	International Conference on Nutrition (Rome, December 1992, FAO and WHO)

IDA	iron-deficiency anaemia
IDD	iodine deficiency disorder
IFPRI	International Food Policy Research Institute
IGT	impaired glucose tolerance
IIPS	International Institute of Population Sciences
INEGI	National Institute of Informatics, Statistics and Geography (Mexico)
INP	India Nutrition Profile
ISCC	inter-sectoral coordinating committee/council
IUGR	intrauterine growth retardation
LAC	Latin America and the Caribbean (region)
LBW	low birth weight
LPE	Lipid Profile among Egyptians
MCDS	Mexican Chronic Diseases Survey
MDG	Millennium Development Goal
MECC	Middle East Cancer Consortium
MHIES	Mexican Household Income and Expenditure Survey
MHS	Mexican Health Survey
MISS	Mexican Institute of Social Security
MNE	multinational enterprise
MNS	Mexican Nutrition Survey
MOHP	Ministry of Health and Population (Egypt)
MPCE	monthly per capita expenditure
MTPPAN	Medium-Term Philippine Plan of Action for Nutrition

NAP	National Agricultural Policy (India)
NCD	non-communicable disease
NCHS	National Center for Health Statistics
NCI	National Cancer Institute (Egypt)
NCPR	National Cancer Registry Programme (India)
NFCS	National Food Consumption Survey (South Africa)
NFHS	National Family Health Survey (India)
NFI	Nutrition Foundation of India
NGO	non-governmental organization
NHP	National Hypertension Project (Egypt)
NIN	National Institute of Nutrition (India)
NNC	National Nutrition Council (the Philippines)
NNI	National Nutrition Institute (Egypt)
NNMB	National Nutrition Monitoring Board (India)
NNS	National Nutrition Survey (China, the Philippines)
NPNL	non-pregnant, non-lactating
NSSO	National Sample Survey Organization (India)
OECD	Organisation for Economic Co-operation and Development
PA	physical activity
PAHO	Pan-American Health Organization
PBMI	percentile body mass index for age
PDS	public distribution system
PEM	protein-calorie malnutrition

PHS	Philippine Health Statistics
PPP	purchasing power parity
PPY	percentage points a year
RDA	recommended dietary allowance
RENI	recommended energy and nutrient intake
RGI	Registrar General of India
RHU	rural health unit (the Philippines)
RNI	recommended nutrient intake
SADHS	South African Demographic and Health Survey
SAMRC	South African Medical Research Council
SANBDS	South African National Burden of Disease Study
SAVACG	South African Vitamin A Consultative Group
SR	serum retinol
STD	sexually transmitted disease
TB	tuberculosis
TGR	total goitre rate
TPDS	targeted public distribution system
U5MR	under-five mortality rate
UIE	urinary iodine excretion
UNDP	United Nations Development Programme
UNESCAP	United Nations Economic and Social Commission for Asia and the Pacific
UNICEF	United Nations Children's Fund
UNU	United Nations University

USDA   United States Department of Agriculture

VAD   vitamin A deficiency

WC   waist circumference

WFP   World Food Programme

WHO   World Health Organization

WHR   waist-to-hip ratio

YLL   year of life lost

YRBS   Youth Risk Behaviour Study (South Africa)

Assessment of the double burden of malnutrition in six case study countries

G. Kennedy, G. Nantel and P. Shetty, Nutrition Planning, Assessment and Evaluation Service, Food and Agriculture Organization of the United Nations

INTRODUCTION

The concepts of nutrition transition and the double burden of malnutrition have been introduced over the past decade. There is documentation of the occurrence of each in many developing countries that are in rapid economic transition (Shetty and Gopalan, 1998; Shetty and McPherson, 1997; *Public Health Nutrition*, 2002; Gillespie and Haddad, 2003) This paper draws on evidence from six countries (China, Egypt, India, Mexico, the Philippines and South Africa) to document the nutrition transition and the double burden by summarizing the trends in dietary changes and accompanying changes in nutritional status and disease burden experienced in the past 20 years. Many contributory factors have influenced these processes, including urbanization, demographic shifts, sedentary lifestyles and the liberalization of markets. In-depth discussion of these drivers has been reviewed extensively in recent literature (FAO, 2004; *Development Policy Review*, 2003).

Double burden of malnutrition

The double burden of malnutrition refers to the dual burden of under- and overnutrition occurring simultaneously within a population. Historically, undernutrition has been associated with higher prevalence of infectious diseases; as populations move into epidemiologic and demographic transition, increases in overweight and obesity begin to appear, while undernutrition and infectious disease become past problems. Today, the burden of disease and malnutrition does not fit neatly into the classic stages of transition, but reflects a modified pattern referred to as the protracted-polarized model, where infectious and chronic diseases coexist over long periods of time (Frenk *et al.,* 1989 in Chopra, 2004a). Evidence of this has been documented in countries as diverse as China (Cook and Dummer, 2003) and South Africa (Chopra, 2004a).

The protracted-polarized model represents a change in the documented pattern of the epidemiologic transition that occurred in Europe and North America in the nineteenth century. The classic pattern of "epidemiologic transition" constitutes a shift from high mortality and fertility patterns to lower mortality followed by lower fertility. Improvements in water and sanitation, and more effective public health services such as immunization result in an associated shift in disease burden from high rates of infectious disease to increasing non-communicable disease (NCD). In tandem with this shift, life expectancy increases and the demographic profile shifts towards lower child-to-adult dependency ratios and greater numbers of elderly in the population, with NCD becoming more predominant as longevity increases.

Underweight and obesity are both among the top ten leading risk factors for the global burden of disease (WHO, 2002). The current double burden of malnutrition seen in many developing countries is brought about by a coupling of risk factors. Progress in improving water and sanitation systems has been slow and the development of sound public health systems weak, thwarting efforts to reduce undernutrition. At the same time, increasing urbanization and changing dietary patterns and lifestyles are contributing to a rapid rise in overweight and diet-related chronic diseases.

Although there seems to be clear evidence of a double burden of malnutrition and disease at the global level, it is not clear how critical the issue is at the national level and to what extent developing countries need to concern themselves with the seemingly incongruous problems of under- and overnutrition and infectious and chronic disease. Some countries, such as South Africa and the United Republic of Tanzania, report no decline in numbers of cases of infectious diseases including tuberculosis (TB), malaria and HIV/AIDS, while the incidences of coronary heart disease (CHD), diabetes and stroke are on the rise (Kitange, no date). The protracted-polarized model of epidemiologic transition has been documented in South Africa, with poor people suffering increased mortality from infectious, chronic and accidental/violent causes (Chopra, 2004b). Regarding malnutrition, there is increasing documentation of rising rates of overweight and obesity among children and adults, and slow progress in reducing undernutrition, particularly in children under five years of age. This paper attempts to summarize and evaluate the problem of the double burden of malnutrition and disease as reported in the six country case studies, and discusses potential options for addressing both sides of the problem.

Characteristics of the nutrition transition

The nutrition transition refers to changes in the composition of the diet, usually accompanied by changes in physical activity levels. Popkin (2003) has characterized the nutrition transition into three stages: receding famine, degenerative disease, and behavioural change. In the first stage, diets are primarily derived from plant-based food sources, tend to be monotonous and are based more on home food production that requires high levels of physical activity related to planting, harvesting and processing. The second stage encompasses dietary changes that generally include more animal source foods, higher intakes of fat – both vegetable oils and saturated fat from animal products – increased use of sugar and other sweeteners, and higher reliance on food produced and processed outside the home or immediate community. Mandatory physical activity to produce food and procure water and fuelwood, including agriculture-based labour and household labour, is often also reduced. The final stage involves a shift to a diet with less saturated fat and decreasing reliance on processed foods. Typically, this stage encompasses increased intakes of whole grains, fruits and vegetables and decreased consumption of saturated fat, with a preference for animal source foods with lower saturated fat content (fish and poultry). Intensive physical labour related to agricultural production is not reintroduced, but non-obligatory physical activity is increased.

In which populations is the nutrition transition occurring?

The diets of most of the world's population lie somewhere between the first and second stages of nutrition transition, while subsections of populations in North America and northern and southern Europe may be moving into the third stage. In most of the case study countries there is evidence of a rapid movement from primarily plant-based diets to diets with greater proportions of energy derived from meat, milk products, animal fats and vegetable oils.

Urban populations are typically the first to begin incorporating more fats, animal source foods and processed products into the diet. Dietary changes are not however limited to urban areas, nor to wealthier population groups. Research by Mendez, Du and Popkin (2004) on dietary transition in China used a scale of "urbanicity", which considered access to health care, housing, communications and transport in urban and rural areas. They found increasing intakes of animal source foods and edible oils in low urbanicity urban areas and more urbanized rural areas. In low-income areas of Brazil, processed bakery products, processed meat products, sweets and soft drinks were among the most commonly consumed foods (Sawaya, Martins and Martins, 2004). Falling prices are another stimulus for dietary changes. A high-fat diet is much more affordable today than it was 30 years ago (Popkin, 2002). In China, over a period of six years in the 1990s, the relative prices of fish, pork and oil all decreased (Mendez, Du and Popkin, 2004).

KEY DEVELOPMENT INDICATORS AND LINKAGES TO THE DOUBLE BURDEN OF MALNUTRITION IN THE CASE STUDY COUNTRIES

Economic, health and social indicators for each of the case study countries are presented in Table 1. Rapid urbanization has been linked to dietary change and obesity in developing countries (Mendez and Popkin, 2004). There is a wide range in the proportions of urban population among the case study countries, with Mexico being the most urbanized and India the least. Low birth weight (less than 2 500 g) has been identified as a risk factor for developing NCDs in later life (Barker, 2004). Among the case study countries, India has the highest percentage of infants born with low birth weight, followed by the Philippines and South Africa. The demographic transition, particularly the ageing of the population and longer life expectancy, can also contribute to increased incidence of NCD. Of the case study countries, China appears to be ageing the fastest, with the largest percentage of adults aged 65 years and older and the smallest of children up to 14 years. High adult literacy rates and improvements in water and sanitation contribute to decreasing undernutrition, particularly among children under five years of age. Mexico, the Philippines and China have adult literacy rates of more than 90 percent, infant mortality rates of less than 35 per 1 000 live births, and life expectancy of more than 70 years. HIV prevalence is a grave public health concern in South Africa and is reflected in this country having the lowest life expectancies for both men and women.

TABLE 1
Economic, health and social development indicators

Indicator	China	Egypt	India	Mexico	Philippines	South Africa
Annual population growth rate (%)	1.2	2.2	1.9	2.0	2.3	2.0
Percentage urban population	37.7	42.1	28.1	75.2	60.2	56.5
Population aged 0–14 years (%)	23.7	35.2	33.3	32.8	36.6	33.2
Population aged ≥ 65 years (%)	7.1	4.6	5.1	5.0	3.7	3.9
Infants with low birth weight (%)	6	12	30	9	20	15
Infant mortality rate (per 1 000 live births)	31	35	67	24	29	52
HIV prevalence (%)	.01	< 0.1	0.4-1.3	0.3	< 0.1	21.5
Life expectancy (overall)	71	68.8	63.9	73.4	70	47.7
Life expectancy (female)	73.2	70.8	64.4	76.3	71.9	51.9
Life expectancy (male)	68.8	66.6	63.1	70.3	67.9	46
Adult literacy (%)	90.9	55.6	61.3	90.5	92.6	86
Population with access to improved sanitation (%)[1]	40	98	28	74	83	87
Population with access to an improved water source (%)[2]	75	97	84	88	86	86
GDP per capita (US$)	989	1 354	487	6 320	975	2 299
GDP per capita (PPP US$)	4 850	3 810	2 670	8 970	4 170	10 070
Population with less than US$1/day (%)	16.6	3.1	34.7	9.9	14.6	7.1

[1] Access to safe sanitation is defined as access to adequate excreta disposal facilities such as a connection to a sewer or septic tank system, a pour-flush latrine, simple pit latrine or ventilated improved pit latrine. An excreta disposal system is considered adequate if it is private or shared and if it can prevent human, animal and insect contact with excreta.
[2] Access to safe water is defined as reasonable access to any of the following water supplies used for drinking: household connection, public standpipe, borehole, protected well, protected spring and rainwater collection.
Source: UNDP, 2004.

REVIEW OF TRENDS IN FOOD AVAILABLE FOR CONSUMPTION IN THE SIX CASE STUDY COUNTRIES
Trends in food availability using FAOSTAT data
The Food and Agriculture Organization of the United Nations (FAO) maintains a comprehensive database of food production from 1960 to the present. Country-specific food balance sheets provide information on the supply and utilization of many different commodities. Factors accounting for food supply include production, imports, stock changes and exports. The per capita supply of energy, protein and fats for many food commodities can be calculated by extrapolating from these data.

When analysing FAO food supply statistics it is important to consider the application of the per capita measurements. These figures are based on population totals for all ages and represent *average, not actual,* per capita availability. Actual food availability may vary by region, socio-economic level and season. Certain difficulties are encountered when estimating trade, production and stock changes on an annual scale. In order to reduce these errors, three-year averages should be calculated. This paper uses three-year averages for 1970–1972, 1980–1982, 1990–1992 and 2000–2002.

Trends in availability of dietary energy
Between 1970 and the present, per capita dietary energy supply increased in all the case study countries (Figure 1), although rates of growth were different. The largest absolute increase in caloric availability was in Egypt, and the largest percentage increase over the period from 1970–1972 to 2000–2002 occurred in China (49 percent). Over the same period, Egypt and the Philippines experienced increases of 41 and 30 percent, respectively.

The slowest growth in per capita dietary energy supply over the past 30 years was in South Africa. However, of the six countries analysed, South Africa started with the highest per capita dietary energy supply and its still remains higher than India's and the Philippines'.

FIGURE 1
Trends in dietary energy availability, 1970 to 2000

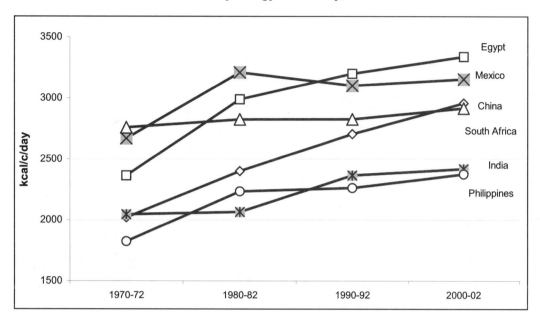

Commodity trends

Food availability and the percentages of dietary energy derived from basic food groups were calculated for 1970–1972 and 2000–2002 (Tables 2 to 4). Per capita supply of cereals and starchy staples has increased in all but one of the countries, but their percentage contribution to total energy supply has generally declined. Legumes, pulses and nuts have mainly remained stable or declined in terms of both quantity and percentage of dietary energy supplied. Oils, fats and animal products have increased in all case study countries, with the exception of fats/oils in Egypt. Fruits and vegetables have increased in most countries, as has percentage of energy from fruits and vegetables. The World Cancer Research Fund (1997) recommends that at least 7 percent of dietary energy be supplied from fruits and vegetables and, based on food balance sheet data, this goal would be achievable (assuming equitable distribution) in three countries. Sugar and sweeteners increased in all countries except South Africa, but the proportion of energy derived from sugar has not increased as dramatically as those from animal source foods and oil.

TABLE 2
Trends in food supply of different commodities (kg/capita/year), 1970–1972 and 2000–2002

Food group	China		Egypt		India		Mexico		Philippines		South Africa	
	1970	2000	1970	2000	1970	2000	1970	2000	1970	2000	1970	2000
Cereals, roots and tubers	266	251	185	257	164	179	179	192	142	168	195	215
Legumes, pulses and nuts	12	10	12	17	22	19	21	17	5	7	5	6
Oils and fats	3	11	10	8	5	12	8	13	5	7	10	14
Meat, fish, poultry	15	80	15	40	7	11	49	74	51	60	46	51
Milk	2	11	34	50	33	64	85	114	17	20	84	53
Eggs	2	17	1	2	0.5	2	6	16	3	6	4	6
Vegetables	45	246	130	183	44	69	33	57	66	62	46	43
Fruit	5	45	38	92	25	38	81	116	78	100	35	37
Sugar and sweeteners	3	7	48	75	29	38	37	49	22	30	40	33
Other	2	27	2	3	2	34	31	53	14	18	74	81

TABLE 3
**Percentage of dietary energy supply from major food groups, 1970–1972
and 2000–2002**

Food group	China		Egypt		India		Mexico		Philippines		South Africa	
	1970	2000	1970	2000	1970	2000	1970	2000	1970	2000	1970	2000
Cereals, roots and tubers	82.1	57.7	66.8	64.8	67.6	60.8	54.9	46.8	59.0	56.1	54.7	59.6
Legumes, pulses and nuts	5.3	3.5	4.5	4.6	9.2	6.2	7.5	5.1	1.3	1.9	1.7	2.0
Oils and fats	2.9	8.7	9.4	5.9	5.8	11.6	6.6	9.0	6.6	6.9	7.9	12.1
Meat, fish, poultry	4.8	15.4	2.5	3.7	1.1	1.4	6.0	9.9	10.7	11.2	8.8	8.6
Milk	0.2	0.7	1.9	2.2	3.0	4.2	4.9	5.4	1.2	1.0	4.5	3.0
Eggs	0.4	2.3	0.2	0.3	0.1	0.2	0.8	1.8	0.7	1.1	0.5	0.8
Vegetables	1.7	5.2	3.6	3.3	1.4	1.9	0.7	1.2	2.7	2.0	1.3	1.3
Fruit	0.3	1.8	3.0	4.7	1.5	2.0	3.3	3.6	5.5	5.6	1.4	1.5
Sugar and sweeteners	1.4	2.2	10.5	10.1	9.5	10.2	13.6	15.0	10.4	11.7	14.1	11.5
Other	0.7[1]	2.4[1]	0.3	0.4	0.8	1.4	1.7	2.2	1.9	2.6	5.1	5.4

[1] In China, the majority of the "other" category represents alcoholic beverages.

In terms of qualitative changes to the diet, China, India and Mexico exhibit the same pattern of declining per capita intakes of cereals and legumes and pulses and nuts, and increasing intakes of all the other food groups (Table 4). South Africa exhibits the most widely divergent pattern of increasing cereal and pulse intakes and decreasing intakes of meat, fish and poultry and sugars and sweeteners. Per capita supply of oils and fats has risen in all the countries except Egypt.

TABLE 4
Direction of the shift in percentage dietary energy from food groups, 1970–2000

Food group	China	Egypt	India	Mexico	Philippines	South Africa
Cereals, roots and tubers	⇓	⇓	⇓	⇓	⇓	↑
Legumes, pulses and nuts	⇓	↑	⇓	⇓	↑	↑
Oils and fats	↑	⇓	↑	↑	↑	↑
Meat, fish, poultry	↑	↑	↑	↑	↑	⇓
Milk	↑	↑	↑	↑	⇓	⇓
Eggs	↑	↑	↑	↑	↑	↑
Vegetables	↑	⇓	↑	↑	⇓	–
Fruit	↑	↑	↑	↑	↑	↑
Sugar and sweeteners	↑	⇓	↑	↑	↑	⇓
Other	↑	↑	↑	↑	↑	↑

Shaded arrows highlight declining trend.

FIGURE 2
Percentages of daily energy supply from fat, sugar and alcohol, 2000–2002

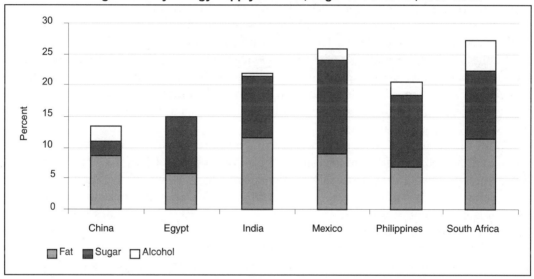

In Mexico and South Africa, more than one-quarter of the dietary energy available per capita is assigned to sugar, fat or alcohol (Figure 2). In three of the six countries analysed, sugars and sweeteners account for more than 10 percent of daily energy supply,[1] and in South Africa alcohol accounts for 5 percent of total dietary energy supply. WHO/FAO set a population nutrient intake goal of 15 to 30 percent of energy from fat (WHO/FAO, 2003). Extrapolating from FAOSTAT data, consumption of fat remains below the recommendation of 15 to 30 percent of total dietary energy intake in the case study countries.

---

[1] The food balance sheet data from which the figure is derived are not representative of actual food energy intake (food consumption) but indicate overall availability, and are generally thought to be an overestimation of actual consumption. This note of caution should be kept in mind when comparing the data with dietary goals.

DIETARY INTAKE DATA

Dietary intake survey data provide a more precise measure of the food consumption habits of households and individuals. These data can be used to look at differences in consumption by such characteristics as income, gender and place of residence.

Most of the dietary intake data from the case study countries come from nationally representative surveys that use a variety of methodologies and capture different age groups. Although it is not appropriate to compare these data with data from FAOSTAT, trends from both could be expected to go in the same direction, but this is not always the case.

Trends in dietary energy intake

Nearly all the case study countries show a trend towards declining energy intake (measured as kilocalories [kcal] per capita per day) (Table 5). This pattern has also been observed in other developing countries, leading to debate over the seemingly paradoxical increase in overweight and obesity at lower reported dietary energy intakes (Stubbs and Lee, 2004; Heini and Weinsier, 1999; Prentice and Jebb, 1995). The declining trend in dietary energy intake also contrasts with FAOSTAT data on total dietary energy availability. The real picture of what is happening appears to lie somewhere in between.

Some researchers support their intake data with the theory that there have been large declines in energy expenditure. Thus, increasing overweight is possible even at lower intakes because there is a greater energy imbalance (India case study). Others conclude that the declining trend reflects problems with data collection and the well-documented tendency of underreporting and systematic bias in intake measures, with heavier persons consistently underreporting more frequently than individuals of normal weight (Mexico case study; Livingstone and Black, 2003).

Both of these explanations may be true. Underreporting of energy intake is one of the major limitations of dietary intake studies (Livingstone and Black, 2003). At the same time, energy expenditures have fallen dramatically as a result of the modernization of agriculture and the increased use of motor vehicles, computers and labour-saving technologies. Recent evidence from the United States, where obesity rates have risen from 15 to 31 percent, has reversed the idea of the "American paradox" in which reported energy intakes were falling while obesity rates climbed. Reports for recent years show increases in reported energy intakes for both men and women (*MMWR Weekly*, 2004).

These findings highlight a need for better dietary intake instruments and training of the staff who carry out dietary intake studies, as well as a critical need for more and better information on energy expenditure. Information on energy expenditure is not routinely included in most national-level surveys. However, if energy expenditure is believed to be a major factor in rising obesity and risk of NCD, measurement instruments and collection of energy expenditure data need to be improved and supported.

TABLE 5
Trends in dietary energy intake from household surveys

	Kcal/c/day (year)	Kcal/c/day (year)	Kcal/c/day (year)	Trend	Comments
China	3 006 (1989)	2 635 (1993)	2 467 (2000)	Decreasing	Adults 20–59 yrs: 24-hr recall
Egypt		2 602 (2000)	1995 (2004)	Decreasing	Mothers: 24-hr recall
India	2 340 (1975–79)	2 283 (1988–90)	2 255 (2000–01)	Decreasing	Rural areas only
Mexico		1 624 (1988)	1 471 (1999)	Decreasing	Females 12–49 yrs: 24-hr recall
Philippines	1 808 (1982)	1 684 (1993)	1 905 (2003)	Increasing	1993 unusual year of economic crisis. One-day household food weighing. Total amount consumed by all household members
South Africa			1 128 (1999)		Children 1–6 yrs. Unweighted average of age groups 1–3 and 4–6

Energy density of the diet

One apparently consistent trend is that of increased energy density of diets. The percentage of energy derived from fat has increased in all the case study countries, especially China where it rose by nearly 10 percent over the past decade. The highest percentage of dietary energy from fat (31 percent) is in Mexico, and the lowest in India (14 percent). The low meat consumption in India is a likely explanation for this low figure.

TABLE 6
Trends in percentage of dietary energy from fat

	Percentage of energy from fat (year)			Trend	Comments
China	19.3 (1989)	22.2 (1993)	28.9 (2000)	Increasing	Adults
India	9 (1979)		14 (2001)	Increasing	Rural areas only, not all states
Mexico		25.8 (1988)	31.3 (1999)	Increasing	Females 12–49 yrs
Philippines	15 (1987)	15 (1993)	18 (2003)	Increasing	
South Africa	17 (1962)		25.8 (1999)	Increasing	Black schoolchildren in urban Gauteng

Trends in dietary intake by food group

FAOSTAT data are used to show changes in food intake in much of the initial work on the occurrence of a nutrition transition in developing countries (Popkin, 1994). There is fairly good concordance between commodity trends using FAOSTAT data and trends in consumption of different food groups using dietary intake data.

The five case study countries for which trend data on dietary intake by food group are available show much the same pattern of dietary changes. The main trends observed from intake data are:

- decreasing intakes of cereals, roots and tubers;
- decreasing intakes of legumes, nuts and seeds (except in China);

- no change or an increase in intakes of edible fats and oils;
- large increases in intakes of fish, meat and poultry (except in India);
- increasing intakes of sugars and sweets;
- increasing intakes of fruits and vegetables (except in rural China and the Philippines).

Beneficial and detrimental aspects of observed changes

The adverse effects of the observed patterns of dietary change, including the increases in saturated fat, cholesterol and dietary energy density, have been the subject of much recent literature, while the positive effects have largely been overlooked. Transition from a predominantly cereal-based diet to one that includes more meat and dairy products should have a positive impact on the intakes of high-quality protein and several micronutrients. In particular, intakes of vitamin A and iron, two of the most widespread micronutrient deficiencies worldwide, should show improvement.

The crossover from beneficial to detrimental is experienced when intakes of commodities (sugar, alcohol) or dietary components (saturated fat, salt) reach levels known to create disease risk factors. These levels have been reviewed recently in the WHO/FAO report on diet, nutrition and the prevention of chronic disease, which forms the basis for the population nutrient intake goals listed in Table 7 (WHO/FAO, 2003). The Philippines case study highlights the beneficial effects of the dietary changes, which are reflected by an increased proportion of people consuming the recommended percentages of energy from carbohydrates and fat. However, decreasing consumption of fruits and vegetables in the Philippines and China is reflected in lower percentages of the population with recommended intakes of these commodities (Table 7).

TABLE 7
Trends in achievement of population nutrient intake goals

Country	Year	% of population with 15–30% energy intake from fat	% of population with < 10% energy intake from free sugars	% of population with 55–75% energy intake from carbohydrate	% of population consuming ≥ 400g/day fruits and vegetables
China	1989	43.9	99.6	56.3	29.3
	2000	44.3	97.8	54.8	21.3
Mexico	1988	40.9		44.2	
	1999	39.6	97.4	44.3	9.3
Philippines	1993	37.6	94.3	53.0	11.5
	2003	46.2	92.1	57.9	8.2

The impact of changes in dietary patterns on micronutrient intake

Given the increasing intake of animal source foods, and in some countries the increased intake of fruits and vegetables, a trend towards improved intakes of micronutrients (particularly iron and vitamin A) could be expected. Data from Mexico, China and the Philippines indicate that there is a marginal positive trend towards increased consumption of iron in the diets of children (Table 8). Intakes of vitamin A also increased for children in the Philippines and China, while vitamin C intake decreased slightly in China but increased in the Philippines.

In the Philippines, adult intake of vitamin A has increased, but intakes of iron and vitamin C have not shown any change. In Mexico, adult intake of vitamin A has increased, but intake of iron has decreased.

The trends among children are encouraging, and indicate that dietary changes are having a positive impact on micronutrient intakes. Changes among adults are less dramatic, and do not indicate much of a positive trend, except in the case of vitamin A. Given the large increase in meat, fish and poultry consumption, an improvement in the iron intake of adults could be expected, but this is not observed. This seemingly contradictory pattern could be the result of:

• changes in consumption patterns within animal source foods – the Philippines consumes more pork, which has lower iron content than beef;
• revisions in food composition tables – again in the Philippines, where the tables now include more processed and canned fish products, which contain less iron than the values used previously.

TABLE 8
Percentage changes in intakes of iron, vitamin A and vitamin C

Country	Iron intake		Vitamin A intake		Vitamin C intake		Comments
	Children	Adults	Children	Adults	Children	Adults	
China	+ 3%		+ 4%		- 4%		1991 and 2000: children 2–5 yrs
Mexico		- 30%		+ 193%			1988 and 1993: females 12–49 yrs
Philippines	+ 3%	0	+ 35%	+ 16%	+ 28%	0	1993 and 2003: adults < 20 yrs, children 3–59 months (1993) and 6–59 months (2003)

TRENDS IN NUTRITIONAL ANTHROPOMETRY AND MICRONUTRIENT DEFICIENCIES AMONG CHILDREN AND ADULTS

Caution is needed regarding inter-country comparisons of data related to trends in nutritional anthropometry and micronutrient status of adults and children, because years, age groups and cut-off points may not be consistent. An effort was made to document such differences among the countries.

Trends in the nutritional status of children

Some progress in reducing child undernutrition has been achieved in all of the case study countries. The differing biological significance of anthropometric indicators of child growth is an important consideration in the current analysis. Stunting is a deficit in gain in length/height caused by deficits of a chronic nature. Wasting reflects short-term deprivation. Underweight is a combination of the two indicators, and has been termed "overall malnutrition". In situations of improving food security and improvements in health, water and sanitation, wasting prevalence should decrease rapidly. Stunting prevalence will be slower to improve, as the indicator is cumulative of past deprivation. Prevalence of underweight will usually decline at a faster rate than that of stunting.

China's progress between 1992 and 2000 has been the most rapid of the case study countries, with rates of stunting falling by 55 percent, from 31 to 14 percent, prevalence of underweight declining 42 percent, from 17.4 to 10 percent, and wasting decreasing by 35 percent, from 3.4 to 2.2 percent. Progress has been slower in all the other countries, with prevalence rates of stunting declining 38 percent in Egypt, 13 percent in the Philippines and 22 percent in Mexico (calculation of percentage changes was not possible for India and

South Africa because of differences in age groups). Reductions in the prevalence of underweight have been faster, with reductions of more than 30 percent in Egypt and Mexico, but only 5 percent in the Philippines. Wasting prevalence is now very low in Mexico and Egypt, but has increased in the Philippines from 5.6 to 6.5 percent.

The Center for Disease Control classifies rates of stunting of more than 30 percent, underweight of more than 20 percent and wasting of more than 10 percent as high prevalence (Epi-info Manual), indicating the level of public health significance. In India, all three nutritional anthropometric measures are still at high levels. In the Philippines, stunting and underweight are classified as high, while wasting has fallen to less than 10 percent. In the other case study countries, prevalence levels of stunting, underweight and wasting are classified as medium or low, at least at the nationally aggregated level. Nationally aggregated data hide disparities within regions and among different ethnic and socio-economic groups. For example, in poor, rural areas of China, stunting prevalence is 29 percent. In Mexico, it is more than 30 percent for children aged one to four years in rural areas, the south region and the lowest socio-economic bracket. Clearly, child growth remains an important public health problem.

The use of resources to ensure appropriate foetal and early child growth is justified, not only by the direct cost of undernutrition in terms of loss of life and diminished mental and physical potential, but also by more recent evidence of links between suboptimal foetal and early child growth and later problems with NCDs, particularly cardiovascular disease (CVD), type-2 diabetes and hypertension (Delisle, 2002).

Overweight in children is an emerging concern in many of the case study countries. In Egypt, prevalence of overweight among children is higher than prevalence of underweight and stunting, signalling an urgent need for Egypt to develop strategies to address this new problem. Increasing rates of overweight and obesity in children signal a very alarming trend. Half of the children who are obese at six years of age will go on to become obese adults (Georgetown University Center for Aging, 2002). Obesity is a risk factor for a range of chronic health problems, including type-2 diabetes, coronary heart disease, hypertension and some types of cancers (WHO, 1997). Early onset of obesity confers higher risk of developing these obesity-related chronic diseases.

TABLE 9
Trends in child anthropometry

	China		Egypt		India		Mexico		Philippines		South Africa	
	1992	2000	1990	2000	1991/ 1992	1998/ 1999	1988	1999	1989/ 1990	1998	1986	1999
Stunting	31.4	14.2	30.0	18.7	61.2	44.9	22.8	17.7	37.2	32.1	24.5	24.9
Under-weight	17.4	10.0	10.4	4.0	61.0	46.7	14.2	7.5	33.5	31.8	8.4	11.5
Wasting	3.4	2.2	3.5	2.5	18.9	15.7	6.0	2.0	5.6	6.5	1.8	3.4
Over-weight	4.3	2.6		11.7		2.2	3.7	5.3		1.0		6.2
Age range	0–4.99 yrs		0–4.99 yrs		0–4.99 yrs	0–2.99 yrs	0–4.99 yrs		0–4.99 yrs		0–4.99 yrs (rural only)	1–4.99[1] yrs

[1] Oversampling of low socio-economic groups
Source: WHO Global Database on Child Growth.

Trends in nutritional status of adults

The prevalences of under- and overweight among adults are strikingly different from those of children (Table 10). Overweight is more prevalent than underweight in adults in China, Egypt, Mexico and the Philippines. Overweight prevalence has been increasing in all countries, while underweight is on the decline.

Data presented at the national level hide large disparities in prevalence rates among regions and socio-economic classes. For example, in India, 23.5 percent of women 15 to 45 years of age living in urban areas have a body mass index (BMI) ≥ 25, and in Delhi more than 40 percent of women have a BMI above 25. In the highest socio-economic classes, obesity rates of more than 50 percent for females and 32 percent for males have been reported (Shetty, 2002). In Mexico, there are important differences between northern and southern regions; 31 percent of adults living in the north are obese (BMI > 30), compared with 24 percent in the south.

TABLE 10
Trends in adult anthropometry

	Underweight (%)		Overweight (%)		Comments
	Female	**Male**	**Female**	**Male**	
China					
1998	8.9	8.4	11.5	6.5	
2000	7.1	6.4	24.1	21.1	
% Δ	- 20	-24	+109	+224	
Egypt					
1995	1.6		51.8		
2004	0.4	2.0	89.3	66.9	
% Δ	-75		+72		
India					
1989/90	49.3	49.0	4.1	2.6	Rural only
2000/01	39.3	37.4	8.2	5.7	
% Δ	-20	-24	+100	+119	
Mexico					
1994	1.5	1.9	59.5	52.0	
2000	1.7	1.8	67.6	62.3	
% Δ	+13	-5	+14	+20	
Philippines					
1993	16.1	11.5	18.6	14.4	
2003	14.2	10.6	27.3	20.9	
% Δ	-12	-8	+46	+45	
South Africa					
1980	18.0			14.7	Whites only
2000	25.5			20.8	
% Δ	+42			+41	

Micronutrient deficiencies

In addition to the double burden of under- and overnutrition, which is demonstrated principally in differences in the prevalence of undernutrition among preschool children and of overweight in adults, many of the case study countries continue to have high prevalence rates of micronutrient deficiencies. Approximately one-third of women and children in China and the Philippines are anaemic, and a staggering 90 percent of women and children in India are diagnosed with anaemia (Table 11). Persistently high levels of anaemia in the

Philippines are attributed to poor child feeding and weaning practices and poor compliance with iron supplementation programmes (Philippines case study). In India, the dietary intakes of iron and folate are low, and there are high rates of blood loss from malaria and parasitic infections (India case study).

TABLE 11
Prevalence of anaemia in women and children (last available year)

	Women (%)	Children (%)	Comment
China	18.8	24.2	Rural women, children 0–2 yrs (2002)
Egypt	26.3	29.9	Women 15–49 yrs, children 6–71 months (2000)
India	88	90	Pregnant women, preschool children (2002/03)
Mexico	20.8	27.2	NPNL women 12–47 yrs, children 0–5 yrs (1999)
Philippines	43.9	29.1	Pregnant women, children 1–5 yrs (2003)
South Africa		11	Children 6–71 months (1994)

Large percentages of the populations in the case study countries are also suffering from vitamin A deficiency (VAD). Few countries have trend data for VAD, but the Philippines recorded a higher prevalence of children with VAD in 2003 compared with ten years earlier. VAD among children in China differs according to residence. The prevalence of low serum retinol among children aged three to 12 years is 3.0 percent in urban and 11.2 percent in rural areas.

TABLE 12
Prevalence of vitamin A deficiency[1] in children and adults

	Adults (%)	Preschool children (%)	School-age children (%)	Comment
China			9.3	Children 3–12 yrs
Egypt	20.5		26.5	Adults 20+ yrs, children 11–19 yrs (2004)
Philippines	17.5	40.1		Adults, pregnant women only, children 6–60 months
South Africa		39		0–71 months (1994)

[1] Serum retinol < 20 μg/dl.

BURDEN OF DISEASE

Although the classic definition of the double burden of malnutrition is concerned primarily with the dual burden of over- and undernutrition, it is also useful to examine morbidity and mortality trends given the close links among disease, disability and under- and overnutrition.

Disability-adjusted life years (DALYs) report on the time lived with a disability and the time lost because of premature mortality. Globally, the proportion of DALYs lost to NCD has been increasing, while DALYs from communicable disease, including nutritional disorders, are declining (Figure 3).

FIGURE 3
Trends in DALYs by disease category

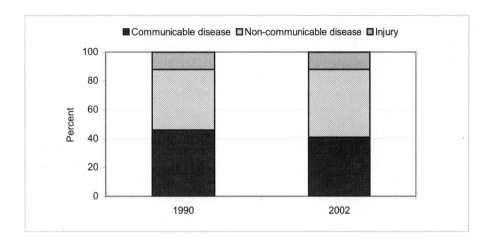

In its annual publication *State of the world's health,* the World Health Organization (WHO) reports data on DALYs from specific diseases by region and mortality stratum (Table 14). The double burden of disease is most clearly evident in the proportional DALYs of the Southeast Asia and Eastern Mediterranean regions, with high DALYs lost from both communicable and non-communicable diseases. The regions of the Americas and Western Pacific are moving away from high levels of communicable disease, while malaria, HIV and respiratory infection remain high in the Africa region.

TABLE 13
DALYs lost from communicable and non-communicable diseases and injuries

	World	Africa	Americas	Southeast Asia	Eastern Mediterranean	Western Pacific
Communicable diseases	**41.0**	**74.8**	**20.0**	**45.6**	**52.1**	**21.5**
Tuberculosis	2.3	2.7	.62	3.0	2.5	2.4
HIV	5.7	24.5	2.0	2.9	1.2	.92
Diarrhoeal diseases	4.2	5.8	1.8	5.2	7.0	2.7
Malaria	3.1	10.3	.11	.62	1.9	.18
Respiratory infections	6.3	8.3	2.3	8.6	8.9	3.3
Nutritional deficiencies	2.3	2.6	1.3	2.9	3.4	1.7
Non-communicable conditions	**46.8**	**17.3**	**63.5**	**41.4**	**36.8**	**64.3**
Malignant neoplasms	5.1	1.3	5.6	2.9	2.5	8.9
Diabetes mellitus	1.1	.29	2.2	.98	.73	1.2
Hypertensive heart disease	0.5	.16	.71	.31	.56	.89
Ischaemic heart disease	3.9	.78	3.3	4.9	3.4	2.7
Cerebrovascular disease	3.3	.95	3.1	2.4	1.7	6.5
Injuries	**12.2**	**7.9**	**16.4**	**13.0**	**11.1**	**14.2**
Traffic accidents	2.6	1.8	3.2	2.1	2.4	3.5
Intentional (violence, war, self-inflicted)	3.3	2.9	8.1	2.6	2.6	3.5

Data estimates from 2002. Africa: high child/very high adult mortality stratum; Americas: low child/low adult mortality stratum; Southeast Asia: high child/high adult mortality stratum; Eastern Mediterranean: high child/high adult mortality stratum; Western Pacific: low child/low adult mortality stratum.
Source: WHO. *World Health Report 2004.* Geneva.

NCDs and NCD risk factors

In addition to obesity, diabetes, CVD and some cancers are also related to diet and lifestyle (WHO/FAO, 2003), as are certain risk factors including high blood pressure, increased cholesterol and elevated blood sugar.

For most of the case study countries, monitoring the incidence and prevalence of NCDs and associated risk factors is relatively new, so examination of trends is not possible. Some of the case study countries do not yet have nationally representative monitoring systems in place, and data on the magnitude of the problem of NCDs have to be inferred from various small studies.

In the four case studies with data, more than 20 percent of adults have high blood pressure, a risk factor for CVD. In Egypt and Mexico, prevalence of diabetes is nearly 10 percent (Table 14). In China, prevalence rates of diabetes in people over 60 years of age reach as high as 17 percent.

TABLE 14
Prevalence of hypertension and diabetes

	Hypertension	Diabetes	Comment
China	20.2/18.0	2.6	Adults male/female (2002)
Egypt	26.3	9.3	Adults > 25 yrs (1995)
Mexico	39.2/30.9	7.6/8.3	Adults male/female(2000)
Philippines	22.5	3.4	Adults > 20 yrs (2003)

Physical activity

Trend data on physical activity are weak or non-existent in most of the case study countries. China is the exception, and has information from 1989 to 2000 on light, moderate and heavy physical activity. The data show a 20 percent decrease in people reporting heavy activity and a 46 percent increase in people reporting light physical activity.

Double burden of malnutrition

The data presented in this section clearly demonstrate that most countries in the study are struggling to some degree with the double burden of malnutrition. The countries were classified into the following three typologies based on predominant health and nutrition problems.

Typology one: (India and the Philippines)
- High prevalence of undernutrition in both children and adults.
- Emerging problems of overnutrition, diabetes and high blood pressure, mainly in urban areas.
- High prevalence of micronutrient deficiencies.

Typology two: (South Africa)
- Stunting at levels of public health significance, but declining underweight and wasting.
- In adults, overweight/obesity more of a problem than underweight.
- Rising incidence of NCD, particularly CVD, diabetes and cancer.
- Rise in some infectious diseases, notably TB and HIV.
- High prevalence of micronutrient deficiencies.

Typology three (China, Egypt and Mexico)
- Both stunting and overweight appear as public health problems in children.
- Low prevalence of underweight and wasting in children.
- Underweight in adults no longer of public health significance, but prevalence of overweight high and/or rapidly increasing.
- Iron and vitamin A deficiencies remain public health problems.
- Diabetes and coronary heart disease are increasing, while infectious disease is decreasing (although certain diseases such as TB and HIV remain high in China and Egypt).

In many of the case study countries there is a striking discrepancy in anthropometric outcomes between children and adults. For example, in the Philippines, 27 percent of children under five years of age are underweight, while 27 percent of women are overweight or obese. It seems that there are environmental and biological factors leading to such extreme outcomes. There is also evidence of increased risk of adult obesity when undernutrition occurs during childhood (Delisle, 2005). Poverty is a main driver of stunting (UN Millennium Project, 2005), but the inverse is not necessarily true for overweight. In many countries, the urban poor and undereducated have high prevalence rates of overweight (Mendez and Popkin, 2004).

The different typologies suggest that country programmes should focus on different areas. For example, in India and the Philippines, reducing child and adult undernutrition and micronutrient deficiencies should remain a top priority, and efforts to limit the rise of overweight/obesity and diet-related chronic diseases should be initiated. In Egypt, Mexico and, to a lesser degree, China and South Africa, overweight and obesity among adults is already widespread and the problem is becoming more significant among children. In these countries, in addition to prevention efforts, more focus needs to be directed to early detection and treatment.

CONCLUSIONS

Noticeable changes in dietary patterns have occurred in all of the case study countries; these changes have not necessarily corresponded to increased intakes of total dietary energy, but have corresponded to increased fat content of diets. The most striking changes have been increases in pork, poultry and beef, sugar and sweet products, and – in most countries – fats and oils.

Some of the dietary changes have brought welcome improvements to nutritional status, contributing to reduced child undernutrition and improved micronutrient intake in some countries. However, the combination of an energy-dense diet with low physical activity has contributed to an increasing prevalence of overweight adults. This pattern will probably continue, given that current economic and social trends are conducive to widespread changes in lifestyle.

Although some progress has been made in reducing undernutrition of children, national and regional efforts to improve child growth need to continue and should not be overshadowed by the need to address NCD among adults. It is worth bearing in mind the continuing evidence generated by the Barker hypothesis, which links undernutrition in foetal and early life to greater risk of NCD in adulthood.

Dietary and lifestyle choices, including food choice, smoking, physical inactivity and alcohol consumption, are some of the most strikingly modifiable risk factors. The challenge is to develop effective programmes and policies aimed at both prevention and control. Developed countries have attempted to tackle these problems for many years, but with little success. Ideally, strategies that are effective in ameliorating both under- and overnutrition should be identified and developed. In the shorter term, priority should be given to preventive action by addressing undernutrition of infants, children and pregnant women, thereby circumventing the risks predicted by the Barker hypothesis.

REFERENCES

Barker, D.J.P. 2004. The developmental origins of adult disease. *Journal of the American College of Nutrition,* 23(6): 588S–595S.

Chopra, M. 2004a. From apartheid to globalization: Health and social change in South Africa. *Hygiea Internationalis,* 4(1): 153–174.

Chopra, M. 2004b. Globalization, urbanization and nutritional changes in South Africa. *In* FAO. *Globalization of food systems in developing countries: impact on food security and nutrition,* pp.119–133. FAO Food and Nutrition Paper No. 83. Rome, FAO.

Cook, I. & Dummer, T. 2003. Changing health in China: re-evaluating the epidemiological transition model. *Health Policy,* 67: 329–343.

Delisle, H. 2002. *Programming of chronic disease by impaired foetal nutrition. Evidence and implications for policy and intervention strategies.* WHO/NHD/02.3. Geneva, WHO Department of Nutrition for Health and Development.

Delisle, H. 2005. Early nutritional influences on obesity, diabetes and cardiovascular disease risk. International Workshop, 6–9 June 2004, Montreal University, Quebec, Canada. *Maternal and Child Nutrition,* 1(3), 128–129.

Development Policy Review. 2003. Issue September/November 2003.

FAO. 2004. *Globalization of food systems in developing countries: impact on food security and nutrition.* FAO Food and Nutrition Paper No. 83. Rome.

Georgetown University Center on Aging. 2002. *Childhood obesity. A lifelong threat to health.* Data profile March 2002. Institute for Health Care Research and Policy, Georgetown University. Available at: http://hpi.georgetown.edu/agingsociety/pdfs/obesity.pdf.

Gillespie, S. & Haddad, L. 2003. *The double burden of malnutrition in Asia. Causes, consequences and solutions.* Washington, DC, International Food Policy Research Institute. Sage Publications. pp. 236.

Heini, A. & Weinsier, R. 1997. Divergent trends in obesity and fat intake patterns: the American paradox. *The American Journal of Medicine,* 102: 259–264.

Kitange, H. The worst of two worlds. Adult mortality in Tanzania. Available at: www.id21.org/zinter/id21zinter.exe?a=0&i=insightshealth%231art3&u=41fe3e16.

Livingstone, M.B. & Black, A. 2003. Markers of the validity of reported energy intake. *Journal of Nutrition,* 133: S895–S920.

Mendez, M., Du, S. & Popkin, B. 2004. Urbanization, income and the nutrition transition in China: a case study. *In* FAO. *Globalization of food systems in developing countries: impact on food security and nutrition,* pp.169–194. Rome, FAO.

Mendez, M. & Popkin, B. 2004. Globalization, urbanization and nutritional change in the developing world. *In* FAO. *Globalization of food systems in developing countries: impact on food security and nutrition,* pp.55–80. FAO Food and Nutrition Paper No. 83. Rome, FAO.

MMWR Weekly. 2004. Trends in intake of energy and macronutrients in the United States, 1971–2000. *MMWR weekly,* 53(04): 80–82.

Popkin, B. 1994. The nutrition transition in low-income countries: an emerging crisis. *Nutrition Reviews,* 52(9).

Popkin, B. 2002. The shift in stages of the nutrition transition in the developing world differs from past experiences. *Public Health Nutrition,* 5(1A): 205–214.

Popkin, B. 2003. The nutrition transition in the developing world. *Development Policy Review,* 21(5–6): 581–597.

Prentice, A. & Jebb, S. 1995. Obesity in Britain: Gluttony or sloth? *British Medical Journal,* 311: 437–439.

Public Health Nutrition. 2002. Volume 1(A), 2002.

Sawaya, A., Martins, P. & Martins, V. 2004. Impact of globalization on food consumption, health and nutrition in urban areas: a case study of Brazil. *In* FAO. *Globalization of food systems in developing countries: impact on food security and nutrition,* pp. 253–274. FAO Food and Nutrition Paper No. 83. Rome, FAO.

Shetty, P. 2002. Nutrition transition in India. *Public Health Nutrition,* 5(1A): 175–182.

Shetty, P. & Gopalan, C., eds. 1998. Diet, nutrition and chronic disease: an Asian perspective. London, Smith-Gordon and Co.

Shetty P. & McPherson, K., eds. 1997. *Diet, nutrition and chronic disease: Lessons from contrasting worlds.* Chichester, UK, John Wiley and Sons.

Stubbs, C. & Lee, A. 2004. The obesity epidemic: both energy intake and physical activity contribute. *Medical Journal of Australia,* 181(9): 489–491.

UNDP. 2004. *Human Development Report, 2004. Cultural liberty in today's diverse world?* New York, United Nations Development Programme (UNDP). Available at: http://hdr.undp.org/reports/global/2004/.
UN Millennium Project. 2005. *Halving hunger: It can be done.* Task Force on Hunger. London, Earthscan.
WHO. 1997. *Obesity – preventing and managing the global epidemic.* Report of a WHO Consultation on Obesity. Geneva.
WHO. 2002. *World Health Report 2002. Reducing risks, promoting healthy life.* Geneva.
WHO/FAO. 2003. *Diet, nutrition and the prevention of chronic diseases.* Report of a Joint WHO/FAO expert consultation. WHO Technical Report Series No. 916. Geneva, WHO.
World Cancer Research Fund. 1997. *Food nutrition and the prevention of cancer: a global perspective.* Washington, DC, American Institute for Cancer Research.

The double burden of malnutrition in China, 1989 to 2000

Fengying Zhai and Huijun Wang, Institute of Nutrition and Food Safety, Chinese Center for Disease Control and Prevention, Beijing, China

INTRODUCTION

Twenty-five years ago, China introduced sweeping structural reforms to the rural economy, family planning programme and financial accountability of its enterprises and service sector organizations. A rapid rise in economic productivity has resulted in continuing increases in income and changes to the traditional Chinese diet. These changes have been accompanied by shifts in the patterns of mortality and disease risk factors, and are occurring at markedly different rates across the country. A post-reform China in the new millennium faces a range of challenges in health, nutrition and family planning. Income disparities have increased as coastal areas have become wealthier, while the 300 poorest counties – most of which are in western China – suffer stagnation. The ageing of the population and increased life expectancy have contributed to an inevitable increase in the demand for long-term care.

This case study assesses trends in the Chinese dietary intake and reviews changes in nutritional status, morbidity and mortality.

Demographic and health indicators

Over the past three decades, the Chinese population has expanded from 987 million to 1.267 billion (Table 1). There has also been an increasing trend towards urbanization, with the urban proportion of the population growing from 19 to 36 percent. Birth and death rates have been declining, while the natural growth rate has remained relatively stable (Figure 1). Additional demographic and development indicators are presented in Table 2. The declining birth and death rates of the past 20 years are causing the Chinese population to become older, with a decreased percentage in the 0 to 14 years age group and increases in the percentages of adults (15 to 64 years) and elderly (65 years and more). Population health indicators have improved over the past 30 years, and 90 percent of Chinese adults are literate. Although the proportion of population with access to safe sanitation has increased, it remains low, at less than 50 percent (State Statistical Bureau, 2002).

TABLE 1
Trends in population by residence and gender, 1980 to 2000

Year	Total population, millions (at year-end)	By sex		By residence	
		Male (%)	Female (%)	Urban (%)	Rural (%)
1980	987	51.45	48.55	19.39	80.61
1985	1 058	51.70	48.30	23.71	76.29
1990	1 143	51.52	48.48	26.41	73.59
1995	1 211	51.03	48.97	29.04	70.96
2000	1 267	51.63	48.37	36.22	63.78

Data include military personnel of the Chinese People's Liberation Army, but not the populations of Hong Kong, Macao and Taiwan.
Source: State Statistical Bureau, 1980 to 2002.

FIGURE 1
Trends in birth, death and natural growth rates in China, 1980 to 2000

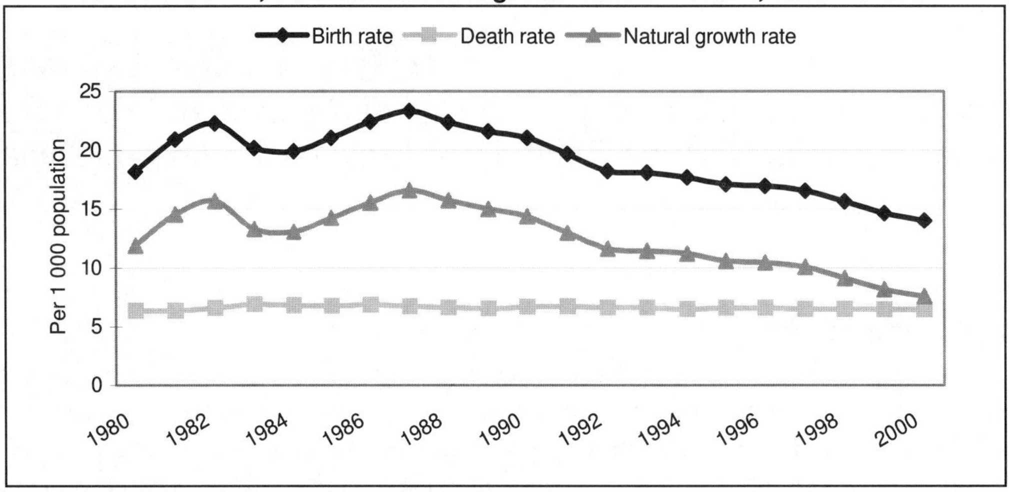

Source: State Statistical Bureau, 1980 to 2002.

TABLE 2
Trends in population structure and selected health and education indicators, 1980 to 2000

Indicator	Year			Source
	1980	1990	2000	
Population 0–14 years (%)	35.5	27.7	22.9	UNESCAP, 2004
Population 15–64 years (%)	59.8	66.9	70.2	UNESCAP, 2004
Population ≥ 65 years (%)	4.7	5.4	7.0	UNESCAP, 2004
Annual population growth rate (%)	1.2	1.4	0.8	UNESCAP, 2004
Infant mortality rate (per 1 000 live births)	41	33	28	UNESCAP, 2004
Overall life expectancy (years)	67.8 (1981)	68.6	71.4	Chinese population census
Female life expectancy (years)	69.3 (1981)	70.5	73.3	Chinese population census
Male life expectancy (years)	66.4 (1981)	66.9	69.6	Chinese population census
Adult literacy (%)		78.3	90.9 (2002)	UNDP, 2004
Population with access to improved sanitation (%)		29	40	UNDP, 2004
Population with access to an improved water source (%)		71	75	UNDP, 2004

Employment and economy

The Chinese economy has experienced exponential growth in the past decade, with per capita gross domestic product (GDP) rising from 460 yuan in 1980 to 7 084 yuan in 2000 (Figure 2). Since 1990, per capita GDP has grown by an average of 8.6 percent per year (UNDP, 2004). Although the number of employed people has been rising in the past decade, the number and percentage of unemployed people indicate a need for increased focus on job creation (Table 3) (State Statistical Bureau, 2002).

FIGURE 2
Trends in per capita GDP (yuan), 1980 to 2002

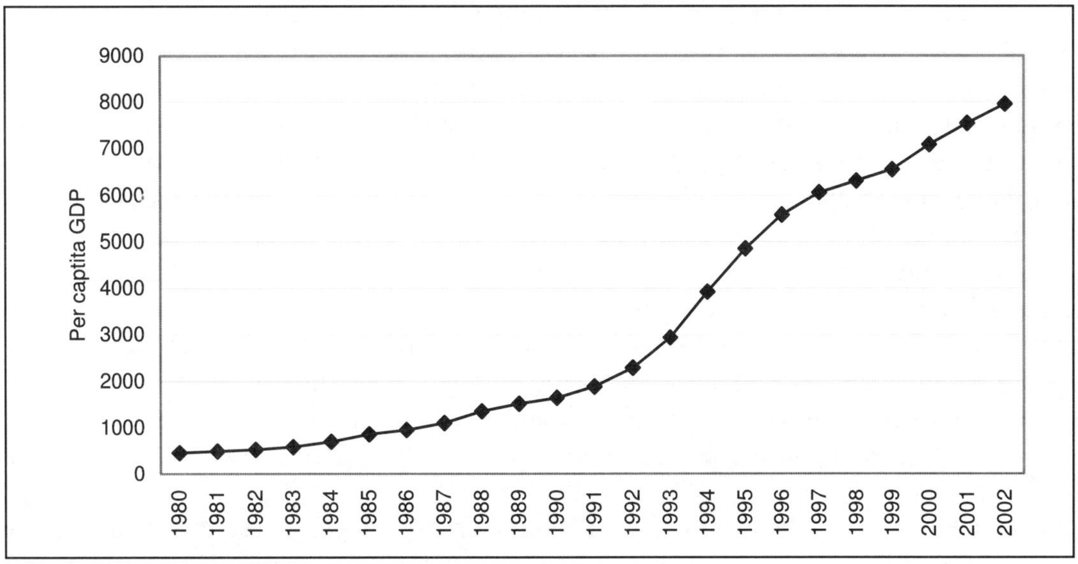

Source: State Statistical Bureau, 1980 to 2002.

TABLE 3
Trends in unemployment in China, 1991 to 2001

Indicator	1991	1995	2000	2001
Total number of employed people (10 000s)	58 360	67 947	72 085	73 025
Number of registered unemployed people in urban areas (10 000s)	288	520	595	681
Registered unemployment rate in urban areas (%)	2.3	2.9	3.1	3.6

Source: State Statistical Bureau, 1990 to 2002.

DATA SOURCES FOR DIETARY INTAKE, NUTRITION AND HEALTH INDICATORS

Three main data sources were used to analyse the trends in diet, nutritional status and disease burden in the Chinese population. The primary source of data on dietary intake is the China Economic, Population, Nutrition and Health Survey (CHNS), which was conducted in 1989, 1991, 1993, 1997 and 2000. The National Nutrition Survey (NNS) was conducted in 1992 and 2002 – this report uses only the data on chronic disease risk factors from NNS. The third data source is the China Disease Surveillance System. An outline of each of these sources is given in the following subsections

China Economic, Population, Nutrition and Health Survey

CHNS covers nine provinces that vary substantially in geography, economic development, public resources and health indicators (Figure 3). It is not nationally representative however. A multistage, random cluster sample is used to draw the sample surveyed in each of the provinces. Counties in the nine provinces are stratified by income (low, middle and high) and a weighted sampling scheme is used to select four counties randomly in each province. The provincial capital and lower-income cities are selected when feasible. Villages and townships in the counties and urban and suburban neighbourhoods in the cities are selected randomly. From 1989 to 1993, there were 190 primary sampling units; a new province (and its sampling units) was added in 1997, and currently there are about 3 800 households in the overall survey, representing 16 000 individuals of all age groups. The data can be stratified by region, gender and province.

Follow-up levels are high, but families that migrate from one community to another have not been followed.

CHNS collects information on all the individuals living in a household. A complete household roster is used as a reference for subsequent blocks of questions on time allocation at home (e.g., child care, elderly care and other key home activities) and on economic activities. Questions concerning income and time allocation aim to take into account all the activities that each person could have engaged in during the past year, both in and out of the formal market. Information on water sources, construction and housing conditions and ownership of consumer durables is gathered from respondents. Three days of detailed food consumption information is collected by combining household- and individual-level data. Household food consumption is determined by a detailed examination of changes in inventory between the start and end of each day for three consecutive days, in combination with a weighing technique. Dietary intake at the individual level is surveyed by 24-hour recalls for the same three consecutive days by asking individuals to report all their food consumption for each day, both away from and at home.

Recent CHNS have used food composition tables from 1992 to determine the nutrients consumed. In addition, individual dietary intake is collected for each household member for three consecutive days, irrespective of age or relationship to the household head. Adults and children receive detailed physical examinations that include weight, height, arm and head circumference, mid-arm skin fold and blood pressure (adults only) measurements. Limited clinical nutrition and physical functioning data were collected in 1993, 1997 and 2000. In 1997, the survey added daily living activities, related information for older adults and a new set of physical activity and inactivity data for all respondents.

FIGURE 3
Map of the CHNS survey regions[1]

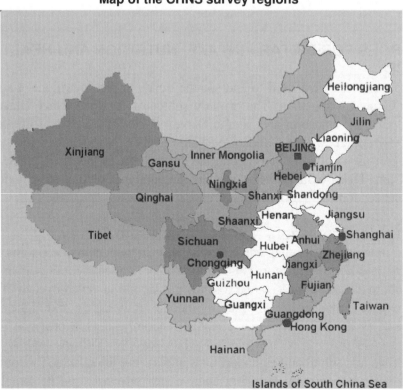

[1] Light shaded regions included in CHNS

National Nutrition Survey (NNS) of China

The third NNS of China was conducted in 1992 and the fourth in 2002. In 1992, a stratified multi-stage cluster random sampling method was used. The survey covered the residents of sample units selected from 30 provinces. The sample size was 32 sites, including 960 households for each province, metropolis and autonomous region. Adjustments were made in some provinces to provide a total sample of 28 000 households in 30 provinces.

The fourth NNS of 2002 was China's first comprehensive nutrition and health survey. It systematically integrated several previous, separately organized surveys on nutrition, hypertension, diabetes, etc. into one survey and included some new indicators related to social and economic development. Cities were classified as large, medium or small according to their level of economic development. Beijing, Shanghai, Tianjin and Chongqing were included in the total of 18 large cities. Rural areas were classified as first, second, third or fourth class, based on economic level and population size. First class rural areas were the richest, and fourth class the poorest.

A stratified multi-stage cluster random sampling method was adopted to sample 71 971 households (24 034 urban and 47 937 rural) chosen from 132 counties in the 31 provinces, autonomous regions and municipalities directly under the central Government of China. The data can be stratified by urban and rural residence, gender and age. The survey covered diet, nutrition and a range of diet-related non-communicable disease (DR-NCD) risk factors, including hypertension, diabetes, obesity and abnormal blood lipid levels.

China Disease Surveillance System

The China Disease Surveillance System was established in 1989. A multistage, randomized cluster process was used to draw the sample. The first layer was based on geographic representation, the second on urban and rural areas, and the third on economic and development levels and demographics. Cities were classified as large, medium and small. Rural areas were classified into four classes according to socio-economic status, population and the index of death, which were obtained from the Chinese population census of 1982. The four classes were (a) the richest rural areas, (b) the richer rural areas, (c) the poor rural areas, and (d) the poorest rural areas.

The survey covered 10 million people, about 1 percent of China's population. In 1989, 9 261 436 people were chosen for the sample, 2 253 963 from the cities and 7 007 473 from rural areas. A survey was conducted on this sample every year to collect data on demographics, births and deaths, infectious disease, smoking and other lifestyle factors. This report uses data from the period 1990 to 2002 to describe trends in the burden of disease.

TRENDS IN DIETARY INTAKE

This case study uses data from NNS and CHNS to identify trends in the food consumption of the Chinese population. In the period 1989 to 2000, total dietary energy intake decreased for all age groups – in adults 20 to 59 years of age by 39 kcal per day. However, the percentage of dietary energy derived from fat increased for all age groups, reaching 30.9 percent in people aged 60 years and over and 29.8 percent in children under nine years.

FIGURE 4
Total energy intake and dietary energy from fat in China, 1989 to 2000

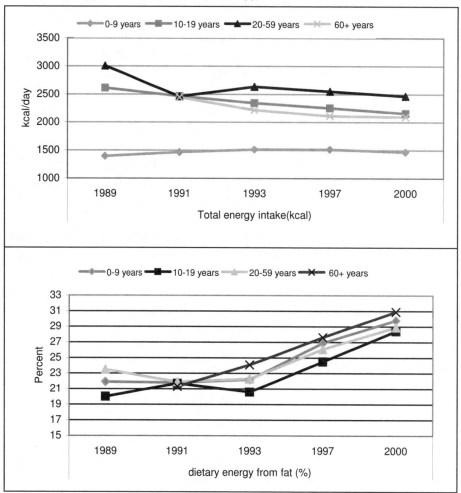

TRENDS IN THE INTAKES OF CHILDREN AGED TWO TO FIVE YEARS

Over the past ten years, children's intakes of cereals and tubers declined from 240 to 205 g and from 64 to 40 g per day, respectively (Figure 5). The intake of vegetables remained relatively stable, while fruit intake decreased from 33 to 17 g per day. During the same period, the consumption of animal food increased – meat by 80 percent, and eggs by 75 percent (Figure 6). From 1997 to 2000, the consumption of milk increased from 10 to 15 g, which may signal an increasing trend in dairy consumption. Total energy intake decreased slightly, but the diet became proportionately richer in fat, which rose from providing 22 percent of dietary energy in 1989 to 31 percent in 2000 (Table 4). These trends generally represent positive developments in children's diets, indicating greater dietary variety, intake of high-quality protein sources and increases in essential micronutrients, including calcium, iron and zinc. However, in addition to the rapidly escalating percentage of dietary energy derived from fat, two other alarming trends are decreasing intakes of vitamins A and C, most likely resulting from decreased intake of fruits, which are good sources of these nutrients.

FIGURE 5

Trends in per capita intakes of vegetable products among children aged two to five years, 1989 to 2000

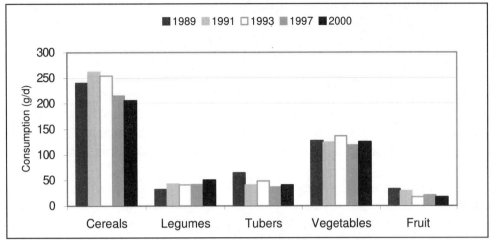

Sample sizes: 1989, 1 009; 1991, 1 086; 1993, 982; 1997, 514; 2000, 437.
Source: CHNS.

FIGURE 6

Trends in per capita intakes of animal products among children aged two to five years, 1989 to 2000

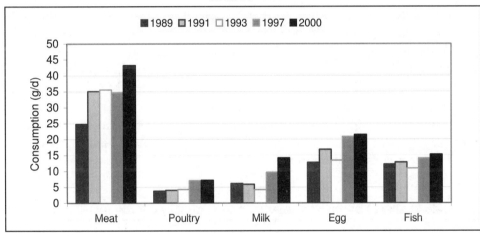

Sample sizes: 1989, 1 009; 1991, 1 086; 1993, 982; 1997, 514; 2000, 437.
Source: CHNS.

TABLE 4

Trends in intakes of nutrients in children aged two to five years, 1989 to 2000

Year	Nutrients									
	Energy (kcal)	Protein (g)	Fat (g)	Calcium (mg)	Iron (mg)	Zinc (mg)	Vitamin A(ug)	Vitamin B1(mg)	Vitamin B2(mg)	Vitamin C(mg)
1989	1 240	36.8	30.1	212.5	11.2	5.7	304.9	0.6	0.4	56.5
1991	1 363	41.6	37.1	215.5	12.8	6.3	286.5	0.7	0.5	47.0
1993	1 264	39.4	32.5	209.8	11.7	6.1	268.8	0.6	0.4	52.3
1997	1 179	36.1	37.5	220.4	11.8	5.9	243.3	0.5	0.4	39.8
2000	1 225	38.3	42.8	246.3	13.2	6.3	298.7	0.6	0.5	44.9

Sample sizes: 1989, 1 009; 1991, 1 086; 1993, 982; 1997, 514; 2000, 437.
Source: CHNS.

Trends in the dietary intake of adults

The shift in the Chinese diet follows a classic pattern of Westernization. Economic progress, linked in part to the liberalization of food production controls and the introduction of a free market for food and food products, is connected to these important shifts in diet. Both the NNS and CHNS data show that intakes of cereals and tubers have decreased considerably during the past two decades, in both urban and rural areas and among all income groups. The results are shown in Tables 5 and 6 and Figure 8. The total intake of vegetables decreased and the intake of fruits remained stable over these years. At the same time, the daily intake of animal foods showed a large increase, with pork and eggs increasing far more rapidly than the others. Urban residents' per capita daily intake of animal foods was higher than rural residents' (Table 5). The intake level of animal foods for the high-income group was almost twice that for the low-income group (Figure 9).

Over the past decade, the proportion of dietary energy derived from fat in the adult diet increased dramatically from 19 to 28 percent, mainly owing to the replacement of dietary energy from carbohydrates (Figure 7). The food group changes that accompanied this trend in increasing fat intake included an increased consumption of meat, especially pork, poultry and milk. Surprisingly, the consumption of animal fats and vegetables oils did not increase, in either urban or rural areas (Table 5). However, about one-half of dietary fat came from edible oil, while the consumption of refined animal fat decreased. The pace of this trend is alarming and signals a need to slow the population's intake of fats, which will soon exceed recommended levels. Decreasing consumption of vegetable oil, pork and pork products is critical in controlling the fat intake in the Chinese diet.

An analysis of current trends in intakes of the major food groups, stratified by income and urban/rural residence, provides some interesting insights. Certain trends in intake (e.g., increased fruit, vegetables and milk) seem to be dominated by residence location, with urban consumers more likely to have increased intakes of fruit and milk, and rural consumers more likely to consume more vegetables. Income can be seen as driving the intake of sugar, while a combination of residence location and income seems to be significant in meat consumption trends.

FIGURE 7
Trends in shares of macronutrients in total dietary energy intake, 1989 to 2000

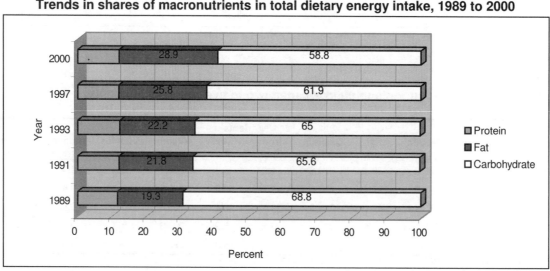

TABLE 5
Trends in intakes (g/day) of food groups among adults (18 to 45 years) by residence, 1989 to 2000

Food	Total					Rural					Urban				
	1989	1991	1993	1997	2000	1989	1991	1993	1997	2000	1989	1991	1993	1997	2000
Cereals															
Rice	348	337	320	297	274	362	338	335	312	290	316	336	284	262	237
Wheat	190	196	199	181	152	193	196	211	193	154	183	194	169	153	146
Maize	44	25	21	20	14	60	28	27	25	16	18	6	6	6	7
Other	19	10	11	8	6	26	9	12	9	6	5	11	6	6	7
Tubers															
Potato	18	26	23	28	27	22	28	27	32	30	9	23	12	19	19
Sweet potato	58	24	13	10	6	75	26	16	13	7	21	18	6	4	3
Other	71	44	53	45	40	77	41	55	46	41	58	50	48	44	48
Meat															
Beef	3	4	6	7	7	2	4	5	5	5	5	5	10	11	11
Pork	52	59	62	60	69	44	59	52	49	60	71	59	89	86	91
Poultry	7	7	9	12	14	4	7	6	10	12	7	7	14	17	19
Eggs	11	14	15	24	26	9	13	12	20	23	16	15	22	33	32
Other	2	1	1	2	2	2	1	1	1	1	2	1	2	5	4
Fish	24	21	22	28	26	22	21	20	25	25	27	22	28	35	30
Dairy															
Fresh milk	1.2	1.8	2.1	1.5	3.8	0.1	1.3	0.8	0.5	1.7	3.5	2.9	5.3	3.9	9.3
Powdered milk	0.1	0.2	0.1	0.3	0.3	0.1	0.2	0.1	0.1	0.0	0.3	0.3	0.2	0.8	0.8
Legumes															
Pulses	79	80	77	81	96	78	80	77	79	96	80	80	78	87	95
Nuts	3	3	2	2	4	3	3	2	3	4	5	3	3	2	3
Vegetables															
Green leafy	227	181	178	172	159	242	181	188	183	169	182	151	148	133	163
Vegetables	53	84	94	98	98	53	86	102	98	100	53	79	76	97	92
Other	16	13	12	10	8	19	16	13	11	8	8	8	10	9	7
Fruit															
Citrus	2	1	1	2	1	1	1	1	1	1	3	2	2	3	2
Other	12	8	11	8	11	13	7	10	5	7	11	10	14	17	20
Fats and oils															
Animal fat	18	13	10	10	12	19	14	11	10	12	15	12	9	9	12
Vegetable oil	32	22	22	31	30	30	22	21	30	30	37	22	26	34	30
Sugar															
Soft drinks	0.1	0.1	0.1	0.4	0.3	0.1	0.1	0.1	0.1	0.2	0.1	0.1	0.2	1.1	0.4
Confectionary	2.6	1.8	2.0	2.5	2.0	2.3	1.8	1.4	2.3	1.9	3.5	1.8	3.3	3.0	2.3
Other foods	54.1	32.8	31.4	38.5	39.8	51.1	33.6	31.0	38.3	40.1	60.8	31.2	32.2	39.0	38.8

Sample sizes: 1989, 5 789; 1991, 5 838; 1993, 5 468; 1997, 5 334; 2000, 4 831.
Source: CHNS.

TABLE 6
Food consumption in rural and urban areas of China (g/day), 1992 and 2002

Foods	Total		Rural		Urban	
	1992	2002	1992	2002	1992	2002
Rice	226.7	238.3	255.8	246.2	223.1	217.8
Wheat	178.7	140.2	189.1	143.5	165.3	131.9
Other cereals	34.5	23.6	40.9	26.4	17.0	16.3
Tubers	86.6	49.1	108.0	55.7	46.0	31.9
Green leafy vegetables	102.0	90.8	107.1	91.8	98.1	88.1
Other vegetables	208.3	185.4	199.6	193.8	221.2	163.8
Fruit	49.2	45.0	32.0	35.6	80.1	69.4
Nuts	3.1	3.8	3.0	3.2	3.4	5.4
Meat	58.9	78.6	37.6	68.7	100.5	104.5
Eggs	16.0	23.7	8.8	20.0	29.4	33.2
Fish	27.5	29.6	19.2	23.7	44.2	44.9
Dairy	14.9	26.5	3.8	11.4	36.1	65.8
Vegetable oil	22.4	32.9	17.1	30.1	32.4	40.2
Animal fat	7.1	8.7	8.5	10.6	4.5	3.8
Sugar and starch	4.7	4.4	3.0	4.1	7.7	5.2
Salt	13.9	12.0	13.9	12.4	13.3	10.9
Sauce	12.6	8.9	10.6	8.2	15.9	10.6

Source: NNS.

FIGURE 8
**Trends in cereal consumption in adults (18 to 45 years) by income group and residence,
1989 to 2000**

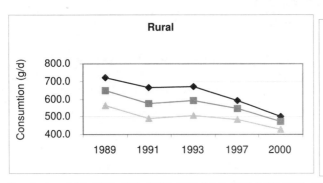 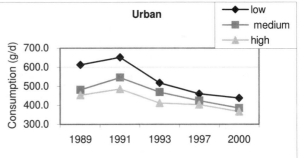

Sample sizes: 1989, 5 789; 1991, 5 838; 1993, 5 468; 1997, 5 334; 2000, 4 831.
Source: CHNS.

FIGURE 9
**Trends in consumption of meat in adults (18 to 45 years) by income group and residence,
1989 to 2000**

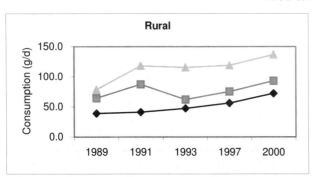 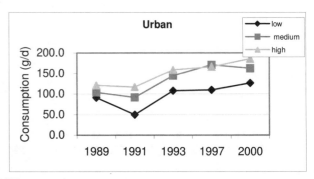

Sample sizes: 1989, 5 789; 1991, 5 838; 1993, 5 468; 1997, 5 334; 2000, 4 831
Source: CHNS.

Trends in the achievement of various population nutrient intake goals are shown in Table 7. The percentage of dietary energy derived from fat increased in all age groups. The dietary fat intake in suburban and town areas increased rapidly. The proportion of energy from fat reached 30 percent in suburban and town areas, and 35 percent in urban ones. The percentage of people consuming at least 400 g of fruits and vegetables a day dropped for all age groups, while those consuming less than 5 g of sodium chloride also decreased. In 1997, urban adults' intake of cholesterol reached 361.6 mg/d, exceeding the recommended daily allowance (RDA) of 300 mg/d. The cholesterol intake of 54 percent of urban adults was more than 300 mg/d. The cholesterol intakes of suburban and town residents increased to 250 mg/d and 270 mg/d, respectively, but that of rural residents remained stable at a lower level of 150 mg/d. High intakes of dietary fat, sodium and cholesterol increase the risk of chronic diseases such as obesity, diabetes, cardiovascular disease (CVD) and some cancers, especially in middle-aged and elderly populations.

TABLE 7
Achievement of population nutrition intake goals

Age (yrs)	Year	% energy intake from fat			55–75% energy intake from carbohydrate (%)	< 5 g sodium chloride per day (%)	< 10 % energy intake from sugars (%)	≥ 400 g/day fruit and vegetables
		< 15	15–30	> 30				
10–19	1989	43.0	35.5	21.5	52.7	37.0	100.0	23.1
	1993	34.8	45.4	19.8	57.1	22.5	99.9	23.1
	2000	12.3	45.7	42.0	57.1	18.6	97.7	15.3
20 - 59	1989	28.1	43.9	28.0	56.3	27.9	99.6	29.3
	1993	28.3	47.9	23.8	57.6	17.0	99.9	26.0
	2000	11.3	44.3	44.4	54.8	13.9	97.8	21.3
≥ 60	1991	29.4	51.1	19.5	60.8	16.6	99.8	18.8
	1993	23.3	47.1	29.6	58.1	22.7	99.7	16.2
	2000	9.2	37.7	53.1	46.9	14.6	98.4	15.4

TRENDS IN NUTRITIONAL STATUS

This case study used the CHNS and NSS data to describe trends in the nutritional status of children and adults in China. Data from CHNS are preferred as they cover five points in time from 1989 to 2000. Unfortunately, CHNS surveyed very few children under two years of age and so cannot be used to provide information about trends in the prevalence of malnutrition for children in that age group. NNS, which provides data for 1992 and 2002, was used to examine changes in prevalence of stunting and underweight among children up to five years of age.

Trends in the nutritional status of children aged two to five years

The analysis results of CHNS showed that dramatic improvements in the nutritional status of Chinese children aged two to five years occurred between 1989 and 2000 (Figure 10). The prevalence of stunting decreased from 33 to 10 percent overall, from 17 to 3 percent in urban areas, and from 30 to 14 percent in rural ones. The height for age Z-score also increased, from –0.72 to 0.54 in urban areas, and from –1.28 to –0.27 in rural ones. There was also a sustained decrease in the prevalence of underweight children, from 16 to 6 percent overall, 11 to 3 percent in urban areas and 15 to 7 percent in rural ones. The weight-for-age Z-score increased from –0.36 to 0.32 in urban areas and from –0.71 to –0.35 in rural ones. Over the same period, the prevalence of overweight children increased from 2.6 to 8.2 percent.

FIGURE 10
Trends in the nutritional status of children aged two to five years, 1989 to 2000

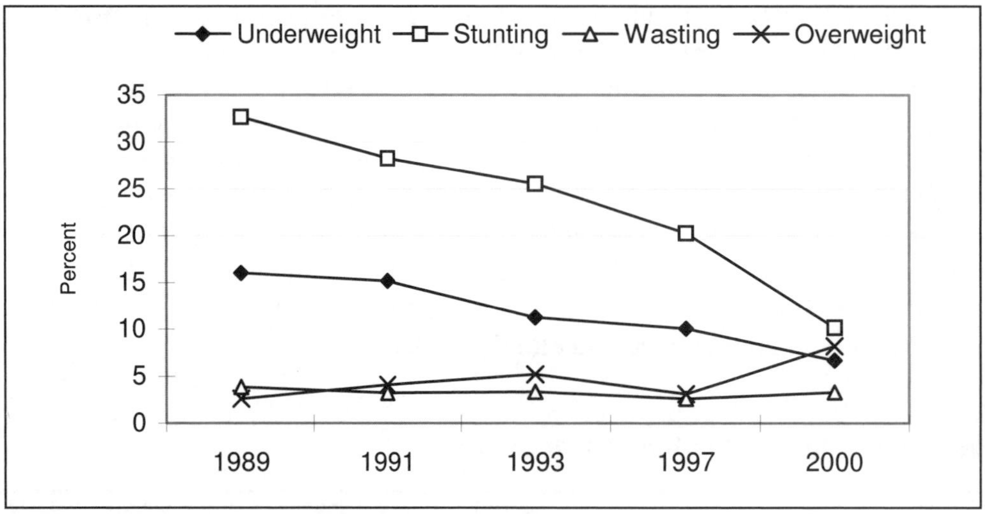

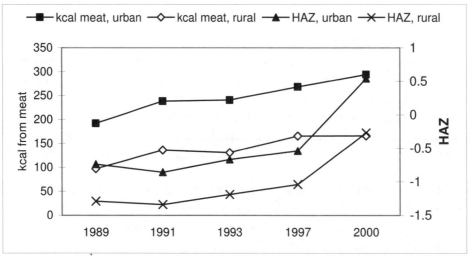

Sample sizes: 1989, 699; 1991, 721; 1993, 651; 1997, 325; 2000, 451.
CHNS growth references: underweight = weight-for-age < -2SD; wasting = weight-for-height < -2SD; stunting = height-for-age < -2SD; overweight = weight-for-height > 2SD.
Source: CHNS.

The results of many investigations have shown that in developing countries, energy intake plays an important role in the long-term development of children (Zhai *et al.,* 2004; Chang *et al.,* 1996). When nutritional status and energy intake improve, the increase in the percentage of energy intake from animal protein becomes a key contributor to child development. The data from CHNS show that the height gain of children is positively correlated with the percentage of energy they derive from animal food (Figure 11).

FIGURE 11
Trends in energy supply from animal foods and mean height-for-age Z scores, 1989 to 2000

Sample sizes: 1989, 699; 1991, 721; 1993, 651; 1997, 325; 2000, 451.
Source: CHNS.

Trends in the nutritional status of children up to five years of age

Tables 8 and 9 show data for stunting and underweight by age and residence. In rural areas, stunting prevalence is 17.3 percent, compared with 4.9 percent in urban ones. The prevalence of underweight is lower than that of stunting, but differences by residence remain. A further disaggregation by economic status and residence (not shown) indicates that the prevalence rates of stunting and underweight in poor rural areas in 2002 were 29.3 and 14.4 percent, respectively. The prevalence of stunting and underweight were lowest among the one-year age group, at 8.0 and 2.6 percent, respectively. The highest prevalence of stunting in 2002 was in the 12 to 23-month age group, after which age prevalence decreased slightly.

TABLE 8
Trends in prevalence of stunting (percentage) by age and residence, 1992 and 2002

Age	Urban		Rural		Total	
	1992	2002	1992	2002	1992	2002
0–11 months	10.7	3.9	15.2	9.2	14.4	8.0
12–23 months	19.9	8.6	37.3	20.9	33.8	18.0
24–35 months	17.2	8.0	33.0	17.3	30.3	15.1
36–47 months	19.0	3.3	41.0	19.0	36.6	15.2
48–59 months	24.8	4.9	40.6	19.6	37.4	16.1
Overall	19.1	4.9	35.0	17.3	31.9	14.3

Reference: WHO Growth Reference.
Source: NNS.

TABLE 9
Trends in prevalence of underweight (percentage) by age and residence, 1992 and 2002

Age	Urban		Rural		Total	
	1992	2002	1992	2002	1992	2002
0–11 months	8.7	1.7	10.0	2.9	9.7	2.6
12–23 months	9.8	4.6	21.8	9.6	19.3	8.4
24–35 months	10.6	5.1	21.0	11.2	19.2	9.8
36–47 months	8.5	2.4	23.8	11.7	20.7	9.4
48–59 months	12.4	3.4	19.5	11.5	18.1	9.6
Overall	10.1	3.1	20.0	9.3	18.0	7.8

Reference: WHO Growth Reference.
Source: NNS.

Trends in the nutritional status of adults

CHNS and NNS provided detailed anthropometric data that made it possible to analyse the trends in adult nutritional status. The CHNS data were used to describe the trends in body mass index (BMI) distribution among adults aged 18 to 45 years. The World Health Organization (WHO)-defined cut-offs were used to classify adults as underweight, normal weight or overweight. Underweight was defined as BMI less than 18.5 kg/m^2. BMI of more than 25 kg/m^2 was classified as overweight/obese.

Figures 12 and 13 show trends in the BMI distribution of males and females aged 18 to 45 years. The shape of the BMI distribution curves of males and females changed over the 11 years from 1989 to 2000. The main characteristic of the change is a shift to the right for both the male and the female curves. For males, mean BMI increased from 21.3 to 22.4 kg/m^2; for females, it increased from 21.8 to 22.5 kg/m^2. At the same time, the dispersion of BMI distributions widened. For males, the standard deviation increased from 2.3 to 3.1, for females, from 2.7 to 3.2. When the male and female BMI distribution curves from 1989 to 2000 are compared, the mean BMIs for females in 1989 and 1997 are significantly higher than those for males. The difference in BMI distribution between genders disappeared in 2000, because the change was significantly higher in males than in females.

In 2002, the total prevalence of overweight and obesity was 22.7 percent; however, 6.8 percent of adults aged 18 to 45 years were underweight. The prevalence of adult obesity was 7.1 percent. It is estimated that 200 million Chinese adults are overweight, and 60 million obese. The prevalence rates of overweight and obesity among adults in large cities were 30.0 and 12.3 percent, respectively.

FIGURE 12

Trends in under- and overnutrition in adults (18 to 45 years) by residence and gender, 1989 to 2000

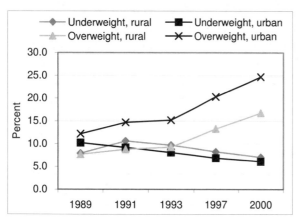
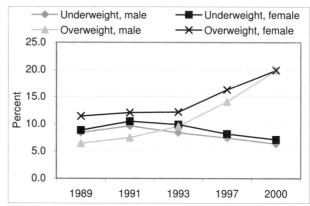

Sample sizes: 1989, 4 527; 1991, 7 204; 1993, 7 621; 1997, 7 969; 2000, 7 862.
Source: CHNS.

FIGURE 13

Changes in BMI distribution curves for males and females, 1989 to 2000

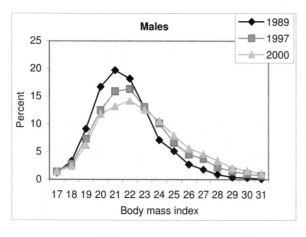
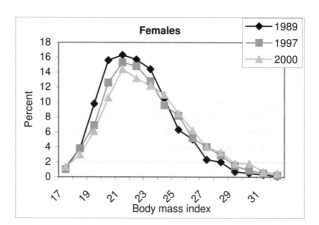

Survey population: adult males 18 to 45 years; adult females 20 to 45 years.
Sample sizes: 1989, 4 527; 1991, 7 204; 1993, 7 621; 1997, 7 969; 2000, 7 862.
Source: CHNS.

TABLE 10
Prevalence of overweight and obesity in China (percentages), 2002

Age (years)	Overweight	Obesity	Overweight and obesity
0–6	3.4	2	5.4
7–17	4.2	1.8	6
18 and over	18.9	2.9	21.8
Overall	14.7	2.6	17.3

Sample size: 209 849.
Reference: WHO reference.
Source: NNS.

Trends in micronutrient deficiencies

Although the prevalence rates of micronutrient deficiencies, including iron and vitamin A, have declined in the past ten years, they are still common problems in China.

Anaemia

The NNS data from 1992 and 2002 were used to analyse changes in the prevalence of anaemia among the Chinese. The WHO and United Nations Children's Fund (UNICEF) cut-offs of 2001 were used to define the prevalence of anaemia. The results showed that prevalence decreased slightly in the period 1992 to 2002 (Table 11). In adults, the prevalence of anaemia in urban males declined from 15.2 to 12.0 percent, and in urban females it declined from 25.8 to 20.1 percent. The prevalence among rural males remained at 18 percent, and among rural females at 24 to 25 percent. The prevalence rates of anaemia among infants and children under two years of age, people over 60 years of age and child-bearing women were 24.2, 21.5 and 20.6 percent, respectively. Anaemia is still a public health problem in China.

TABLE 11
Changes in the prevalence of anaemia (percentages) by gender and residence, 1992 and 2002

Age (years)	Urban male		Rural male		Urban female		Rural female	
	1992	2002	1992	2002	1992	2002	1992	2002
0–1	23.0	29.9	29.5	33.9	28.8	24.5	30.0	32.8
2–4	13.3	7.2	18.1	15.6	12.8	5.8	16.9	13.3
5–11	14.8	8.4	14.7	14.0	15.7	9.0	17.0	13.3
12–17	12.9	11.2	16.5	16.2	22.7	13.0	16.3	19.0
18–44	11.9	10.9	14.4	14.6	26.5	23.7	24.7	27.2
45–59	16.3	13.1	20.6	21.5	29.1	21.1	27.2	28.0
60 and more	26.2	18.3	34.1	31.9	31.5	20.9	32.9	31.3
Overall	15.2	12.0	17.8	18.0	25.8	20.1	23.3	24.9

Source: NNS.

Vitamin A deficiency

In 2002, the prevalence of vitamin A deficiency (VAD) (measured as serum retinol < 20 µg/dl) among children aged three to 12 years was 9.3 percent, in urban areas it was 3.0 percent, and in rural ones 11.2 percent. The prevalence of marginal VAD (measured as serum retinol between 20 and 29µg/dl) was 45.1 percent, with a prevalence in urban areas of 29.0 percent and in rural areas of 49.6 percent.

Iodine deficiency

The prevalence of goitre among children eight to ten years of age declined from 20 percent in 1995 to 6 percent in 2002; in 2002 it was less than 5 percent in 12 provinces, between 5 and 10 percent in 14 provinces, and more than 10 percent in five provinces.

TRENDS IN CHRONIC DISEASE RISK FACTORS
Hypertension

The 2002 NNS data and the 1991 National Sample Hypertension Survey data were used to study the prevalence of hypertension. Hypertension was defined as a mean systolic blood pressure of $\geq$ 140 mm Hg, mean diastolic blood pressure of $\geq$ 90 mm Hg, or both, when taken at two ambulatory visits five to 14 days apart. The prevalence of hypertension in people over 18 years of age increased from 11.9 percent in 1991 to 18.8 percent in 2002. It is estimated that more than 160 million people in China have hypertension. Compared with 1991, the prevalence of hypertension increased by 31 percent, and there have been more than 70 million new hypertension patients in the past decade. The prevalence of hypertension in rural areas also increased rapidly; there is no significant difference between urban and rural prevalence rates.

TABLE 12
Trends in the prevalence of hypertension in adults, 1991 and 2002

Gender	1991	2002
Male	12.3	20.2
Female	11.5	18.0
Overall	11.9	18.8

Sources: NNS, 2002; National Hypertension Survey, 1991.

Diabetes

It is estimated that there are more than 20 million diabetic patients in China. In 2002, the prevalence of type-2 diabetes among adults over 18 years of age was 2.6 percent, and among those over 60 years of age living in large cities it was 16.97 percent. The prevalence of diabetes is significantly higher in urban than in rural areas; in 2002, the prevalence in large cities was three times as much as it was in rural areas.

There are insufficient history data on diabetes to allow the change in prevalence of type-2 diabetes in China to be described. However, data from urban areas in the National Diabetes Survey in 1996 and the NNS in 2002 can be compared (Table 13). The prevalence of type-2 diabetes in large cities increased from 4.58 to 6.07 percent during the 1996 to 2002 period.

TABLE 13
Trends in the prevalence of type-2 diabetes among adults in China, 1996 and 2002

Age (years)	1996		2002		
	Large city	Small city	Large city	Small city	Rural
18–44			3.13	1.45	0.98
45–59			9.88	6.88	2.96
$\geq$ 60			16.97	11.37	4.41
Overall	4.58	3.37	6.07	3.74	1.83

Sources: NNS, 2002; National Diabetes Survey, 1996.

Blood lipids

The 2002 NNS was the first survey to provide national information about abnormal blood lipid levels in China. Hypercholesterolaemia was defined as blood cholesterolaemia of ≥ 5.72 mmol/l, while blood cholesterolaemia between 5.20 and 5.71 mmol/l was defined as borderline high cholesterol. Low serum HDL cholesterol was defined as serum HDL ≤ 0.91 mmol/l, and hypertriglyceridaemia as serum triglyceridaemia ≥ 1.70 mmol/l. A person who has one of these conditions is regarded as being in the abnormal blood lipids group.

The results show that the problem of abnormal blood lipid levels in China requires close attention. The prevalence of abnormal blood lipid levels among adults over 18 years of age was 18.6 percent – 22.2 percent among males and 15.9 percent among females. In 2002, it was estimated that 160 million people suffered from abnormal blood lipid levels. The prevalence rates of various types of abnormalities were: hypercholesterolaemia, 2.9 percent overall, 2.7 percent in males, and 2.9 percent in females; hypertriglyceridaemia, 11.9 percent overall, 14.5 percent in males, and 9.9 percent in females; and low blood HDL cholesterol, 7.4 percent overall, 9.3 percent in males, and 5.4 percent in females. An additional 3.9 percent of survey subjects had borderline high cholesterol levels. There was no significant difference in the prevalence of abnormal blood lipid levels between middle-aged and elderly subjects, nor any significant difference between urban and rural populations.

Physical activity levels

Large changes in technology at the workplace and in leisure activities are linked to rapid declines in physical activity. Economic activities are shifting towards the service sector, particularly in urban areas.

Data from CHNS for the last decade show a remarkable downward shift for the proportion of adults aged 18 to 45 years whose daily activity profile (based on occupation) would put them into a heavy activity category, compared with those in the light and medium categories.

The ownership of television sets has increased considerably over the past 20 years, especially in rural areas and among lower-income groups. In 2000, more than 90 percent of Chinese households owned a television. Television ownership represents a major potential source of inactivity.

TABLE 14
Trends in physical activity levels among Chinese adults (percentages), 1989 to 2000

Activity level	1989	1991	1993	1997	2000
Light	16.5	16.2	16.2	13.8	24.1
Moderate	18.9	19.0	18.9	21.3	25.2
Heavy	64.6	64.8	64.9	65.0	50.7

Classifications: light physical activity = working in standing position (e.g., office worker, watch repairer, salesperson, laboratory technician, teacher); moderate physical activity (e.g., student, driver, electrician, metal worker); heavy physical activity (e.g., logger, miner, stonecutter, farmer, dancer, steelworker, athlete).
Source: CHNS.

TRENDS IN MORBIDITY AND MORTALITY FROM CHRONIC AND INFECTIOUS DISEASE

In the past 20 years, the prevalence rates of chronic diseases have increased rapidly in China, while mortality from infectious disease has declined (Figure 14 and Table 15). China has shifted from infections and malnutrition to diseases related to hypertension, coronary heart disease

(CHD) and cancers. Chronic diseases have become the main cause of death in China. In 2000, the leading cause of death was cancer, followed by cerebral-vascular disease and CHD. Although infectious diseases are no longer the main causes of death, the morbidity levels from hepatitis, tuberculosis and dysentery remain high, and the burden of infectious diseases is still very high.

FIGURE 14
Trends in mortality from chronic disease in urban and rural areas, 1980 to 1999

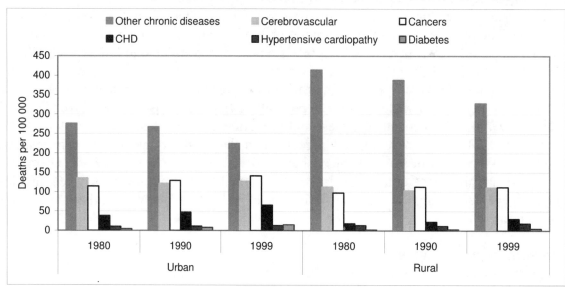

Source: Ministry of Health of China.

TABLE 15
Trends of morbidity and mortality rates to infectious disease (per 100 000 population), 1990 to 2002

Year	Hepatitis		Tuberculosis		Dysentery		Malaria		HIV	
	Morbidity	Mortality	Morbidity	Mortality	Morbidity	Mortality	Morbidity	Mortality	Morbidity	Mortality rate
1990	117.57	0.16			127.44	0.17	10.56	0.00		
1991	116.87	0.14			115.58	0.10	8.88	0.00		
1992	109.12	0.12			79.55	0.06	6.40	0.00		
1993	88.77	0.10			54.50	0.04	5.05	0.00		
1994	73.52	0.09			74.84	0.02	5.29	0.00		
1995	63.63	0.09			73.30	0.04	4.19	0.00		
1996	63.41	0.08			66.31	0.03	3.08	0.00		
1997	66.05	0.09	39.21	0.07	59.69	0.03	2.87	0.00	0.15	0.00
1998	65.78	0.07	34.69	0.07	55.34	0.03	2.67	0.00	0.10	0.00
1999	71.68	0.06	41.72	0.07	48.30	0.02	2.39	0.00	0.18	0.00
2000	64.91	0.07	43.75	0.03	40.79	0.01	2.02	0.00	0.20	0.00
2001	65.46	0.06	44.89	0.03	39.86	0.01	2.15	0.00	0.30	0.00
2002	66.10	0.08	43.58	0.08	36.23	0.02	2.65	0.00	0.33	0.00

Source: China Disease Surveillance.

POLICIES AND PROGRAMMES

China is undergoing a remarkably – and undesirably – rapid transition towards a stage of the nutrition transition characterized by high rates of DR-NCDs. Some public sector organizations in China have combined their efforts in the initial stages of systematic attempts to reduce these problems. Such efforts, which focus on both under- and overnutrition, include the new Dietary guidelines for Chinese residents, the Chinese Pagoda and the National Plan of Action for Nutrition in China, which has been issued by the highest body of the government – the State Council. Apart from some activities in the agriculture sector, few systematic efforts are having an impact on behaviour. In the health sector, efforts to reduce hypertension and diabetes are increasing, but limited work is being done in the nutrition sector. There is a need for nutrition education activities and dissemination to promote the principles of the Dietary guidelines for Chinese residents, as well as more guidance on increased physical activity and its benefits (Zhai *et al.,* 2002b).

CONCLUSION

The nutrition and health status of Chinese people has improved significantly in the past 20 years. China is one of the world's most rapidly developing countries. Over the past two decades, the annual gross domestic product (GDP) growth rate was more than 8 percent, the highest in recent world history (World Bank, 2002). As a result, the proportion of the absolutely poor population in China decreased sharply from 80 percent in 1978 to less than 12 percent in 1989; the proportion of the extremely poor decreased from 20 to 6 percent over the same period (State Statistical Bureau, 2002). China has achieved remarkable economic progress and high levels of education, and a rapid evolution of the Chinese diet has accompanied these economic shifts and related social changes.

Historically, the Chinese diet has been primarily plant-based. The classic diet includes cereals and vegetables, with few animal foods. Many experts consider such a diet to be very healthy when adequate levels of intake are achieved (Du *et al.,* 2002; Campbell, Parpia and Chen, 1998). The fat intake of the Chinese population remained at a low level for a relatively long time. Since the 1990s, however, there have been noticeable changes in the Chinese dietary pattern resulting from rapid economic development, an adequate food supply and changes in consumption patterns. With income increases, the consumption of animal food – particularly meat and eggs – has grown dramatically, while consumption of cereals and tubers has decreased.

The quality of the average diet in China has improved significantly. Energy and protein intakes among both urban and rural populations have been basically satisfactory, consumption of meat, poultry, eggs and other animal products has increased significantly as has the percentage of good-quality protein in the diet. In general, the changes have improved the quality of the Chinese diet, but there are some alarming trends in the proportional intake of energy from fat, the increased consumption of saturated fat and cholesterol and the decreasing consumption of fruits and vegetables. Many, but not all, of these changes are more pronounced in urban areas (Du *et al.,* 2002; Campbell, Parpia and Chen, 1998; Zhai *et al.,* 2002a; Wang *et al.,* 2003; Popkin and Du, 2003; Popkin, Lu and Zhai, 2002), and dietary patterns among urban residents are not entirely satisfactory. Meat and oil consumption is too high, and cereal consumption is at a relatively low level. Low consumption of dairy products remains a common problem in China.

China is facing simultaneous challenges of malnutrition and overnutrition. The growth of children and teenagers has improved steadily. The prevalence of malnutrition and nutrition deficiencies such as stunting and underweight in children under six years of age, has decreased continuously (UNESCAP, 2004; UNDP, 2004; Du *et al.,* 2002; Campbell Parpia and Chen, 1998; Chang *et al.,* 1996; Zhai *et al.,* 2004; Wang, Monteiro and Popkin, 2002). Deficiencies of micronutrients such as iron and vitamin A are still important public health problems in both urban and rural populations. The prevalence of malnutrition is still high: in 2002, 14.3 percent of preschool children were stunted, while 7.8 percent of preschool children and 6.8 percent of adults were suffering from underweight (NNS, 2005). On the other hand, the prevalence of overweight and obesity has risen at a relatively high degree, and stood at 22.7 percent for the overall population in 2002 (NNS, 2005).

Mortality from infectious diseases such as hepatitis, dysentery and malaria has been controlled in the past 20 years. Meanwhile, however, China is shifting remarkably quickly to a stage of the nutrition transition dominated by high intakes of fat and animal food, and an increasing prevalence of DR-NCDs such as obesity, diabetes mellitus, cardiovascular disease and cancer. The overweight and obesity prevalence and the morbidity to NCDs such as hypertension and type-2 diabetes have increased significantly in the past 20 years (Popkin *et al.,* 2001; Wang *et al.,* 2004). High dietary energy, high dietary fat and reduced physical activity are closely related to the occurrence of overweight, obesity, diabetes and abnormal blood lipid level. High salt intake increases the risks of hypertension. It should be emphasized that those with higher levels of fat intake and lower physical activity are at the highest risk of these chronic diseases (Popkin, 2001). Overweight, obesity and related chronic diseases have increased in both children and adults in the past 20 years and are now a major public health problem in China. In view of China's rapid nutrition transition, it is necessary to provide better guidance to the public to enable them to make rational dietary choices and take measures to control their high intakes of dietary fat and cholesterol – factors that are very significant in the prevention and control of chronic diseases.

REFERENCES

Bell, A.C., Ge, K. & Popkin, B.M. 2002. The road to obesity or the path to prevention: motorized transportation and obesity in China. *Obesity Research,* 10: 277–283.

Campbell, T.C., Parpia, B. & Chen, J. 1988. Diet, lifestyle, and the etiology of coronary artery disease: the Cornell China study. *Am. J. Cardiol.,* 82: 18–21T.

Chang, S.Y., Chang, Y., Fu, Z.Y. & He, W. 1996. Multiple factor analysis of the nutrition status of children in poor rural counties of China. *Hygiene Research,* 25(Suppl.): 83–86.

Du, S., Lu, B., Zhai, F. & Popkin, B. 2002. A new stage of the nutrition transition in China. *Public Health Nutrition,* 5(1A): 169–174.

National Hypertension Survey of China. 1991 and 1993. Informal reports. (unpublished)

NNS. 2005. *The synthetical report of the National Nutrition Survey of China 2002.* Public Health Press.

Popkin, B.M. 2001. Nutrition in transition: The changing global nutrition challenge. *Asia Pac. J. Clin. Nutr.,* 10: S13–S18.

Popkin, B.M. & Du, S. 2003. Dynamics of the nutrition transition toward the animal foods sector in China and its implications: a worried perspective. *J. Nutr.,* 133: 3898S–3906S.

Popkin, B.M., Lu, B. & Zhai, F. 2002. Understanding the nutrition transition: measuring rapid dietary changes in transitional countries. *Public Health Nutr.,* 5: 947–953.

Popkin, B.M., Horton, S., Kin, S. & Gao, J. 2001. Trends in diet, nutrition status, and diet-related non-communicable disease in China and India: the economic costs of the nutrition transition. *Nutrition Reviews,* 59(12): 379–390.

State Statistical Bureau. 1980 to 2002. *China Statistical Yearbook.* China Statistic Press.

State Statistical Bureau. 2002. *China Statistical Yearbook 2001.* China Statistic Press.

Stookey, J.D. 2001, Energy density, energy intake and weight status in a large free-living sample of Chinese adults: exploring the underlying roles of fat, protein, carbohydrate, fiber and water intakes. *Eur. J. Clin. Nutr.,* 55: 349–359.

UNDP. 2004. *Human development report, 2004.* New York, United Nations Development Programme (UNDP). Available at http://hdr.undp.org/reports/global/2004/.

UNESCAP. 2004. *Asia Pacific in Figures.* United Nations Economic and Social Commission for Asia and the Pacific (UNESCAP). 70 pp. Available at: www.unescap.org/stata/data/apif/index.asp.

Wang, Y., Monteiro, C. & Popkin, B.M. 2002. Trends of obesity and underweight in older children and adolescents in the United States, Brazil, China and Russia. *Am. J. Clin. Nutr.,* 75: 971–977.

Wang, H., Zhai, F., Du, S., Ge, K. & Popkin, B.M. 2003. The changing trend of dietary fat intake of Chinese population: an eight provinces case study in China. *Acta Nutrimenta Sinica,* 25(1): 234–238.

Wang, H., Zhai, F., He, Y., Du, S. & Hao, H. 2004. Trends in overweight among Chinese adults in some provinces from 1989 to 2000. *Acta Nutrimenta Sinica,* 26(5): 329–332.

World Bank. 2002. *World development report, 2002.* New York.

Zhai, F., Wang, H., Du, S., Ge, K. & Popkin, B.M. 2002a. The changing trend of dietary pattern of Chinese population: an eight provinces case study in China. *Acta Nutritimenta Sinica,* 24(4): 6–10.

Zhai, F., Fu, D., Du, S., Ge, K., Chen, C. & Popkin, B.M. 2002b. What is China doing in policy-making to push back the negative aspects of the nutrition transition? *Public Health Nutr.,* 5: 269–273.

Zhai, F., Wang, H., Chang, S., Fu, D., Ge, K. & Popkin, B.M. 2004. The current status, trend, and influencing factor to malnutrition of infants and children in China. *J. Community Nutrition,* 6(2): 78–85.

Assessment of dietary changes and their health implications in countries facing the double burden of malnutrition: Egypt, 1980 to 2005

H. Hassan, W. Moussa and I. Ismail, National Nutrition Institute

INTRODUCTION[1]

Egypt lies in the northwest corner of Africa and has the largest population of the Arab countries – 68.6 million people – according to population estimates made in 2004 (CAPMAS, 2004). The total land area is approximately 1 million km^2, only 6 percent of which is inhabited. Population density in the inhabited areas (primarily the Nile valley and delta) is therefore very high

DEMOGRAPHY AND URBANIZATION

The Egyptian population is estimated to have increased from 40.5 million in 1980 to 68 million in 2003. The average annual growth rate during the period 1976 to 1986 was 2.75 percent, decreasing to 2.08 percent in 1986 to 1996, and then increasing slightly again to 2.3 percent (Figure 1).

FIGURE 1
Average population growth rates (percentage), 1897 to 2002

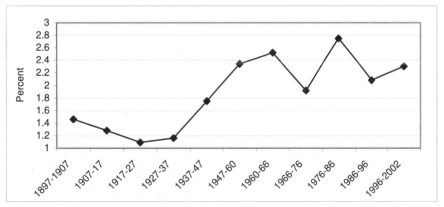

Sources: CAPMAS, 2004; EHDR, 2004.

The urban population has been growing rapidly since the early and mid-1980s, and now constitutes somewhat more than 40 percent of the total, with a decreasing growth rate that the most recent estimates put at 1.8 percent per annum (Figure 2). The declining growth rate of the urban sector may reflect the greater success of family planning efforts in urban than in rural

---

[1] This section was investigated by A. El-Hady Abbas, S. Khairy and M. Shehata.

areas. However, the urban population density has increased as a result of internal migration and the transformation of many villages into semi-urban areas (EHDR, 2004).

FIGURE 2
Urban population (as percentage of total), 1960 to 2002

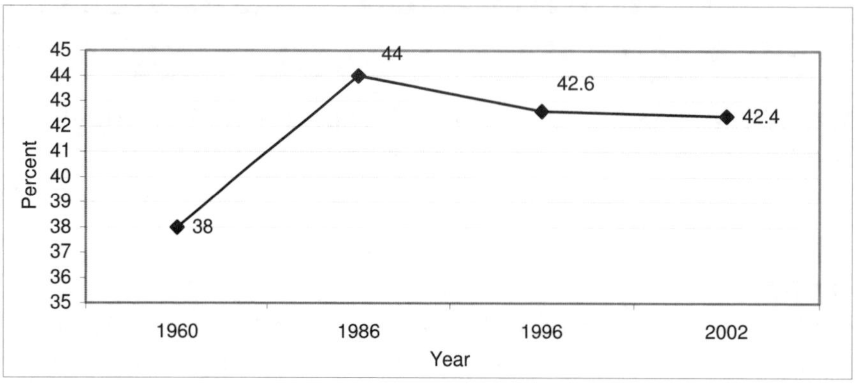

Source: EHDR, 2004.

Economy

The government adopted an Arab socialist orientation during the period 1960 to 1970, which resulted in a fairly closed economy until 1974, when Egypt moved to an open market economy. The economy expanded rapidly during the 1990s, with gross national product (GNP) almost doubling between 1993 and 1997 and the rate of inflation decreasing to 3.6 percent (EDHS, 2000).

Gross domestic product (GDP) was 354 563.6 million Egyptian pounds (LE) in 2001/2002, increasing to 365 541.1 million LE in 2002/2003, with an annual growth rate of 3.1 percent. Over the last decade, there has been a gradual increase in annual per capita income, from 4 822.4 LE in 1998/1999, to 5 537.6 LE in 2000/2001 and 5 652.8 LE in2002/2003 (CAPMAS, 2004).

Indicators of quality of life in Egypt
Health indicators

Egypt was one of the first countries in the region to set up a comprehensive, nationwide health system with a relatively well-established network of health facilities in rural and urban areas. Nearly all of the Egyptian population has access to health care services. An illustrative indicator is the current complete immunization rate for children of 88 percent.

Childhood mortality rate. The 2003 Egypt Interim Demographic and Health Survey (EIDHS, 2003) estimates that childhood mortality is becoming increasingly concentrated in early infancy. For the five-year period before the survey, the under-five mortality rate was 46 per 1 000 births, and the infant mortality rate 38 per 1 000 births. More than 80 percent of early childhood deaths in Egypt were occurring in infants under the age of one year. Neonatal and post-neonatal mortality rates (23 and 15 per 1 000, respectively) show that three-fifths of infant deaths occur within the first month of life. Estimates of childhood mortality trends over the last 40 years (1964 to 2003) show a substantial decrease. Overall, the probability of dying before the age of five years has fallen by about 80 percent, from 243 deaths per 1 000 live births in the period 1964 to 1969, to 46 in the period 1998 to 2003 (Figure 3).

FIGURE 3
Trends in early childhood mortality rate, 1964 to 2003

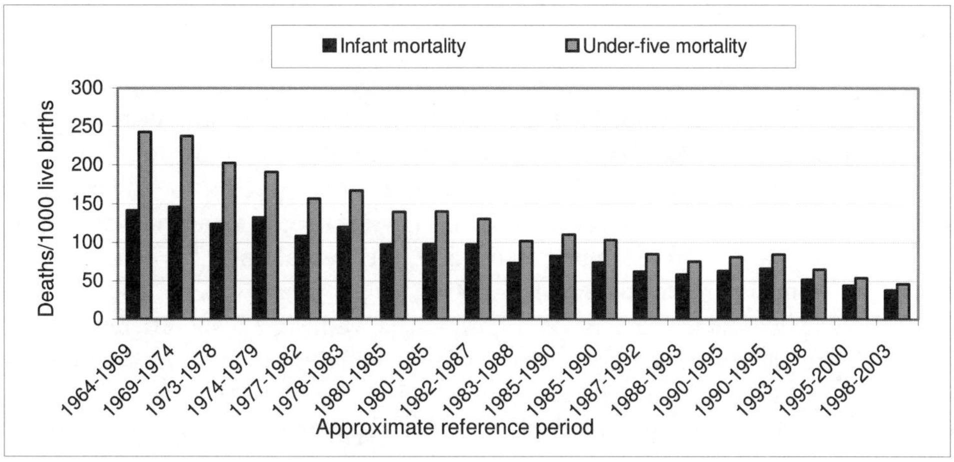

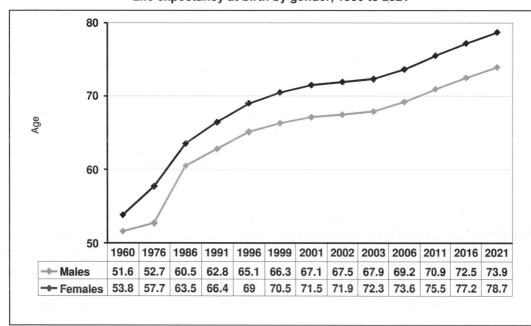

Source: EIDHS, 2003.

Life expectancy. Life expectancy increased for males from 52.7 years in 1976 to 67.9 in 2003, and for females from 57.7 years in 1976 to 72.3 in 2003 (Figure 4). Life expectancy is anticipated to reach 73.9 and 78.7 years for males and females, respectively, in 2021 (CAPMAS, 2004).

FIGURE 4
Life expectancy at birth by gender, 1960 to 2021

	1960	1976	1986	1991	1996	1999	2001	2002	2003	2006	2011	2016	2021
Males	51.6	52.7	60.5	62.8	65.1	66.3	67.1	67.5	67.9	69.2	70.9	72.5	73.9
Females	53.8	57.7	63.5	66.4	69	70.5	71.5	71.9	72.3	73.6	75.5	77.2	78.7

Education and literacy

Enrolment in secondary education rose from 42 to 86 percent between 1960 and 2001. A similar trend also occurred in primary school enrolment, which increased from 68.6 to 91.4 percent during the same period. Literacy in the adult population (aged 15 years and over) grew from 25.8 percent in 1960 to 65.6 percent in 2001 – a significant increase that demonstrates the relative success of the government's education policy to eliminate illiteracy; this is one of the major factors in Egypt's transition into the "medium level of development" category.

Water and sanitation

More than eight out of ten Egyptian households have access to piped water, mainly within their dwellings. Urban households have almost universal access to safe drinking-water; 99 percent of them have piped water in their residences, and most of the remaining households obtain water from a public tap. In rural areas, access to safe water is less widespread, with 74 percent of rural households having access to piped water, 6 percent obtaining drinking-water from public taps and the remaining 20 percent obtaining drinking-water from covered wells (EIDHS, 2003).

Two out of five households have modern flush toilets, with significant differences according to residence. More than two-thirds (68 percent) of urban households have modern flush toilets, compared with only 13 percent of rural households. In Upper Egypt, 80 percent of households in the urban governorates have modern flush toilets, compared with 8 percent in rural areas (EIDHS, 2003).

DIET AND DIETARY TRENDS[2]

There are two main sources of national-level food consumption data for Egypt. The first of these is a series of national surveys conducted by the National Nutrition Institute (NNI). In the early 1980s, a national food consumption survey was conducted in urban and rural areas of six governorates – Cairo, Alexandria, Sharkia, Souhag, Fayoum and Beheira; this covered 6 300 households, representing 35 334 individuals (Aly *et al.*, 1981). In 1995, an assessment of vitamin A status was conducted on children aged six months to six years. In 2000, another national survey was carried out to obtain up-to-date information on the national food consumption pattern; this covered 1 669 households, representing 9 134 individuals, which were randomly selected from the governorates that were studied in 1981 (Hassanyn, 2000). In 2004, a national survey was carried out to assess osteoporosis among adolescents and adults in Egypt (Hassan *et al.*, 2004). Dietary data for these surveys were collected by the food frequency of households method, and 24-hour recall and sample weighing of individuals' food intakes (Annexes 1 and 2). In the 1981 and 2000 surveys, 24-hour recall was used to calculate the mean daily per capita energy and protein intakes. For this case study, dietary data for the 1981 and 1995 surveys were derived from tables presented in the final reports, while those for the 2000 and 2004 surveys were reanalysed.

The second source of food consumption data is a series of surveys conducted by the Food Technology Research Institute, Agriculture Research Centre (FTRI/ARC) of the Ministry of Agriculture. These were first made in 1993/1994 (Khorshed, Ibrahim and Galal, 1995; Khorshed *et al.*, 1998), with subsequent rounds in 1999 and 2001/2002 (ARC, 2001/2002; Ibrahim, Youssef and Galal, 2002). The FTRI/ARC surveys were designed to create a system for monitoring the food consumption of Egyptian populations. With the exception of Khorshed *et al.*, 1998 – which is published in English and summarizes the first round of the FTRI/ARC surveys – the results of these surveys are available only in the form of final reports, and some are in Arabic only.

The NNI and FTRI/ARC surveys used different methods for analysing food intake data. In NNI surveys, data were converted into nutrient intake using Egypt's Food Composition Table, which is maintained by NNI and was compiled in 1996. To analyse the adequacy of nutrient

---

[2] This section was investigated by A. Tawfik, M. Mattar and D. Shehab.

intake, the NNI surveys use the recommended dietary allowances (RDAs) from FAO, the World Health Organization and the United Nations University (FAO/WHO/UNU, 1985) for protein and energy, from WHO (1989) for iron and from FAO/WHO (1975) for vitamins A and C, except the 2004 survey data, for which the FAO/WHO (2002) recommendations were utilized for vitamins and minerals.

The FTRI/ARC surveys conducted since 1993 used a rotating sampling scheme. The first and largest round drew its sample from rural and urban areas in Cairo, Aswan, New Valley, Ismalia and Dakhalia governorates. Subsequent rounds utilized some overlapping and some different governorates, which were selected to include a large urban centre and governorates representing the Nile Delta and Upper Egypt. Data on adult women and on children aged two to six years were collected by the household food frequency method and quantitative 24-hour recall, with collection of detailed household recipes for prepared foods and the modelling survey methodology or that used in the United States National Nutrition Monitoring System surveys. Food intake data were converted to nutrient intakes using a modification of the United States Department of Agriculture's (USDA) standard reference database (Food Intake and Analysis System, Version 2.3, University of Texas), which was adjusted to remove the influence of enrichment/fortification and to include more than 1 000 Egypt-specific recipes (Khorshed *et al.,* 1998). Nutrient intake adequacy was expressed using the extant versions of the United States RDAs (published by the National Academy Press since 1989). The quality of the first round of these data was investigated with regard to completeness and underreporting (Harrison *et al.,* 2000) and it was found that the degree of apparent underreporting was far lower than it was in surveys of adult American women conducted with a similar methodology.

Because of important methodological differences between the surveys conducted by NNI and by FTRI/ARC, this case study presents each separately. However, both used internally consistent methodology so that trends over time in the data are reliable.

Trends in dietary energy and macronutrient intake

Data from NNI national surveys conducted in 1981 and 2000 show that the mean per capita calorie intake decreased from 3 057 kcal in 1981 to 2 460 kcal in 2000 (Aly *et al.,* 1981; Hassanyn, 2000) (Figure 5).

FIGURE 5
Mean per capita calorie intake, 1981 and 2000

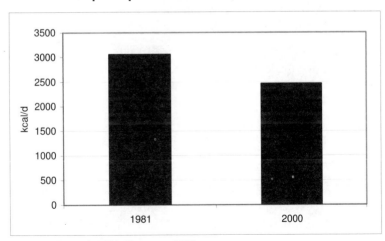

Sources: Aly *et al.,* 1981; Hassanyn, 2000.

The changes in consumption patterns of Egyptian populations shown in the data from these two surveys can be explained by changes in socio-economic status, feeding habits, urbanization and globalization. The per capita consumption of cereals decreased from 1 980 kcal in 1981 to 1 266 kcal in 2000; cereals accounted for 61.2 percent of the total energy intake in 1981, and only 52 percent in 2000. Sugar's share of total consumption also decreased, from 10.1 percent of total energy intake in 1981 to 7.7 percent in 2000. Over the same period, per capita consumption of items in the meat group increased from 163 kcal, representing 5.6 percent of total energy intake, to 298 kcal – 10.9 percent of total energy intake. The per capita consumption of items in the milk group increased from 74 kcal and 2.5 percent of total energy intake, to 177 kcal and 7.0 percent of total energy intake. This means that the percentage contribution of animal protein to total energy increased from 8.1 percent in 1981 to 19 percent in 2000 (Figure 6).

FIGURE 6
Percentage contributions of selected food groups to total energy intake, 1981 and 2000

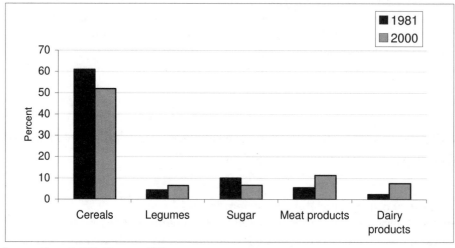

Sources: Aly *et al.,* 1981; Hassanyn, 2000.

Regarding the per capita consumption of protein, the protein intake from cereals decreased from 61.2 g/day and 54.9 percent of total protein intake in 1981, to 52 g/day and 48.2 percent of total protein intake in 2000. Per capita consumption of protein from meat increased from 16.3 g/day and 18.8 percent of total protein intake, to 25.5g/day and 26.8 percent of total protein intake (Figure 7).

FIGURE 7
Percentage contributions of selected food groups to total protein intake, 1981 and 2000

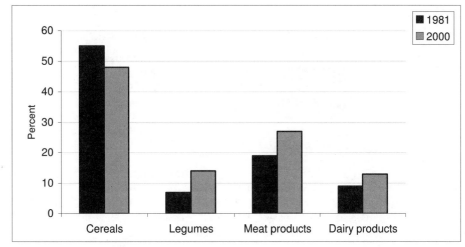

Sources: Aly et al., 1981; Hassanyn, 2000.

In order to compare the national dietary surveys conducted in 2000 and 2004, the dietary intakes of mothers were reanalysed to provide more comprehensive results. Table 1 and Figure 8 show the contributions of different food groups to the total energy intakes of mothers in 2000 and 2004. The total energy intake of mothers decreased from 2 602 kcal in 2000 to 1 995 kcal in 2004. The contribution of cereals to the total energy intake of mothers decreased from 1 349 to 1 066 kcal.

TABLE 1
Contributions of selected food groups to the total energy and protein intakes of mothers, 2000 and 2004

Food group	Energy (mean kcal/day)		Protein (mean g/day)	
	2000	2004	2000	2004
Cereals	1 349	1 066	41.4	32.7
Legumes	173.8	152	12.6	10.9
Tubers	134	110	2.0	1.7
Sugar	222	150	0.0	0.0
Fat and oils	280	195	0.0	0.0
Fruits	134	106	1.5	1.3
Vegetables	110	77.0	5.8	4.0
Meat group	291	245	23.5	21.9
Milk group	173	151	10.8	9.7
Total	**2 602**	**1 995**	**91.5**	**73.5**
Median	**2 442**	**1 944**	**88.3**	**71.5**
Number	**835**	**1 090**	**835**	**1 090**

FIGURE 8
Percentage contributions of selected food groups to the total energy intake of mothers, 2000 and 2004

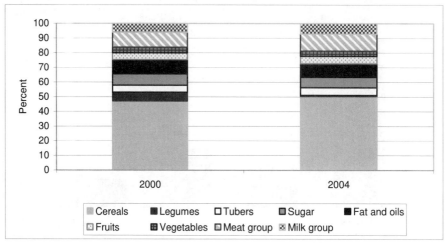

Source: NNI surveys.

Dietary adequacy

Table 2 shows the mean and median intakes of energy and nutrients for mothers in the NNI 2000 and 2004 surveys. As well as a decrease in their mean energy intakes, mothers' intakes of all macro- and micronutrients also decreased, especially those of plant protein, animal fat and calcium.

TABLE 2
Mean intakes of macro- and micronutrients among mothers, 2000 and 2004

Nutrient	2000 (n = 835)		2004 (n = 1 090)	
	Mean ± SD	Median	Mean ± SD	Median
Energy (kcal)	2 602 ± 985.9	2 442.3	1 995 ± 670.9	1 943.5
Protein (g)	91.5 ± 31.3	88.3	73.5 ± 26.7	71.5
Animal source (g)	27.4 ± 20.6	24.2	24.2 ± 18.3	21.3
Plant source (g)	64.1 ± 23.8	60.9	49.3 ± 20.9	47.1
Fat (g)	70.6 ± 53.9	64.0	53.3 ± 25.1	50.1
Animal source (g)	32.5 ± 50.5	24.5	23.5 ± 20.9	19.7
Plant source (g)	38.1 ± 23.3	33.2	29.8 ± 17.3	26.9
Iron (mg)	27.8 ± 14.7	24.0	21.1 ± 9.8	19.4
Animal source (mg)	3.2 ± 4.8	2.2	2.8 ± 3.1	2.0
Plant source (mg)	24.6 ± 13.6	21.3	18.3 ± 9.4	16.7
Vitamin A (µg)	517.3 ± 415.6	416	483.8 ± 380.2	384.1
Vitamin C (mg)	98.5 ± 102.9	72.3	92.8 ± 73.4	73.8
Calcium (mg)	626 ± 407	510.1	494.9 ± 292.3	432.8
Iodine (µg)	59.2 ± 33.3	52.8	51.1 ± 35.1	45.3

Data from ARC surveys conducted between 1995 and 2002 show the percentages of mothers and children aged two to five years who consumed less than 50 percent of the United States RDAs of selected macro- and micronutrients (Figures 9 and 10). The percentage of mothers with inadequate intakes of several nutrients decreased over time, but there are still notably high percentages of women with low intakes of vitamins A and C and calcium. The iron intake data shown here are not adjusted for bioavailability.

FIGURE 9
Percentages of mothers consuming < 50 percent of RDA of selected nutrients, 1995 to 2002

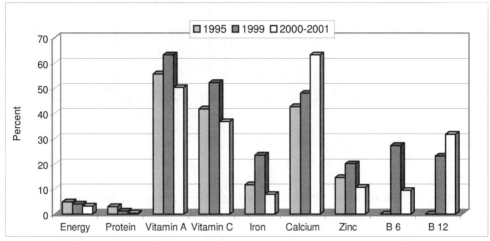

Source: ARC surveys.

FIGURE 10
Percentage of children consuming < 50 percent of RDA of selected nutrients, 1995 to 2002

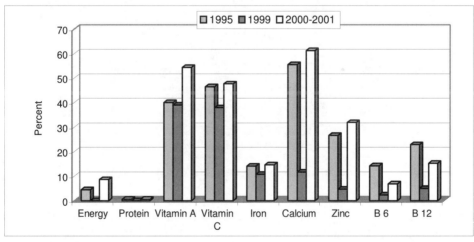

Source: ARC surveys.

ARC used the truncated method of data analysis, whereby all the data that contain consumption of more than 100 percent of RDAs are removed. NNI did not use this method, and its findings regarding the percentages of mothers and children consuming at least 100 percent of the RDAs for selected macro- and micronutrients are shown in Figures 11 and 12.

FIGURE 11
Percentages of mothers consuming ≥ 100 percent of the RDAs for macro- and micronutrients, 1995 and 2004

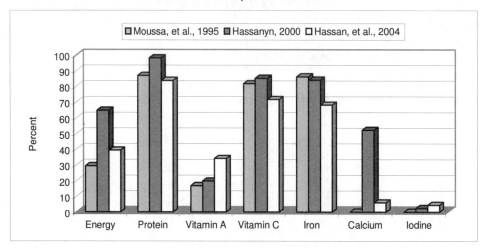

Iron requirements in 1995 and 2000 are based on WHO, 1989; and in 2004 on FAO/WHO, 2002.
Source: NNI surveys.

FIGURE 12
Percentages of children aged two to six years consuming ≥ 100 percent of the RDAs for macro- and micronutrients, 1995 and 2000

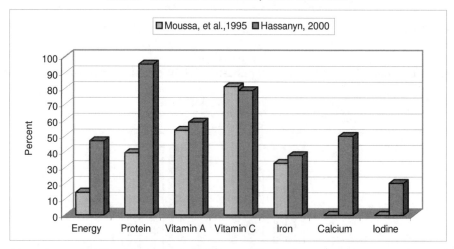

Iron requirements in 1995 and 2000 are based on WHO, 1989; and in 2004 on FAO/WHO, 2002.
Source: NNI surveys.

The special case of iron should be given separate attention. In Egyptian dietary data, the intakes of iron appear to be relatively high and do not take bioavailability into account; however, the prevalence of anaemia is also high in vulnerable populations, and is even increasing. When bioavailability is considered, iron intakes become lower. Table 3 compares the iron intake and the available iron intake calculated from the data of the 1995 FTRI/ARC survey of women. Available iron was calculated using the method of Monsen *et al.,* in which the proportion of iron absorbed is estimated from the amounts of meat, fish, poultry and ascorbic acid – all of which enhance iron absorption – in the diet. It is evident that although the average intake of iron meets or exceeds the RDA, the intake of absorbable iron is insufficient to meet average requirements. Iron bioavailability is compromised by relatively high amounts of fibre, phytate and other inhibitors in the diet, as well as by the even more significant lack of absorption enhancers.

TABLE 3
Total and available iron intakes of Egyptian women, 1995

Governorate	Total Fe (mg)	Available Fe (mg)
Cairo	14.2 ± 6.8	1.2 ± 1.3
Ismailia	15.1 ± 6.3	1.2 ± 1.2
Dhakahlia	15.8 ± 5.3	1.0 ± 1.0
New Valley	20.2 ± 7.3	1.1 ± 1.5

RDA = 15 mg.
Requirement = 1.5 to 2.5 mg.
Source: Harrison, 2000. Calculated from Ministry of Agriculture/FTRI, 1995.

Food intakes in relation to population dietary guidelines
FAO/WHO (2002) provide guidance on population nutrient intake goals for fat, sugar, sodium, fruits and vegetables and fibre, among other foods. These goals include achieving a fat intake that accounts for between 15 and 30 percent of total dietary energy. Between 1995 and 2004, the percentage of total energy provided by fat showed a modest decrease in low-fat intake groups (those for whom fat accounts for < 15 percent of dietary energy) and no change in high-intake groups (for whom it accounts for > 30 percent of dietary energy). In 2004, about 20.5 percent of mothers and more than 30 percent of young children had fat intakes that accounted for more than 30 percent of total energy intake.

The FAO/WHO recommendation on sugar indicates that less than 10 percent of total dietary energy should be derived from free sugars. The intakes of free sugars in more than half of the mothers surveyed in Egypt accounted for less than 10 percent of their total energy intakes. Most of these women lived in urban governorates (Cairo and Alexandria). High sugar intakes, accounting for 10 to 20 percent or ≥ 20 percent of total energy, were markedly more frequent in rural than urban areas and in Upper Egypt than in Middle and Lower Egypt; this is mostly owing to the habit of drinking heavily sweetened strong tea in rural areas (Hassanyn, 2000).

Almost half the survey sample (48.2 percent) reported excess intakes of animal fat (accounting for ≥ 10 percent of total energy). On the other hand, almost three-quarters of mothers consumed less than 300mg/day of cholesterol in their diets, which matches the FAO/WHO population nutrient goal recommended (Hassanyn, 2000).

Infant feeding practices
Infant feeding patterns have important impacts on the health of children. According to the Egypt Demographic and Health Surveys (EDHS) of 1992 and 1995, almost all Egyptian children (about 92 percent) are breastfed for some period, and there was no significant change in this figure between the two studies. Among the children who are breastfed, the percentage of those for whom breastfeeding begins within the first day after birth increased. Exclusive breastfeeding of children up to six months of age also increased between 1992 and 1995, as did the number of children over six months of age who received complementary foods (Figure 13). These positive trends imply that nutrition education programmes for mothers have been well received. The complementary foods that are given along with breastmilk to infants of six to 24 months usually include cereals, cow's milk and products, eggs, meat, vegetables and fruits.

FIGURE 13
Breastfeeding status of children less than 24 months, 1992 and 1995

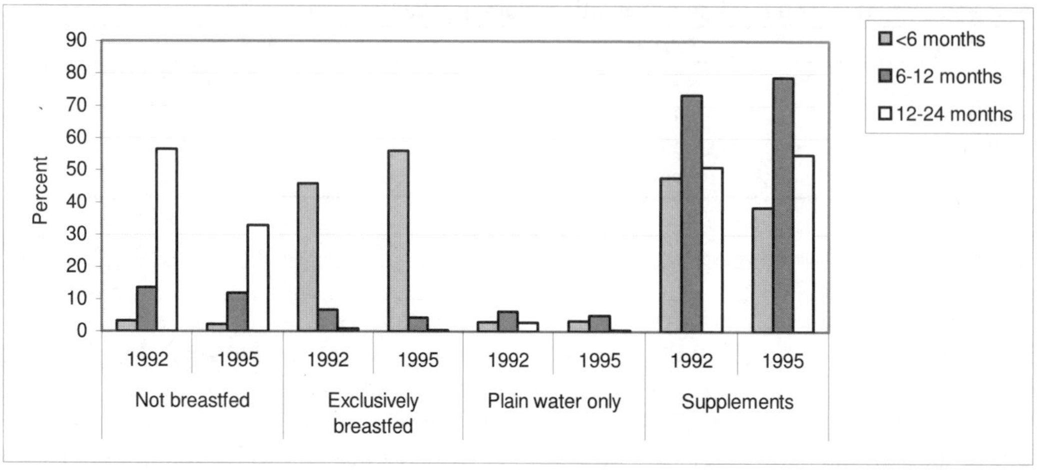

Sources: EDHS, 1992 and 1995

Intra-household food distribution

In Egypt, the prevalence of malnutrition among certain sectors of the population raises concern about intra-household food distribution. A survey studied the intra-household food distribution of 1 470 Egyptian families in three governorates – Cairo, Qualyobia and Beheria – which represent an urban, a semi-urban and a rural community, respectively. The survey included 5 431 target individuals: fathers, mothers, preschool children (aged two to six years), schoolchildren (aged six to 12 years), and male/female adolescents (aged 12 to 19 years). Dietary assessment was carried out on each target individual (using 24-hour recall and the sample weighing method), and a special method of assessing intra-household food distribution was adopted. In this method, the target individual's intakes of energy, protein and selected nutrients (iron, vitamins A and C and calcium) were recorded as percentage shares of the respective total household intake, and then compared with the recommended share for the target individual.

The results showed that fathers' share was almost equal to that recommended; mothers' was much higher than that recommended, especially in urban areas; and preschool and schoolchildren had lower than recommended energy intakes. Fathers consumed more than the recommended shares of iron, vitamin C and calcium, and the recommended share of vitamin A. All other target individuals except mothers consumed less than the recommended shares of calcium. These results were more pronounced in rural than urban communities. (Shaheen and Tawfik, 2000).

Household food security

Khorshed, Ibrahim and Galal (1995) implemented a national food consumption survey in 1994, including 6 000 households in five governorates – Cairo, Ismailia, Dhakahlia, Aswan and New Valley. One of the objectives of this survey was to identify food-insecure households, which were defined as those spending more than three-quarters of their income on food. Food-secure households were defined as those spending less than half of their income on food.

Results of the study revealed that the prevalence of food-insecure households ranged from 4.7 percent in Ismailia to 21.6 percent in Dhakahlia, with New Valley registering a prevalence of 8 percent and Aswan a relatively high 18.6 percent.

Effects of food prices and decreased food subsidies on consumption

Consumers have been affected by increases in food prices resulting from the removal of food subsidies. Galal (2002) reports that when subsidies were removed between 1990 and 1994, food prices increased sharply and at a higher rate than general inflation – three- to tenfold while wages less than doubled. Household food consumption dropped dramatically by about 20 percent during this period. A study by Ibrahim and Eid (1996) to predict the effect of removing food subsidies and applying free market prices concluded that free market prices for cereals, legumes, oils and sugar would increase the cost of energy for the population and reduce the consumption of animal protein, particularly in vulnerable groups.

Hussein *et al.*, (1989) conducted a study of families' behaviour in response to increasing food prices. A sample of 350 households in Cairo, Assuit, Beheira and industrial areas was selected. Results revealed that the rise in income could not cope with that in food costs. Less expensive foods were substituted, and the frequency of meat consumption in particular declined.

In 1994, Khorshed, Ibrahim and Galal (1995) found that 60 percent of surveyed households had changed their pattern of consumption over the previous year, owing to rising food prices. The range went from 35 percent of households in Cairo to more than 85 percent in Aswan and New Valley. About 21 percent of households indicated that they would spend additional income on improving their dietary quality by purchasing more meat, fruit and vegetables.

TRENDS IN NUTRITIONAL STATUS IN EGYPT, 1985 TO 2005[3]
Nutritional status based on anthropometry

Low birth weight

Low birth weight (LBW) is defined as weight at birth of less than 2 500 g, irrespective of gestational age. Prematurity (infants born before 37 weeks gestation) and intrauterine growth retardation (IUGR) are the two main causes of LBW: most LBW in developing countries is the result of IUGR, while in industrialized countries it is caused by pre-term birth. Most of the studies of LBW in Egypt are small-scale or depend on hospital data. The first national study was carried out in 1995 to 1997 and revealed a LBW rate of 12.6 percent of live births (El-Sahn, 2004). This is lower than the average estimated rates of 18 percent for the East Mediterranean Region (EMR) and 15 percent for the Middle East and North Africa. Among countries in the EMR, Egypt's LBW prevalence is lower than the estimated rates in Yemen (32 percent) and the Sudan (31 percent), but higher than those in the Syrian Arab Republic and Lebanon (6 percent) (UNICEF, 2003). It is also higher than the WHO estimate for Egypt (10 percent) and than most of those reported in other surveys (Figure 14). LBW is a significant public health problem in Egypt, and requires considerable attention (El-Sahn, 2004).

---

[3] This section was investigated by A. Tawfik, M. Mattar and D. Shehab.

FIGURE 14
Trends in prevalence of LBW in Egypt, 1972 to 1997

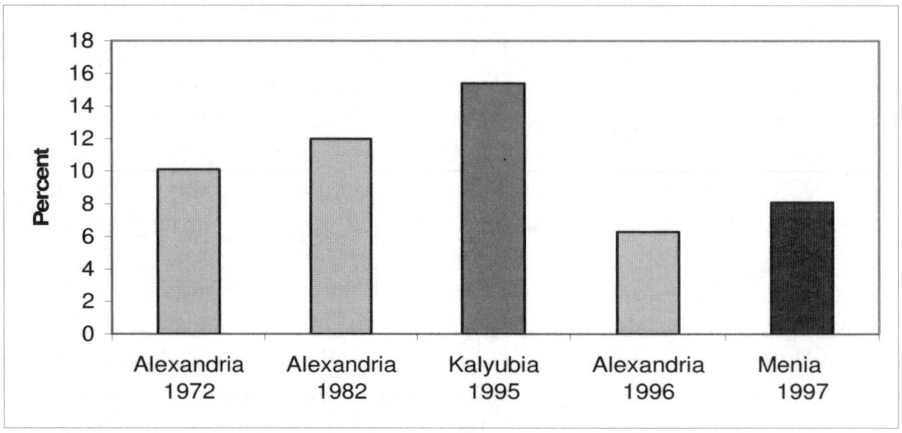

Source: El-Sahn, 2004.

Children under five years of age – Undernutrition

WHO recommends that evaluations of nutritional status be based on three indices: weight-for-age, weight-for-height and height-for-age, using Z-scores in comparison with the reference population median (WHO, 1983; 1995). The reference population of well-nourished children used by most surveys is the international reference population of the National Center for Health Statistics (NCHS), accepted by WHO as the international growth reference.

Since 1978, Egypt has been experiencing decreasing trends in the prevalence of stunted, wasted and underweight children. Between 1978 and 2004, stunting decreased from 40 to 15.8 percent, and underweight from 20.6 to 18 percent. These time series trends should be regarded cautiously as the age range of the children is not consistent across all surveys. Using more recent data from EDHS surveys conducted in 1995 and 2003 (EIDHS, 2003) on children up to 59 months of age, there have been declines in stunting (from 29.8 to 15.6 percent), underweight (12.4 to 8.6 percent) and wasting (4.6 to 4.0 percent) (Figure 15). Boys have a slightly higher prevalence for all indicators. In EDHS 1995, the percentage stunted varied from 18 percent in urban governorates to 40 percent in rural Upper Egypt, while in EDHS 2000 it ranged from 9 percent in urban governorates to 27 percent in rural Upper Egypt. This urban/rural variation is mostly caused by variation in development indicators, particularly education. The general improvement in nutritional status can mainly be attributed to improving socio-economic status, which is reflected in improved health care and quality of food consumed. Nutrition education programmes directed at mothers are contributing factors and are discussed in a later section of this case study.

FIGURE 15

Trends in prevalence of undernutrition among children under five years of age, 1992 to 2003

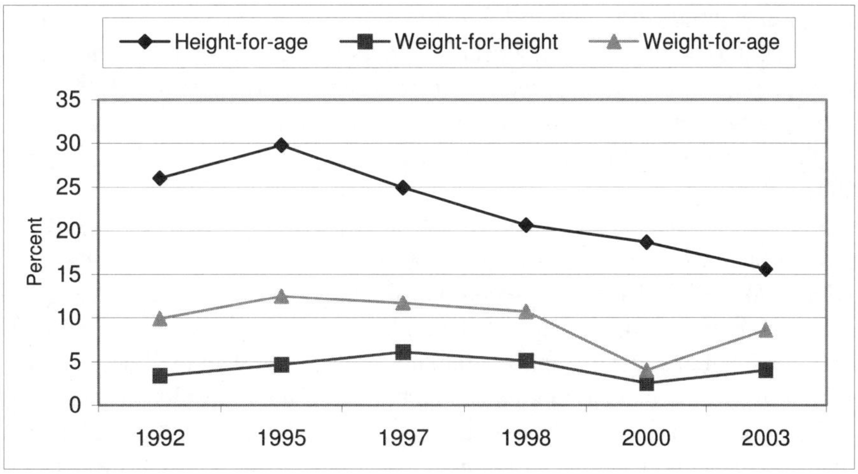

Source: EIDHS, 2003.

Children under five years of age – Overnutrition

Shaheen, Hathout and Tawfik (2004) conducted a national survey to assess prevalence of obesity in children under five years of age. The survey covered a sample of nearly 4 154 children (2 165 males and 1 969 females) in eight governorates – Cairo, Gharbia, Quena, Beni-Suef, Beheira, Suez, Matrouh and El-Wadi El-Gadid – representing six geographic areas: metropolitan, Lower Egypt, Upper Egypt, coastal, canal and frontier. It revealed that almost 8 percent of preschool children were wasted, 3.6 percent were overweight and 2 percent were obese. Obesity was more prevalent in girls (2.6 percent) than boys (1.5 percent). Frontier governorates had the lowest proportions of obese preschool children, followed by the coastal and canal regions. Metropolitan governorates and Lower Egypt had higher proportions of obese preschool children. This could be explained by changes in dietary habits leading to more energy-dense fast food and beverages with high sugar content. Although overweight among children under five years of age cannot yet be considered a public health problem in Egypt at this time, the trend is clearly toward increasing prevalence.

School-age children and adolescents (six to 18 years)

Moussa (1989) reported on the growth of school-age children using data obtained during the Health Examination Survey (HES) of the Health Profile of Egypt (HPE). The sample included at total of 6 004 school-age children (3 119 boys and 2 885 girls) aged six to 18 years from different governorates. The mean weight of boys aged six to eight years is just below the WHO reference mean; among boys of 11 to 18 years it deviates down to lie almost midway between the reference mean and 1 SD below it. The mean weight of girls is close to the reference mean at six years of age, deviates down until the age of 11 – when it is almost 1 SD below the standard mean – then improves and approaches the reference, reaching its closest point at 16 years of age before continuing below the reference mean until 18 years of age. The weights of girls are therefore better than those of boys in the six to 18 years age group. On the other hand, the curves representing mean height for boys and girls are both located below the reference mean, at close to –2SD. Boys show somewhat more relaxation in linear growth than girls, indicating chronic undernutrition.

Between 1998 and 2004, the prevalence of stunting among schoolchildren was essentially stable: 14.5 percent in 1998 and 13.2 percent in 2004. Wasting decreased from 7.8 to 4.1 percent, but underweight increased from 6.65 to 8.8 percent. Thus, the situation with regard to this age group does not seem to be improving noticeably. Underweight and stunting were more prevalent in rural than urban areas, but wasting was more prevalent in urban areas (Hassan *et al.*, 1998). Prevalence of overweight and obesity was slightly higher among school-age than preschool children, so the problem appears to be emerging rapidly in children (Shaheen, Hathout and Tawfik, 2004).

Weight status based on percentile body mass index for age (PBMI) (WHO, 1995) and prevalence of obesity were studied among 6 190 adolescents aged 12 to 19 years (Shaheen, Hathout and Tawfik, 2004). Results revealed that the prevalence of overweight is twice that of obesity among both male and female adolescents. For males the figures are 10.6 percent overweight and 5.8 percent obesity, and for females they are 19.9 and 9.7, respectively. Obesity was observed to be more prevalent in metropolitan areas (Cairo). Results are illustrated in Table 4. The trend is for prevalence of underweight to decrease and overweight and obesity to increase among female adolescents. Clearly, overweight and obesity (combined) are prevalent among Egyptian adolescents of both sexes, and at least for girls the prevalence has increased in the last few years.

TABLE 4
Anthropometric data on adolescents

Source and year of survey	Location	Sample			Underweight/ PBMI	Overweight/ PBMI	Obesity PBMI
		Size	Sex	Age (years)	< 5th	85 ≥ 95	≥ 95
Shaheen and Tawfik, 2000	Cairo, Qualyobia and Beheira	382	Male	10–19	11.8	15.2	5.5
		482	Female	10–19	11.6	17.9	7.6
Shaheen, Hathout and Tawfik, 2004	National	2 702	Male	12–19	10.5	10.6	5.8
		3 488	Female	12–19	3.1	19.9	9.7
Hassan *et al.*, 2004	National	2 039	Male	10–19	14.4	9.9	4.8
		2 021	Female	10–19	5.4	15.7	7.8
Ismail, 2005	National	6 018	Total	10–19	7.3	13.4	7.1
		2 969	Male	10–19	10.2	11.5	6.5
		3 049	Female	10–19	4.6	15.2	7.7

Adults

Several studies obtained information on the heights and weights of female adults as shown in Table 5. Underweight, defined as BMI < 18.5, which denotes chronic energy deficiency (WHO, 1995), is almost non-existent among the adult female population. Prevalence of chronic energy deficiency fell from 3.4 percent in 1995 (Moussa, El-Nehry and Abdel Galil, 1995) to 0.4 percent in 2004 (Hassan *et al.*, 2004). However, there is a trend for increasing prevalence of overweight and obesity among female adults in Egypt. From the earliest available survey year (1995) to the latest (2004), overweight among women decreased from 31.3 to 26.9 percent, while obesity increased from 20.5 to 48.2 percent.

Overweight and obesity prevalence among adults in Egypt is among the highest in the world, and there is evidence that the prevalence is still increasing, at least in women. There is a trend of increasing prevalence of overweight and obesity among female adults in Egypt (Figure 16). Between 1995 and the latest survey year 2004, overweight decreased from 31.3 to 26.9 percent among women, while, obesity has increased from 20.5 to 48.2

percent. Among urban women, data collected on large samples indicated that by 1998 the average BMI for women was in the obese range (30.08) (Galal, 2000). Furthermore, almost 5 percent of women were classified as "severely obese", i.e., BMI > 40. Men have been less studied, but 1998/1999 survey data indicated that 65.3 percent of urban Egyptian men and 34.1 percent of those in rural areas were overweight or obese. These trends can likely be attributed to changes in dietary habits towards higher consumption of energy-dense foods, together with a tendency to sedentary lifestyle particularly in urban areas. Continuous snacking between meals among housewives has been mentioned as another causal factor (Galal *et al.,* 1987). Hussein, Moussa and Shaheen (1993) demonstrate that obesity is a problem in both privileged and underprivileged areas. However, the co-morbidities of obesity are more common among the privileged, which is attributed to the quality of diet. The main source of energy among the rich is animal fat (meat and pastries), while among the poor it is carbohydrate (bread and sugar in tea) and vegetable oil (fried vegetables and tubers). Efforts to reduce weight were more common among the rich than the poor (Hussein, Moussa and Shaheen, 1993).

In the national survey by Shaheen, Hathout and Tawfik (2004), a nationally representative sample of 19 021 adults (aged 20 years and over) was used to assess the prevalence of obesity in Egypt. Results of this study revealed that women had higher overall rates of obesity than men (48.2 and 18.7 percent, respectively), although men had higher rates of overweight (34.5 percent) than women (26.9 percent). Frontier governorates and Upper Egypt had the lowest proportions of overweight and obesity. However, Lower Egypt and the metropolitan region, followed by the canal and coastal regions, had the highest percentages of overweight and obesity. This is also documented by Moussa, El-Nehry and Abdel Galil (1995), who record the highest rates of overweight and obesity in Cairo (70 percent) and the lowest in Upper Egypt (39 percent). Urban areas had higher rates of overweight and obesity than rural ones.

According to Shaheen, Hathout and Tawfik (2004), the prevalence of overweight and obesity among adults aged 20 to 80 years differs according to age. The lowest proportions of overweight and obesity were among the 20 to 30 years age group (27.8 and 8.1 percent, respectively). Prevalence gradually increased with age to reach a peak between the ages of 50 and 60 years, when overweight and obesity among men were 37.2 and 29 percent, respectively, and among women 21.8 and 66.1 percent. After the age of 60 years, the prevalence of overweight and obesity decreased slightly among men; among women obesity decreased, but overweight increased, to reach 35.7 percent at 80 years of age. These findings reflect the behaviour of the population, as consumption of extra quantities of food is usual at younger ages, and low levels of physical activity increase with age.

Although overweight and obesity are still increasing in prevalence in Egypt, and the problem is now receiving attention owing to the global emergence of obesity as a public health problem, the phenomenon has been evident in Egypt for at least 20 years. The 1981 national food consumption survey included measurements of the mothers and fathers of sampled children and reported 63.1 percent of mothers and 14.5 percent of fathers were overweight or obese (i.e., > 110 percent of the standard weight at that time) (Galal, 2000). Thus recent trends toward urban living and an abundant food supply do not by themselves totally explain the phenomenon in Egypt. However, there are many physical and cultural barriers to a physically active lifestyle in Egypt, and there is significant opportunity for the development of effective health promotion programmes to encourage physical activity.

TABLE 5
Anthropometric data on adults

Source and year of survey	Location	Sample			BMI (kg/m²)		Anthropometric status according to BMI (%)				
		Size	Gender	Age (years)	Mean	Median	Chronic energy deficiency			Over-weight	Obesity
							< 16.0	16.0–16.9	17.0–18.5	25.0–29.9	≥ 30.0
EDHS, 1995	Egypt (total)	6 314	Mothers	15–49	26.3		0.2	0.3	1.1	31.3	20.5
Moussa, El-Nehry and Abdel Galil, 1995	Egypt (total)	1 629	Mothers	20–45	26.8	26.1	1	0.4	2.0	33.0	25.5
Hassan, 2000	Egypt (total)	835	Mothers	20–48	30.4	28.7	0.2	0.1	0.7	31.3	42.1
Shaheen and Tawfik, 2000	Sub-national sample	187	Fathers	30–65	26.7	26.4			2.7	41.1	21.1
		1 470	Mothers	20–48	30.6	29.9			0.5	27.7	50.4
EDHS, 2000	Egypt (total)	13 624	Mothers	15–49	29.3		0.0	0.0	0.5	36.4	40.8
Shaheen, Hathout and Tawfik, 2004	National	8 136	Males	≥ 20	23.6	21.4	-	-	2.8	35.4	18.7
		10 885	Females		25.8	24.5	-	-	2.0	26.9	48.2
Hassan et al., 2004	National	2 028	Males	≥ 20	-	-	-	-	2.0	38.3	28.6
		2 446	Females		-	-	-	-	0.4	24.0	63.5

FIGURE 16
Trends in overweight and obesity among females, 1995 to 2004

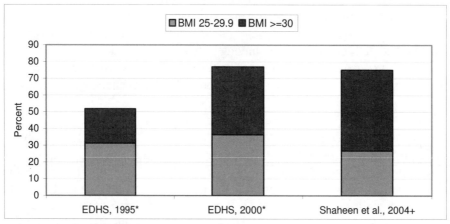

* Women 15 to 49 years in EDHS surveys
+ Women ≥ 20 years in Shaheen *et al., 2004*

Central obesity among adults

Alternative methods to the measurement of BMI are valuable in identifying individuals at increased risk from obesity-related illness owing to abdominal fat accumulation (WHO, 2000). A high waist-to-hip ratio (WHR) (≥ 1 in men and ≥ 0.85 in women) has been accepted as the clinical method of identifying patients with abdominal fat accumulation.

Findings of Shaheen, Hathout and Tawfik (2004) demonstrate that abdominal obesity (high WHR) exists among 20.8 percent of men and 45.3 percent of women. There were significant differences (p = 0.000) in the prevalence of abdominal obesity between men and women in the total sample and between urban and rural areas (p = 0.000), with 41.6 percent of adults in urban and 20.4 percent in rural areas affected. There were also significant differences (p = 0.000) in prevalence of high WHR among different governorates of Egypt.

Recent evidence suggests that waist circumference alone – measured at the midpoint between the lower border of the rib cage and the iliac crest – provides a more practical correlate of abdominal fat distribution and associated ill health (WHO, 2000). This is an approximate index of intra-abdominal fat and total body fat. Furthermore, changes in waist circumference, mainly associated with overweight and class 1 obesity, reflect changes in risk factors for cardiovascular disease (CVD) and other forms of chronic disease. Waist circumferences ≥ 88 cm in women and ≥ 102 cm in men are considered above normal (WHO, 2000).

Results of Shaheen, Hathout and Tawfik (2004) revealed that there was correlation between waist circumference levels and overweight and class 1 obesity in the total sample and in the studied governorates (p = 0.000). Nearly three-quarters of those with class I obesity had central obesity (high waist circumference), except in Beni-Suef where the figure was even higher, at 85 percent. The majority of class 1 obese women (at least 80 percent) in the study governorates and the total sample had high waist circumference, while about one-third of overweight females had high waist circumference. The percentages were lower among men than women.

Stunting and obesity

Many studies document the relation between stunting (< -2 SD height for age) as an indicator for long-standing chronic malnutrition and overweight or obesity (> +2 SD weight for height) due to inadequate intervention programmes early in childhood. There is considerable evidence, mostly from developed countries, that intrauterine growth retardation is associated with an increased risk of coronary heart disease (CHD), stroke, diabetes and raised blood pressure.

Results of Shaheen, Hathout and Tawfik (2004) revealed that 2.3 percent of stunted male and 3.7 percent of stunted female preschool children (aged two to six years) were obese; this is nearly double the prevalence of obesity in children of normal height (1.2 percent of males and 2.1 percent of females). About 6 percent of stunted male and female preschool children were overweight, compared with 2.3 percent of male and 2.9 percent of female normal-height children. This finding also holds true for school-age children: 6.1 percent of stunted male and 5.7 percent of stunted female children were obese, compared with 1.9 and 3.4 percent, respectively, for male and female children of normal height. Nearly 6 percent of stunted male and 8 percent of stunted female school-age children were overweight, while the respective percentage among normal-height school-age children was 3.8 percent for both males and females. There were significant differences in the weight status of both preschool and school-age male and female children depending on their stature levels (p = 0.000).

There was no significant difference in the weight status of either male or female adolescents (12 to 18 years) between the different stature levels. About 5 percent of stunted male and 9.2 percent of stunted female adolescents were obese, compared with 5.3 and 8.5 percent of normal-height male and female adolescents, respectively.

Micronutrient status
Iron deficiency anaemia (IDA)

Table 6 presents a summary of results from different studies on IDA in Egypt. A national survey to assess vitamin A status (Moussa, El-Nehry and Abdel Galil, 1995) recorded haematocrit values for 1 623 preschool children (aged six months to six years) and 762 mothers. Preschool children and pregnant mothers with haematocrit values equal to or less than 33 (11 gm Hb/100 ml) were considered anaemic, as were non-pregnant mothers with haematocrit values equal to or less than 36 (12 gm Hb/100 ml) (WHO, 1989).

EDHS 2000 included direct measurement of haemoglobin levels in a sub-sample of half of all EDHS households for three groups: women aged 15 to 49 years who were or who had been married; children under six years of age; and boys and girls aged 11 to 19 years. Anaemia is classified as mild, moderate or severe depending on the concentration of haemoglobin in the blood. Mild anaemia corresponds to haemoglobin concentration levels of 10 to 10.9 g/dl for pregnant women and young children; 10 to 11.9 g/dl for non-pregnant women, girls aged 11 to 19 years and boys aged 11 to 13 years; and 10.0 to 12.9 g/dl for boys aged 14 to 19 years. For all the tested groups, moderate anaemia corresponds to levels of 7 to 9.9 g/dl, and severe anaemia to levels less than 7 gm/dl.

EDHS 2000 revealed that about three out of ten young children suffer from some degree of anaemia. This is similar to the level that was found among women. Some 11 percent of young children had moderate levels of anaemia, and less than 1.0 percent were classified as having severe anaemia. Children under two years of age were more likely to be anaemic than older children, and rural children were more likely to be anaemic than urban children (33 and 24 percent, respectively). The highest anaemia prevalence (38 percent) was among children aged six to 59 months in rural Upper Egypt and the Frontier governorates, and the lowest (23 percent) was in urban Lower Egypt.

IDA among mothers, whether pregnant, lactating or non-pregnant and non-lactating (NPNL) increased significantly between 1978 (Nassar *et al.,* 1992) and 2000 (EDHS, 2000) (Figure 17).

TABLE 6
Prevalence of IDA in different age groups

Age group	Year	Site	Gender	N	Prevalence (%) < 11g %	< 12 g %	< 13 g %	Source
6–71 months	1978	Universe I	Both	176	37.0			Nassar *et al.*, 1992; NNS
	1980	Universe I	Both	176	39.0			Nassar *et al.*, 1992; NNS
				175	49.0			
	1995 and 1997		Boys[1]	852	25.2			Moussa *et al.*, 1997
			Girls[1]	771	23.7			
			Total	1 623	48.9			
	2000		Both	4 708	29.9			EDHS
6–12 years	1988		Both	3 203		45.0		(Moussa, 1989) HES of HPE
	1998	Primary school	Both	750		42.0		Hassan *et al.*
11–19 years	2000		Both	9 237				EDHS
			Boys	4 835			30.7	
			Girls	4 402		28.9		
	2004		Both	3 721				Hassan, Abdel Galil and Moussa
			Boys	1 896			39.5	
			Girls	1 825		23.0		
20+ years	1978	Community	NPNL			21.0		Nassar *et al.*, 1992; NNS
			Pregnant		22.0			
			Lactating			25.0		
			Total	1 478				
	1995	MCHC	NPNL[2]			11.0		Moussa, El-Nehy and Abdel Galil
			Pregnant[1]		26.0			
			Lactating[2]			19.0		
			Total	803				
	2000	Community	NPNL			26.3		EDHS
			Pregnant		45.4			
			Lactating			31.9		
			Total	7 684				
	2002		NPNL			40.4		El-Sayed *et al.*, 2002
			Pregnant		33.2			
			Lactating			47.0		
			Total	2 961				
	2004	Urban	Adults					Hassan, Abdel Galil and Moussa
			M. adults	692			9.6	
			F. adults	811		23.0		
		Rural	M. adults	297			13.9	
			F. adults	324		22.9		
		Total	M. adults	989			12	
			F. adults	1 135		23.0		
65+ years	2001	Upper Egypt	M. elders	275			46.9	Hassan *et al.*
			F. elders	356		31.5		
			Total	631			36.9	
		Lower Egypt	M. elders	298		19.7		
			F. elders	406				
		Urban governorates	Total	704			33.9	
			M. elders	1 310		22.7		
			F. elders	2 062			32.8	
		Urban sites	Total	3 372		24.9		
			M. elders	1 190			47.1	
			F. elders	1 948		26.2		
		Rural sites	Total	3 138			36.1	
			M. elders	363		25.2		
			F. elders	561				
		Overall total	Total	924				
			M. elders	1 883				
			F. elders	2 824				
			Total					

[1] HCT < 33 percent.
[2] HCT < 36 percent.

FIGURE 17

Trends in prevalence of IDA among pregnant, lactating and NPNL women, 1978 to 2004

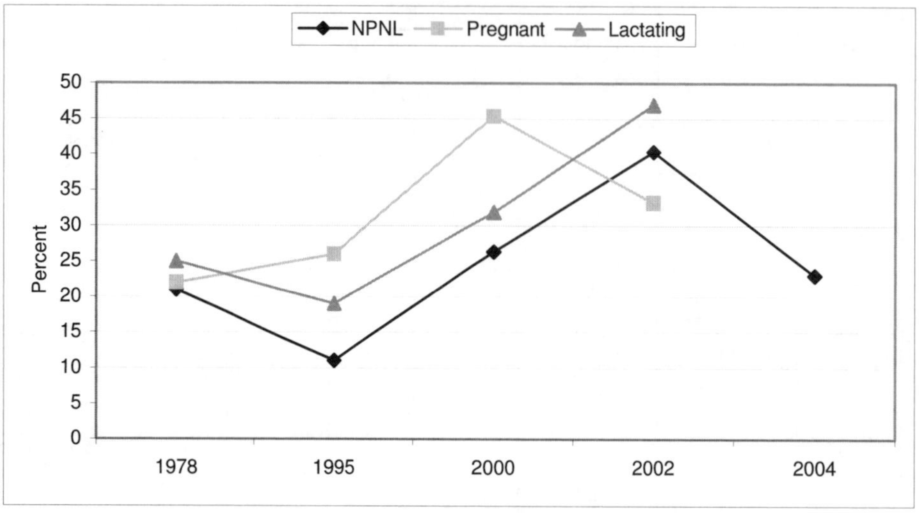

Sources: Nassar *et al.,* 1992 ; Moussa *et al.,* 1997; EDHS, 2000; El-Sayed *et al.,* 2002; Hassan *et al.,* 2004.

Vitamin A deficiency

Values of plasma retinol were available for 1 577 preschool children (aged six to 71 months) in Moussa, El-Nehry and Abdel Galil, 1995 and Moussa *et al.,* 1997. Results denoted that vitamin A deficiency (VAD) is a moderate sub-clinical public health problem in Egypt. In 2002, a national survey to assess the prevalence of vitamin A status after implementation of a vitamin A supplementation programme among children of nine and 18 months revealed that the prevalence of VAD among preschool children (six to 71 months) was 7.2 percent, implying that the vitamin A status of those children had improved.

Results of the survey to assess micronutrient deficiency among primary schoolchildren showed that a higher percentage of girls had low serum retinol levels (< 20 µg/dl) than boys.

A national survey for the determination of bone mass density among adolescents and adults in Egypt (Hassan, Abdel Galil and Moussa, 2004) showed that the prevalence of VAD among adolescents was higher in rural than urban areas. Results for adults showed a similar pattern. Findings are higher than those reported by Moussa, El-Nehry and Abdel Galil (1995) (Figure 22).

TABLE 7
Prevalence of VAD in different age groups

	Year	Site	Gender	N	Serum retinol < 20 µg/dl (%)	Source
6–71 months	1995	Urban	Both	957	11.4	Moussa, El-Nehry and Abdel Galil (national)
		Rural	Both	620	12.7	
		Both	Total	1 577	11.9	
6–11 years	1998	Urban	Boys	272	10.3	Hassan, Abdel Galil and Moussa (national)
			Girls	228	11.0	
			Total	500	10.7	
		Rural	Boys	122	8.2	
			Girls	128	18.0	
			Total	250	13.1	
		Both	Boys	394	9.3	
			Girls	356	14.5	
			Grand total	750	11.9	
6–71 months	2002	Urban	Both	803	8.2	El-Sayed *et al.* (national)
		Rural	Both	2 024	6.8	
		Both	Total	2 827	7.2	
11–19 years	2004	Urban	M. adolescents	1 283	19.7	Hassan, Abdel Galil and Moussa (national)
			F. adolescents	1 381	21.5	
			Total	2 664	20.0	
		Rural	M. adolescents	613	36.0	
			F. adolescents	444	27.0	
			Total	1 057	31.5	
		Both	M. adolescents	1 896	28.0	
			F. adolescents	1 825	24.5	
			Total	3 721	26.5	
20+ years	1995	Urban	F. adults (mothers)	455	11.0	Moussa, El-Nehry and Abdel Galil
		Rural		299	9.0	
		Total		754	10.0	
	2004	Urban	M. adults	692	17.5	Hassan *et al.* (national)
			F. adults	811	18.4	
			Total	1 503	18.0	
		Rural	M. adults	297	23.7	
			F. adults	324	22.1	
			Total	621	22.9	
		Total	M. adults	989	20.6	
			F. adults	1 135	20.3	
			Total	2 124	20.5	
65+ years	2001	Upper Egypt	M. elders	139	11.5	Hassan, Abdel Galil and Moussa (national)
			F. elders	162	12.3	
			Total	301	12.0	
		Lower Egypt	M. elders	106	19.8	
			F. elders	144	16.0	
			Total	250	17.6	
		Urban governorates	M. elders	448	12.3	
			F. elders	595	11.8	
			Total	1 043	12.0	
		Urban sites	M. elders	351	12.3	
			F. elders	470	9.6	
			Total	821	10.7	
		Rural sites	M. elders	161	13.7	
			F. elders	242	15.3	
			Total	403	14.6	
		Overall total	M. elders	512	13.0	
			F. elders	712	12.5	
			Total	1 224	13.3	

TABLE 8
Trends in prevalence of IDD in different age groups

| Age group | Year | Site | Gender | No. | Iodine status | | | Source |
					TGR %	Urinary Iodine (< 100 mg/L)	TSH < 0.39 Mlu / L	
3–<6 years	1995			593				Moussa, El-Nehry and Abdel Galil
		Urban	Boys		7.0			
		Rural	Girls		6.0			
		Total	Both		6.5			
6–11 years	1992	Primary schools		9 538				Hussein *et al.*
			Boys		4.5			
			Girls		6.0			
			Both		5.2			
	1998	Urban schools	Boys	272		27.9		Hassan *et al.*
			Girls	228		27.9		
		Rural schools	Total	500		27.9		
			Boys	122		30.3		
		Both	Girls	128		34.4		
			Total	250		32.4		
			Boys	394		29.1		
			Girls	356		31.2		
			Total	750		30.2		
11–19 years	1992	Preparatory	Both	21				Hussein *et al.*
			Boys	320	4.4			
			Girls		4.6			
					9.5			
11–14 years		Secondary school	Total		8.0			
					7.0			
			Boys		6.3			
			Girls		4.2			
			Total		11.0			
(14–17 years					7.6			
	2004	Urban	M. adolescents	1 283			7.0	Hassan, Abdel Galil and Moussa.
			F. adolescents	1 381			5.5	
			Total	2 664			6.3	
		Rural	M. adolescents	613			10.2	
			F. adolescents	444			12.7	
			Total	1 057			11.5	
		Both	M. adolescents	1 896			8.6	
			F. adolescents	1 825			9.2	
			Total	3 721			8.9	
20+ years	1995	Urban	Mothers	1 629	20.2			Moussa, El-Nehry and Abdel Galil
		Rural			23.1			
		Total			21.4			
	2004	Urban	M. adults	692			7.8	Hassan, Abdel Galil and Moussa
			F. adults	811			4.9	
			Total	1 503			6.4	
		Rural	M. adults	297			11.4	
			F. adults	324			10.5	
			Total	621			11.0	
		Both	M. adults	989			9.6	
			F. adults	1 135			7.7	
			Total	2 124			8.7	

Iodine deficiency disorders

The national survey conducted by NNI in collaboration with WHO (Hussein *et al.*, 1992) found a high prevalence of iodine deficiency disorders (IDDs) manifested by a total goitre rate (TGR) of 6.5 percent. Older adolescents (aged 15 years and over) had a TGR of 7.8 percent, which was higher than the 6.4 percent among younger adolescents (aged 12 years and over). Children of primary school age were the least affected, with TGR of 5.2 percent.

Moussa, El-Nehry and Abdel Galil (1995) also revealed a TGR of ≥ 5 percent among 23.0 percent of mothers in rural and 20.0 percent in urban sites, and in 6.5 percent of children aged six to 71 months. Both surveys denoted the existence of a public health problem among different age groups, particularly older females. Using a cut-off level of < 100 mg/l for urinary iodine excretion, Hassan *et al.* (1998) reported that 30 percent of children in primary schools had iodine deficiency.

Based on serum TSH value < 0.39 ml U/l, the national survey of osteoporosis revealed that nearly 9 percent of adolescents and adults had iodine deficiency (Hassan, Abdel Galil and Moussa, 2004).

Zinc and other micronutrients

Results of the national survey of micronutrient deficiencies among primary schoolchildren (Hassan *et al.*, 1998) showed an overall serum zinc deficiency rate of 15.5 percent, with higher prevalence among boys in rural areas (19.7 percent).

Hassan, Abdel Galil and Moussa's (2004) national survey to determine bone mineral density among Egyptians found that 8.5 percent of adolescents and 5.6 percent of adults had low serum zinc levels, with no significant gender- or area-based differences.

Regarding serum selenium levels, 8.8 percent of primary schoolchildren had low levels (Hassan *et al.*, 1998). Adolescents and adults suffered more from this problem, with low serum selenium rates of 26.0 and 25.0 percent, respectively. Females had higher prevalence than males, regardless of area of residence (Hassan, Abdel Galil and Moussa, 2004).

Calcium, phosphorus and vitamin D data reflect that the problem was mainly related to calcium, with more than 20 percent of adolescents and nearly one-third of adults having low serum calcium. Rural sites showed greater deficiency, particularly among adults, with no apparent gender-based differences. This was mainly related to the higher prevalence of obesity among females on the one hand, and of smoking among males on the other (Hassan, Abdel Galil and Moussa, 2004).

The burden of low serum magnesium (Mg) levels was found to be far higher among adolescents than adults; 22.0 percent of adolescents and 10 percent of adults had low serum Mg. This was mainly explained by the effect of growth on skeletal health and mineral metabolism (Hassan, Abdel Galil and Moussa, 2004) (Table 9).

TABLE 9
Percentage distribution of studied populations according to serum cut-off of micronutrients

Source	Vitamin D (< 14 ng/dl) %	Calcium (< 8.4 mg/dl) %	Selenium[2] (< 9.6 µg/dl) %	Zinc[1] (< 80 µg/dl) %	No.	Gender	Site	Year	Age group
Hassan			11.0	12.0	500		Urban	1998	6–11 years
et al.			6.6	10.7	272	Boys			
			15.4	13.2	228	Girls			
			6.6	18.9	250		Rural		
			6.6	19.7	122	Boys			
			6.6	18.0	128	Girls			
			8.8	15.5	750		Total		
			6.6	15.2	394	Boys			
			11.0	15.6	356	Girls			
Hassan,	4.2	21.6	25.0	8.6	2 664		Urban	2004	>11–19 years[3]
Abdel	5.1	23.2	18.2	7.4	1 283	M. adolescents			
Galil	3.3	20.0	31.9	9.8	1 381	F. adolescents			
and	3.3	23.4	27.3	8.3	1 057		Rural		
Moussa,	4.8	24.5	26.7	7.9	613	M. adolescents			
	1.7	22.3	27.8	8.7	444	F. adolescents			
	3.8	22.5	26.2	8.5	3 721		Total		
	5.0	23.9	22.5	7.7	1 896	M. adolescents			
	2.5	21.2	29.9	9.3	1 825	F. adolescents			
	2.0	25.7	24.6	4.6	1 503		Urban	2004	20+ years[3]
	0.9	25.1	18.6	4.3	692	M. adults			
	3.1	26.2	30.6	4.8	811	F. adults			
	3.8	32.6	26.0	6.6	621		Rural		
	5.2	33.5	16.4	7.5	297	M. adults			
	2.4	31.6	35.8	5.7	324	F. adults			
	2.95	29.1	25.4	5.6	2 124		Total		
	3.1	29.3	17.5	5.9	989	M. adults			
	2.8	28.9	33.2	5.3	1 135	F. adults			

[1] WHO/FAO, 1996 cut-off.
[2] Nelson, 1996 cut-off.
[3] Cut-off of serum zinc is >70 µg/dl, and of serum selenium <7.5 µg/dl (Hassan Abdel Galil and Moussa, 2004).

DIET-RELATED CHRONIC DISEASES[4]

Non-communicable diseases (NCDs) are the primary cause of mortality and morbidity in countries of the Eastern Mediterranean Region (EMR). NCDs are emerging as a major health problem in Egypt, where 41 percent of all deaths are caused by chronic diseases. As life expectancy increases and the elderly population continues to grow, chronic diseases will place an ever-greater burden on society (WHO, 2004).

This section provides a brief overview of trends in the major NCDs (hypertension, diabetes, CVD, cancer and osteoporosis) in Egypt over the last 20 years. Consecutive national surveys are lacking for most diseases, and available data spotlight only the present situation. Data sets on NCDs are shown in Annex 3, and in the tables and figures throughout this section.

Hypertension

Hypertension is considered a major risk factor for CHD, cerebrovascular disease and chronic renal failure. HPE-HES 1987 estimated that the overall prevalence of hypertension among Egyptians over six years of age was 15.8 percent. Systolic hypertension (above 150 mm Hg) was found among 11.3 percent, and diastolic hypertension (above 90 mm Hg)

---

[4] This section was investigated by F. Soliman.

among 4.7 percent of Egyptians. Systolic hypertension was more frequent among urban residents (Said, 1987).

The National Hypertension Project (NHP) of 1995 estimated the overall prevalence of hypertension among Egyptians ≥ 25 years of age at 26.3 percent (Figure 18). High systolic blood pressure (≥ 140 mm Hg) was reported among 17.2 percent, while 13.9 percent had high diastolic blood pressure (≥ 90 mm Hg). Hypertension increased progressively with age, and was slightly more common in women than men. However, younger age groups have shown progressive increases of hypertension over the past 20 years. The NHP results indicated that hypertension is highly prevalent in Egypt, and that awareness, treatment and control of hypertension are relatively limited (Ibrahim *et al.*, 1995).

Adults with high normal blood pressure (130 to 139 mm Hg systolic blood pressure or 85 to 89 mm Hg diastolic blood pressure) are considered to be at high risk of developing hypertension; this group represented 17.5 percent of adults in 1995. The prevalence of hypercholesterolaemia and high levels of LDL-cholesterol was found to be higher among hypertensives than others (Ibrahim *et al.*, 1995).

Preliminary data from a diet, nutrition and prevention of chronic NCDs survey (Ismail, 2005) showed that the crude prevalence of hypertension among adolescents aged ten to 18 years is 1.4 percent (Table 10), with higher prevalence in Upper Egypt than Lower Egypt for both types of hypertension. Females in rural areas reported the lowest prevalence rates of both systolic and diastolic hypertension, while females in urban areas reported the highest prevalence of diastolic hypertension, followed by males of both areas. Generally, males in all age groups had higher systolic hypertension than females (Figure 19), especially in the older age group (16 to 18 years). Females had higher diastolic hypertension, except for in the older age group where both genders were equal. Findings on adolescents with high normal blood pressure denoted that about one-quarter of Egyptian adolescents would develop hypertension over the following few years.

This case study uses studies of the status of hypertension among Egyptians covering the period from 1987 to 2005. They represent different age groups and use different cut-offs for hypertension, so it is not possible to derive trends from them.

Increasing prevalence of overweight and obesity among Egyptians constitutes a risk factor for hypertension. Increasing intakes of animal protein and low intakes of dietary calcium and magnesium probably contribute to the early development of hypertension in Egypt.

FIGURE 18
National estimate of hypertension among Egyptians aged 25 years and more, 1995

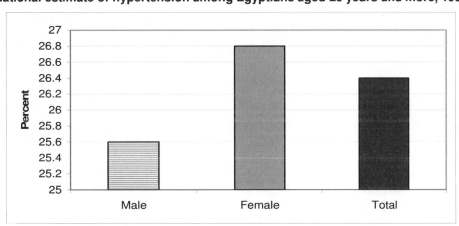

Source: Ibrahim *et al.*, 1995.

TABLE 10
Status of systolic blood pressure and diastolic blood pressure by area and gender among Egyptian adolescents, 2005

	Systolic blood pressure		Diastolic blood pressure	
	% high normal[1]	% high[2]	% high normal[1]	% high[2]
Urban				
Male	13.3	1.6	24.7	1.4
Female	10.7	1.5	28.9	1.7
Rural				
Male	10.5	1.5	22.3	1.6
Female	12.4	0.9	28.4	0.8
Total				
Male	12.0	1.5	23.8	1.2
Female	11.5	1.2	28.7	1.3
Overall total	**11.8**	**1.4**	**26.1**	**1.4**

[1] High normal blood pressure: 90th to < 95th percentile for age.
[2] High blood pressure: 95th to > 99th percentile for age.
Source: Ismail, 2005.

FIGURE 19
Hypertension prevalence among Egyptian adolescents by age group and gender, 2005

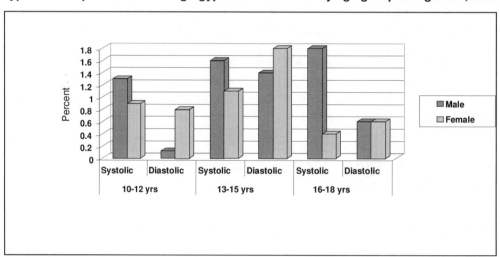

Source: Ismail, 2005.

Diabetes

Diabetes is considered a risk factor for CVD, renal impairment and blindness. In 1987, 1.3 percent of the people interviewed in a survey were aware that they had diabetes. Of these aware diabetics, 19.4 percent in both urban and rural areas were current smokers, and more male than female diabetics smoked. Regardless of area and sex, about half of the smokers smoked ten to 20 cigarettes a day (Said, 1987). In 1992, the overall prevalence of diagnosed diabetes among Egyptians over ten years of age was 4.3 percent, with higher rates among urban populations (Figure 20). Rural desert areas reported the lowest prevalence rate (Moursi, 1992).

In 1995, the combined prevalence of diagnosed and undiagnosed diabetes in the Egyptian population ≥ 20 years of age was estimated to be 9.3 percent (Figure 21). Approximately half of these people were already known to have diabetes, while the other half were discovered to have diabetes during the survey; 9.6 percent had impaired glucose tolerance (IGT). IGT was more prevalent in rural than urban areas and in lower than higher socio-economic groups. As a group, diabetics represent the most obese segment of the population and have the highest WHRs (Hermann *et al.,* 1995).

In 2005, the total prevalence of diabetes among children aged ten to 18 years was 0.7 percent (Table 11). The prevalence was higher among females than males, and equal in urban and rural areas. Children with fasting blood glucose (FBG) levels between 100 and 125 mg/dl were considered pre-diabetic; they represented 16.4 percent of the total sample. Males were more likely than females to be pre-diabetic. The rate differed according to age group, with the older age group (16 to 18 years) showing higher percentages for both sexes. Pre-diabetic males were equally prevalent in urban and rural areas, while there were more pre-diabetic females in rural than urban areas (Ismail, 2005). The high prevalence of pre-diabetic adolescents is an alarming signal for an increase in the incidence of diabetes among Egyptians in the future.

Increasing central obesity among adults (Shaheen, Hathout and Tawfik, 2004) and adolescents (Ismail, 2005) could partially explain the apparent increase in the prevalence of type-2 diabetes.

The National Diabetic Institute of Egypt, in collaboration with the Ministry of Health and Population (MOHP) and WHO, is carrying out a national survey on diabetes in Egypt. Data have not yet been published.

TABLE 11
Prevalence of diabetes and pre-diabetes among adolescents, by age and gender

Age group (years)	Male		Female		Total	
	Diabetic[1] (%)	Pre-diabetic[2] (%)	Diabetic[1] (%)	Pre-diabetic[2] (%)	Diabetic[1] (%)	Pre-diabetic[2] (%)
10–12	0.9	14.9	1.1	15.9	1.0	15.5
13–15	0.5	18.6	0.5	13.7	0.5	16.2
16–18	0.5	21.8	1.2	20.8	0.9	21.1
10–18	0.6	17.9	0.8	15.5	0.7	16.4

[1] FBG $\geq$ 126 mg/dl.
[2] FBG 100 to 125 mg/dl.
Source: Ismail, 2005.

FIGURE 20
Prevalence of diabetes by area at ten years of age and over, 1992

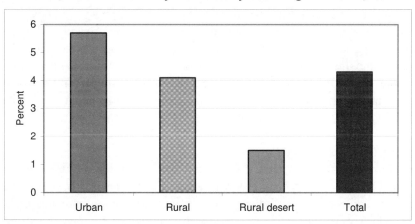

Source: Moursi, 1995.

FIGURE 21
Prevalence of diabetes by area and socio-economic status (SES) at 20 years of age and over, 1995

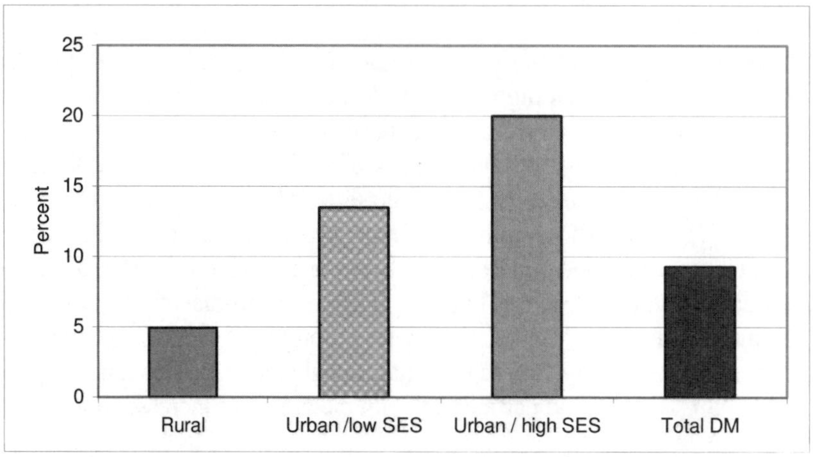

Source: Hermann *et al.,* 1995.

Cardiovascular disease

In Egypt, the prevalence of CVD has multiplied over the last two decades. The possible causes of this increase are the progressive ageing of the population, urbanization, dietary changes, sedentary lifestyles, smoking and stress. Among elderly Egyptians, CVD is the most prevalent chronic disease, followed by rheumatic diseases and diabetes (Hassan *et al.,* 2001).

In September 2000, the Egyptian Central Agency for Public Mobilization and Statistics (CAPMAS) released a report showing that CVD was responsible for 42.6 percent of all deaths. Hospital records of the reasons for admission to the cardiac department of Cairo University in 1984 and 1998 show that the prevalence of CVD increased from 6.9 to 32.9 percent over that period.

NHP data from 1991 to 1994 show that the following cardiovascular risk factors are more frequent in urban than rural Egyptians: hypertension, hypercholesterolaemia, low HDL-cholesterol, obesity, hypertriglyceridaemia, elevated LDL-cholesterol, increased fasting and post-prandial blood sugar, and cigarette smoking (Ibrahim *et al.,* 1995).

The Lipid Profile among Egyptians (LPE) of 1997 to 1999 is Egypt's first national survey of lipid profiles and ischaemic heart disease (IHD) based on a strict probability sample (Abdel-Aziz, 2000). Data from LPE reveal that risk factors varied among geographic areas, between urban and rural sites and between males and females. Lack of exercise and the threateningly high incidence of smoking should receive much attention from all health authorities. The apparently low incidence of smoking among females may not be reliable, as many women who smoke deny doing so. Results from LPE showed that 6 percent of men and 4.7 percent of women had IHD. Almost 40 percent of the whole population have cholesterol levels that are higher than the upper limit of normal (Table 12). There have been gradual increases in serum total cholesterol and LDL-cholesterol, which peak between the ages of 45 and 65 years, and a coincident decline in HDL-cholesterol (Abdel Aziz, 2000).

The Diet, Nutrition and Prevention of Chronic Non-Communicable Disease Survey (Ismail, 2005) is the first national survey to assess risk factors for the development of chronic diseases among Egyptian adolescents. Preliminary data from this survey indicate that the overall proportion of adolescents with high total cholesterol is 6.0 percent; the proportion with high

LDL-cholesterol is 7.0 percent, with high triglycerides 7.8 percent, and with low HDL-cholesterol 40.0 percent (Table 13).

Increasing hypertension, diabetes and central obesity, in addition to dyslipidaemia, should be considered among the risk factors leading to the increase of CVD in Egypt. Decreased intakes of cereals over the last 20 years, with increased consumption of animal protein and trans fat and low intakes of omega 3 fat (Hassanyn, 2000), together with inactivity and smoking (Abdel Aziz, 2000) may all be co-factors for hypercholesterolaemia, which is a leading cause of atherosclerosis and vascular diseases.

TABLE 12
Distribution of total cholesterol, LDL-cholesterol and triglycerides among Egyptian adults

Lipid parameter	Male %	Female %	Total %
Total cholesterol (mg/dl)			
< 200	55.1	53.0	53.8
200–300	39.2	38.1	38.8
> 300	7.7	7.2	7.4
LDL-cholesterol (mg/dl)			
< 150	84.1	78.2	81.6
150–200	16.2	14	15.1
> 200	3.6	3.1	3.3
Triglycerides (mg/dl)			
< 200	83.2	85.0	84.1
200–300	10.5	11.6	11.3
> 300	4.7	4.5	4.6

Source: Abdel Aziz, 2000.

TABLE 13
Distribution of total cholesterol, LDL-cholesterol, HDL-cholesterol and triglycerides among Egyptian adolescents

Lipid parameter	Male %	Female %
Total cholesterol (mg/dl)		
Acceptable: < 170	79.7	73.7
Borderline: –199	14.9	19.2
High: >= 200	5.4	7.1
LDL-cholesterol (mg/dl)		
Acceptable: < 110	85.0	80.9
Borderline: –129	8.6	10.9
High: >= 130	6.9	8.1
HDL-cholesterol(mg/dl)		
Normal: >= 35	60.0	62.2
Risky: < 35	40.0	37.8
Triglycerides (mg/dl)		
Normal: >= 150	91.1	93.3
High: > 150	8.9	6.7

Source: Ismail, 2005.

FIGURE 22
Numbers of cases of NCDs, 2001 to 2003

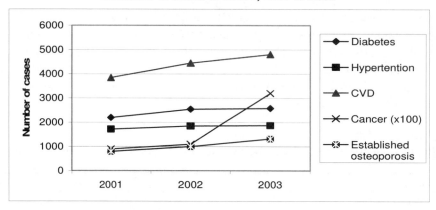

Source: National Centre of Health and Population Information, 2005.

FIGURE 23
Trend in CVD mortality rate in Egypt, 1973 to 1995

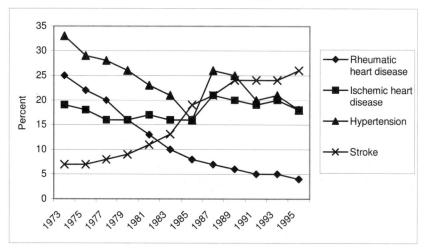

Source: National Centre of Health and Population Information, 2005.

FIGURE 24
CHD crude death rate by gender, 1990 to 1999

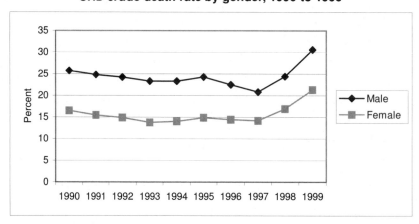

Source: CAPMAS, 2004.

Cancer

In developing countries, cancer is the third most frequent cause of death, after infectious diseases and diseases of the circulatory system; in developed countries it ranks second, after diseases of the circulatory system (WHO/FAO, 2003). Dietary factors account for about 30 percent of all cancers in Western countries, and for up to about 20 percent in developing countries; diet is second to tobacco as a preventable cause. Approximately 20 million people suffer from cancer; a figure that is projected to rise to 30 million within 20 years.

Since 1998, MOHP and the Middle East Cancer Consortium (MECC) have been sponsoring the National Cancer Institute (NCI), which is part of MECC's Joint Cancer Registry. The NCI registry in Cairo is the largest hospital-based cancer registry in Egypt (GPCR Board, 2002).

According to NCI cancer statistics from 2003, the leading cancers in Egyptian patients are those of the breast, gastrointestinal tract, lymphoma and urinary bladder (Table 14). There is male predominance in cancer incidence, with a male–female ratio of 1.4: 1.0 (El-Bolkiny, Nouh and El-Bolkiny, 2005). The increasing prevalence of obesity among females is one of the reasons for increasing rates of breast cancer.

Liver cancer increased markedly from 0.2 percent in the mid-1970s to 7.5 percent in 2003, most probably owing to higher prevalence of hepatitis C infection. Observational data from NCI reveal that lung cancer is increasing, probably because of an increase in smoking. Mesothelloma (cancer of the pleura) is also increasing, which may be owing to asbestos inhalation.

Paediatric cancers are relatively common in Egypt and account for about 10 percent of all cancer cases. In 2003, the most common types of cancer among Egyptian children and adolescents up to 19 years of age where leukaemia (34 percent of cases) followed by lymphoma (17 percent of cases) (El Attar, in press).

TABLE 14
Most common diagnosed types of cancer, 1970 to 2003

Site/type	1970–1985 (%)	1985–1989 (%)	1990–1997 (%)	1997–2001 (%)	2002–2003 (%)
Gastrointestinal tract	17.2	14.3	22.2	18.4	17.0
Urinary bladder	29.9	27.1	32.2	18.2	10.4
Breast	14.0	11.3	13.5	24.3	19
Lymphoma/ leukaemia	12.2	19.2	7.1	9.8	15.6
Data obtained from	In-patient records	Pathology registry records	Pathology registry records	Hospital data base	Hospital data base
Source	Sherif and Ibrahim, 1987	Mokhtar, 1991	El-Bolkiny, Nouh and El-Bolkiny, 2005	NCI, Cancer Statistics, 2002	El Attar, in press

TABLE 15
Most commonly diagnosed types of paediatric cancer, 1997 and 2001

Site/type	NCI, 1997 (%)	NCI, 2001 (%)
Leukaemia	36.7	20.9
Lymphomas	32	15.7
Neuroblastoma	1.6	3.7
Wilm's	3.7	1.6
Soft tissues	9.2	9.4
Bone	8.8	4.9
Liver	0.2	2.5
CNS, brain	1.6	5.5
Retinoblastoma	1.3	3.1

Sources: NCI, Cancer Statistics, 1997; El Attar, in press.

FIGURE 25
Trends in cancer diagnosis among Egyptian adults, 1970 to 2003

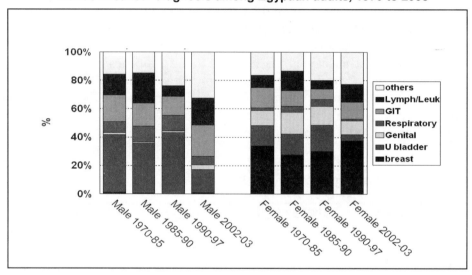

Data obtained from: in-patient records, 1970 to 1985; pathology registry records, 1985 to 1989 and 1990 to 1997; hospital data base, 1997 to 2001 and 2002 to 2003.
Sources: Sherif and Ibrahim, 1987; Mokhtar, 1991; El-Bolkiny, Nouh and El-Bolkiny, 2005; NCI, Cancer Statistics, 2002; El Attar, in press.

Osteoporosis

Osteoporosis is a disease of progressive bone loss associated with an increased risk of fractures. The disease often develops unnoticed over many years, with no symptoms or discomfort until fractures occur (AAOS, 2000). Diagnosis of osteopenia and osteoporosis in this case study is based on WHO 1994 classifications. Data from NNI national surveys to determine bone mass density (BMD) among adolescents and adults in 2004 (Table 16), and among the elderly in 2001 revealed that osteoporosis is a major health problem in Egypt.

About half of male adolescents (aged ten to 19 years) and more than one-quarter of females in the same age group were relatively osteopenic. The prevalence rates of relative osteoporosis were 16.7 and 0.9 percent for males and females, respectively, with no statistical difference between urban and rural areas. There was a statistically significant difference between male and female adolescents, but as age advanced the bone status of male adolescents improved, so that by the age of 18 years only 13 percent still had relative osteopenia. It is reported that nearly 70 to 80 percent of adult BMD is attained by the age of 18 years (Hassan, Abdel Galil and Moussa, 2004).

In the 40 to 50 years age group, 42 percent of females and 43 percent of males had low BMD. At the age of 60 years, about half of the males had osteoporosis, and half of the females had osteopenia, while a third of the elderly population (65 to over 80 years of age) are osteoporotic (Hassan, Abdel Galil and Moussa, 2001).

The unexpectedly high prevalence of low BMD among Egyptians, especially adult men, could be explained by increased smoking, reduced physical activity and increased consumption of soft drinks, in addition to low calcium intake, low omega 3 fat in diets and increasing animal protein intakes.

TABLE 16
Prevalence of osteopenia and osteoporosis among adults, by age and gender

Age group (years)	Gender	Osteopenia[1] %	Osteoporosis[2] %
20–30	Male	0.0	12.5
	Female	5.0	8.6
30–40	Male	11.8	9.5
	Female	5.2	10.6
40–50	Male	13.7	11.8
	Female	7.0	13.8
50–60	Male	15.9	21.9
	Female	11.4	21.3
≥ 60	Male	11.1	55.6
	Female	50.0	0.0
Overall	Male	14.1	14.9
	Female	6.5	12.6

[1] BMD > 1 -< 2.5 SD reference mean.
[2] BMD ≥ 2.5 SD reference mean.
N.B. Osteopenia and osteoporosis are relative in adolescents.
Source: Hassan, Abdel Galil and Moussa, 2004.

COMMUNICABLE DISEASE BURDEN[5]

Table 17 provides numbers of reported cases of the most serious communicable diseases. It is clear from the available data that hepatitis has been the most widespread and serious communicable disease in Egypt over the last 25 years, followed by pulmonary tuberculosis and meningococcal meningitis. There is also high mortality among patients with tuberculosis (TB), meningitis and hepatitis, but the compulsory vaccination programme against hepatitis B and the new prophylactic and therapeutic measures to control the spread of hepatitis C might have diminished the mortality among hepatitis patients (WHO, 2005).

In contrast, the relatively high mortality rate among AIDS patients, which does not correspond to the total of reported cases, may be due to difficulties in identifying cases before they reach their terminal phases when patients are quarantined in fever hospitals. In addition, a high mortality rate for a specific year may include AIDS patients who were infected and diagnosed over many of the previous years.

It is worth mentioning that the success of the Egyptian vaccination programme against diphtheria and poliomyelitis was the main cause of decreases in reported cases over recent years; the programme aims to eradicate these diseases completely (Figure 35).

---

[5] This section was investigated by A. El-Hady Abbas, S. Khairy and M. Shehata.

Malaria is the most widespread and serious communicable disease in the world, and Egypt is among a group of countries with some remaining areas of transmission. The specific target for this disease is to eliminate the few remaining foci of malaria by 2006 (WHO, 2004).

TABLE 17
Numbers of reported cases of communicable diseases in Egypt, 1980 to 2004

Year	Malaria (P)[1]	Diphtheria	Meningococcal meningitis	Poliomyelitis	Pulmonary tuberculosis	HIV/AIDS	Hepatitis
1980	370	333	296	2 006	1 381		
1981							
1982	365	809	2 061	2 113	1 596		18 188
1983							
1984							
1985	72	663	848	564	1 143		17 185
1986							
1987							
1988	225	184	3 327	550	1 231		15 188
1989	192	110	3 894	474	1 394		14 009
1990	75	59	3 976	565	2 740	7	14 209
1991	24	55	1 210	625	1 531	12	
1992	16	44	1 165	584	8 876	23	15 108
1993	17	29	896	150	3 416	29	
1994	527	18	800	120	3 223	22	
1995	313	10	671	47	9 708	16	
1996	25	6	661	100	10 236	14	
1997	11	1	167	14	11 040	25	
1998	13	3	489	35	9 650	33	13 340
1999	61	2	419	9	8 878	34	
2000	17	0	278	4	7 919	44	14 671
2001	11	0	201	5	7 900	33	
2002	10	0	130	7	8 223	47	
2003	45	0		1			
2004	14	0	135	1	5 378		

[1] Malaria P = parasitological confirmed malaria.
Source: WHO, 2005.

FIGURE 26
Numbers of reported cases of diphtheria and poliomyelitis in Egypt, 1988 to 2004

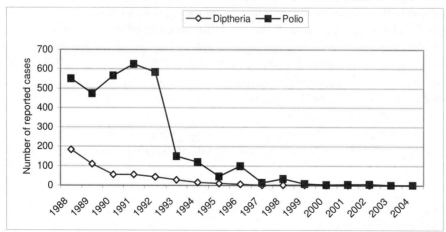

The prevalence of antibody to hepatitis C virus (anti-HCV) was determined in a cross-sectional survey of a village in Upper Egypt (Medhat *et al.,* 2000). Prevalence was higher among males than females, at 11.3 and 6.5 percent, respectively, p < 0.001. It was greater among those over 30 years of age than among those up to 30 years of age (20.0 percent versus 3.6 percent, p < 0.001). Hepatitis C virus RNA was detected in 62.8 percent of the anti-HCV-positive subjects, without significant variation by age, gender, education or marital status.

Abd El-Aziz *et al.* (2000) conducted a cross-sectional survey of the prevalence of anti-HCV in a rural community in the Nile Delta. Overall, 973 (24.3 percent) out of 3 999 residents were anti-HCV-positive, and the age- and gender-adjusted seroprevalence was 23.7 percent. Anti-HCV prevalence increased sharply with age, from 9.3 percent in those aged 20 years and under to more than 50 percent in those over 35 years. Of the 905 anti-HCV-positive samples tested, 65 percent were also positive for HCV-RNA. Active schistosomal infection was not associated with anti-HCV status, but a history of antischistosomal injection therapy was reported by 19 percent of anti-HCV positives.

The population of Egypt has a heavy burden of liver disease, mostly due to chronic infection with HCV. The overall prevalence of anti-HCV in the general population is about 15 to 20 percent. Egyptian parenteral antischistosomal therapy (PAT) mass-treatment campaigns discontinued only in the 1980s, and show a very high potential for transmission of blood-borne pathogens. A cohort-specific exposure index for PAT was calculated and compared with cohort-specific HCV prevalence rates in four regions. The data suggested that PAT had a major role in the spread of HCV throughout Egypt (Frank *et al.,* 2000).

Infections among children

The morbidity load in Egypt, particularly in preschool children, is due mainly to diarrhoea and respiratory tract infections, as shown by statistics from MOHP, as well as many community-based research studies. Detailed studies of urban children under the age of three years revealed that diarrhoea was the cause of morbidity in 37.7 percent of cases in underprivileged areas in Cairo, and of 24.7 percent of cases in Alexandria; respiratory tract infections were responsible for 29.4 and 36.4 percent of cases in the two cities, respectively (Moussa *et al.,* 1983).

Similar studies in rural areas (Galal, 1987) revealed that infants from birth to six months of age were ill for 25 percent of the time observed. Gastrointestinal and respiratory infections constituted, respectively, 37.9 and 31.8 percent of all infant illness. In the same study, toddlers aged 18 to 30 months fell ill an average of almost ten times a year, the total time span of illness averaging 11 percent of the year, but reaching as high as 30 percent. Approximately 40 percent of ailments were gastrointestinal in nature, and one-third respiratory infections.

The National Diarrhoeal Disease Control Programme reported that cases admitted to Bab El-Shaeiria hospitals with acute diarrhoea and dehydration were reduced by 71 percent in 1984 and by up to 75 percent in 1990. Existing data indicate that acute respiratory infection and diarrhoeal diseases were responsible for 30 and 16 percent, respectively, of infant deaths in 1999 (UNICEF, 2003).

Parasitic infestation

Moussa (1989) studied the relation between parasite infestation and malnutrition among schoolchildren aged six to 12 years in different nutritional grades, based on weight-for-age categories. The results revealed that urinary bilharziasis and ancylostoma were most prevalent among the group with third degree undernutrition; ascariasis was highest among the overweight group (but did not exceed 15 percent). Amoebiasis was least prevalent among the group of normal weight-for-age, and most prevalent among the overweight group.

The results of a survey to assess micronutrient deficiencies among primary schoolchildren in three governorates – Cairo, El-Sharquia and Quena – revealed that the highest prevalence of ascaris infestation was among rural boys in El-Sharquia governorate (14.3 percent). Oxyuris infestation was prevalent in the three governorates, with the highest prevalence in El-Sharquia (15.6 percent), followed by Cairo (11.1 percent) and Quena (6.9 percent). The highest prevalence of *Schistosoma hematobium* (urinary bilharziasis) was 10 percent among rural boys in Quena governorate (Hassan *et al.*, 1998).

POLICIES AND STRATEGIES TO IMPROVE NUTRITIONAL STATUS[6]
Ministry of Health and Population strategies
Health strategies

In order to improve the health status of the Egyptian population, MOHP has developed several strategies, including the following:

- *Preventive care system:* the specific areas of intervention are immunization, quarantine measures, safe water supply, food hygiene, public cleanliness, environmental hygiene and infestation control.
- *Primary health care:* through which medical services are provided to the general population and to vulnerable groups (pregnant and lactating mothers and children under five years of age).
- *Curative care services:* where sick people find medical treatment.

Nutrition strategies

Before 1992, ad hoc programmes addressed the problem of malnutrition. Following the International Conference on Nutrition (ICN), held in Rome in December 1992 and sponsored by FAO and WHO, nutrition programmes in Egypt have been enhanced.

Egypt presented a country paper at the conference and took part in post-ICN condensed nutrition activities. A ministerial decree of 1994 formulated a high-level inter-ministerial committee representing the ministries of agriculture, health, planning, information, supply, education and academia. The outcome was the development of the Egyptian National Strategy for Nutrition, which has nine main policy areas. Each policy area includes a problem statement, a goal, measurable objectives, actions, authorities responsible for undertaking the different activities, resources, legislation (if required), and monitoring and evaluation indicators.

The main policy areas are:

- incorporating nutrition objectives, considerations and components into development policies and programmes;
- improving household food security;
- protecting consumers through improved food quality and safety;
- preventing and managing infectious diseases;
- promoting breastfeeding;
- caring for the socio-economically deprived and nutritionally vulnerable;
- preventing and controlling specific micronutrient deficiencies;

---

[6] This section was investigated by A. Gohar and I. Ismail.

- promoting appropriate diets and healthy lifestyles;
- assessing, analysing and monitoring nutrition situations.

Most of the programmes directed at improving the nutritional status of the population fell under the umbrella of this national strategy.

Programmes to improve food security

In addition to health/nutrition care, the availability of food items is also very important in efforts to improve nutrition status. The following are some of the main programmes aimed at increasing food availability in Egypt.

Food ration and subsidy programmes

The main objective of the food subsidy programme was to improve household food security and to prevent malnutrition and chronic energy deficiency. The current food rationing programme was established more than 50 years ago. In addition to price subsidies, specific forms of price intervention include market interventions in the form of subsidized food imports sold through the existing cooperative system. The most recent examples of this are meat imports from the Sudan, which are sold at less than half the price of locally produced meat. According to the present rationing programme, each individual receives – through the family card – a monthly ration of sugar, tea, oil, lentils, broad beans, rice and macaroni that meets a significant proportion of the family's needs. The subsidy of wheat bread is the most important component of this programme, but the food subsidy programme has several drawbacks and constraints as the cost of food price subsidies represents a serious drain on Egypt's national economy and constitutes a major block to the development programme.

Programmes to increase food production

As part of a national land reclamation project, the government has initiated projects all over Egypt. These include the Toshka project in Upper Egypt, which was started in January 1997 and aims to double the area of arable land in Egypt within a period of 15 years. The project's estimated cost was about US$86.5 billion to cover the 20 years from 1997 to 2017.

Programmes to improve nutritional status and to prevent and control malnutrition and morbidity

Programmes to prevent diet-related NCDs

Many programmes have been directed at improving the nutritional status of the Egyptian population and preventing NCDs. These programmes included the following strategies:

- *Nutrition education:* Community nutrition education was carried out through health facilities, schools, non-governmental organizations (NGOs) and the media with the aims of increasing the population's awareness of the programme, enhancing its knowledge and modifying its nutritional behaviours.
- *Food-based dietary guidelines:* With support from the United Nations Children's Fund (UNICEF), NNI produced food-based dietary guidelines for Egypt. These guidelines are directed at educated people, nutrition educators in the health sectors, NGOs and others. They include simple practical messages for healthy eating and lifestyles.

- *Nutrition capacity building:* NNI and MOHP are building capacity through training programmes for health providers, physicians, nurses and community workers.
- *Specialized clinics:* NNI has set up specialized clinics for the prevention, early detection and management of nutritional diseases, particularly obesity, its co-morbidities and stunting.

Programmes for improving nutritional status

Many programmes directed at improving the nutritional status of Egyptian populations have been carried out over the last 20 years. The following paragraphs describe some of these.

The national programme for supporting breastfeeding practices: Exclusive breastfeeding for the first six months of age, continuing breastfeeding up to two years of age, and healthy complementary feeding practices were the main thrusts of breastfeeding promotion activities. Among the many activities implemented to achieve these aims were the formulation of a national committee for the promotion of breastfeeding practices, the establishment of a national policy to support and encourage breastfeeding, implementation of the Baby-Friendly Hospital Initiative in 120 maternity health facilities, and implementation of the international code for the marketing of breastmilk substitutes.

Child Survival and Integrated Management of Childhood Illness: MOHP conducted many projects to improve the health and nutrition status of children under five years of age; these included the Control Diarrhoeal Diseases Programme, Child Survival (1985 to 1995) and Integrated Management of Childhood Illness (1995 to 2005).

The national programme for improving the nutritional status of school-age children: The Ministry of Education implemented school feeding programmes to enhance schoolchildren's physical and mental development. The programmes include the following:

- Iron-fortified biscuits: one packet of 80 g biscuits fortified with iron salt is given to each child in primary schools.
- The School Pie Programme: the ministries of education and agriculture provide pies on 110 days a year to half a million primary schoolchildren in seven governorates (Fayoum, Monofia, Behaira, Port Said, North Sinai, Damitta and Beni Swef). The World Food Programme (WFP) contributes to this programme by extending the period of meal distributions to 150 days.
- Cooked meals: The main target groups for this are handicapped students.
- Cold/dry meals: The main target groups for these are students in secondary, industrial, agricultural, technical and sports schools.

The number of students involved in these programmes increased from 3 019 130 in 1991/1992 to 11 210 258 in 2004/2005. Government contributions and external aid increased from LE 35 806 594 in 1991/1992 to LE 353 600 000 in 2004/2005.

Programmes for the prevention and control of micronutrient deficiencies

The National Programme for the Prevention and Control of IDA: Among MOHP's activities directed at preventing and controlling IDA are:

- health and nutrition education;
- iron supplementation to pregnant women;
- iron supplementation to adolescents and schoolchildren (primary and secondary);
- programmes to prevent and control infection and infestation.

The National Programme for the Prevention and Control of IDD: With support from UNICEF, MOHP and NNI have implemented many programmes to prevent IDD, which is a public health problem in Egypt. These programmes include:

- iodized oil supplementation in New Valley governorate (which has the highest IDD prevalence);
- formation of the National IDD Committee in1993;
- the universal salt iodization programme, launched by MOHP in 1996 with the support of UNICEF;
- four social marketing campaigns to promote iodized salt, which were conducted by NNI, MOHP and UNICEF with the aim of increasing household-level use of iodized salt in governorates where this was low – Gharbia, Fayoum, Quena and Assuit. As a result, household-level use of iodized salt rose from 56 percent in 2000 to 79 percent in 2003 (EIDHS, 2003);
- early detection of neonatal hypothyroidism through a neonatal screening programme that aims to test every child before it reaches one week of age.

The National Programme for the Prevention and Control of Vitamin A Deficiency: After NNI had conducted its national survey of vitamin A status, a national plan to eliminate VAD was implemented. This plan involved the following activities:

- nutrition education and dietary modification;
- the Vitamin A Supplementation Programme for postpartum women;
- vitamin A supplementation to children at ages nine and 18 months.

CONCLUSION[7]

Egypt is a developing country that is facing the double burden of malnutrition. Over recent years, annual per capita income has increased from LE 4 822.4 in 1998/1999, to LE 5 537.6 in 2000/2001 and to LE 5 652.8 in 2002/2003.

Health indicators have also improved over the last 25 years. The under-five mortality rate decreased from 102 per 1 000 live births in 1980 to 1985, to 46 in 1998 to 2003. With infant mortality decreasing from 73 to 38 over the same period. These data indicate that childhood mortality is becoming concentrated in early infancy. Overall, 88 percent of children are immunized against all major preventable childhood diseases. Life expectancy has increased, for males from 52.7 years in 1976 to 67.9 in 2003, and for females from 57.7 years in 1976 to 72.3 in 2003.

The changed consumption patterns of the Egyptian population during the last two decades can be explained as reflecting changes in socio-economic status, changes in feeding habits, urbanization and globalization. The dietary changes that have occurred in Egypt have been associated with increasing proportions of energy-dense foods and saturated fat. Food patterns

---

[7] This section was investigated by A. Gohar and I. Ismail.

have changed towards increasing intakes of fats and oils, high-fat products, sugar, meat and refined carbohydrates, and decreasing cereal consumption.

The total energy intake declined from 3 057 kcal in 1981 to 2 460 kcal in 2000, and the mean protein intake increased from 88.7 g to 91.5 g. In 1981, cereals contributed 61.2 percent of total energy intake, and animal protein only 8.1 percent. In 2000, cereals' contribution had declined to 52.0 percent, while animal protein's had increased to 20 percent. Animal protein's contribution to total protein intake also increased, from 27.7 percent in 1981 to 35.5 percent in 2000. This represents a significant increase in consumption of animal protein, while the contributions of vegetarian food groups to energy and protein intakes are decreasing; this may play a role in the emergence of diet-related chronic diseases in Egypt.

Although mothers' total energy intake decreased from 2 602 kcal in 2000 to 1 995 kcal in 2004, this did not seem to have any influence on the prevalence of obesity among females. This can be explained by the complexity of obesity pathogenesis. Most of the mothers – more than 90 percent – did not practice any regular physical activity.

Food prices and availability have influenced the food consumption of Egyptian populations. Increased income leads to people increasing their consumption of meat and animal protein; after prices increased rapidly following devaluation of the Egyptian pound in 2001, the consumption of all food groups decreased in 2004.

The food adequacy data from NNI national surveys show that the percentage of children receiving more than 100 percent of their energy RDAs increased from about 14 percent in 1995 to about 46.9 percent in 2000. These data, when added to the decrease in physical activity, explain the high prevalence of obesity in adolescence.

Although data show that about 90 percent of children and 70 percent of mothers consume more than 100 percent of the RDA for iron, the prevalence of anaemia in Egypt is still very high. This could be because most of the iron consumed is of plant origin, which decreases the bioavailability of iron.

Changing life styles, with more psychological stress, less physical activity and more high-density food, and changing eating habits, such as eating heavy meals late at night, are leading to increased prevalence of overweight and obesity among Egyptian populations. This in turn is leading to increased prevalence of diet-related chronic NCDs – diabetes, hypertension and certain types of cancer. The alarming results are that diet-related diseases are becoming more prevalent among younger age groups.

It is evident that future surveys should standardize their methodologies, have unified guidelines and be implemented regularly. This will make it easier to analyse, compare and track changes over time.

Changing the conceptual framework for implementing nutrition education programmes so that more attention is paid to raising Egyptians' nutrition awareness could help the prevention of diet-related diseases and their consequences. Such programmes must target adolescents and young adults, especially females, in order to reduce the high prevalence of NCDs in Egypt. Micronutrient deficiencies, especially IDA, still need strategies such as food fortification and nutrition education to increase the bioavailability of iron in foods. It is also recommended that distribution and application of the existing food-based dietary guidelines be strengthened.

Obstacles and constraints faced by this report
The following challenges were encountered during the preparation of this report:

- Raw data from most NNI and ARC surveys were not available, so data had to be obtained from the published reports.

- The NNI and ARC surveys used different types of analysis as regards RDAs, food composition tables and use of the truncated method (removing data pertaining to consumption of > 100 percent RDA). Differences in methodology made it very difficult to compare both sets of data.
- The dietary consumption surveys conducted by NNI had differing objectives and target groups, making it difficult to derive trends in food consumption patterns.

SUMMARY OF THE CAPACITY BUILDING NEEDED TO IMPROVE NUTRITIONAL STATUS IN EGYPT
Institutional needs
National nutrition policy

There is a great need to implement a national nutrition policy with objectives that are modified according to changes in food patterns and food habits. Healthy eating and healthy lifestyles should be addressed in all health facilities and school curricula.

New component in primary health care to address obesity and diet-related NCDs

The role of the primary health care unit in preventing and treating obesity and NCDs must be addressed over the coming years, as the prevalence of diet-related diseases is increasing.

Strengthening of the nutrition surveillance system

A nutrition surveillance system was established in Egypt between 1995 and 1997. There is a great need to redesign and strengthen this system for the early detection and proper management of malnutrition disorders.

Capacity building and training needs

Improving nutrition status requires a well-trained health staff who are capable of communicating with communities to spread information about healthy food and to educate people on the prevention of NCDs. There should be continuous training programmes for health staff, with emphasis on intra- and intersectoral collaboration.

Communication, education and advocacy activities

- Communication programmes are important in supporting strategies to prevent nutrient deficiencies. Information on causes, consequences and measures to control and prevent IDA, IDD and VAD should be disseminated through mother-and-child health centres, primary and secondary schools and the mass media.
- Education and communication programmes are needed to raise awareness of the risks of obesity and diet-related NCDs and to change the health and nutrition behaviour of women. Such programmes should be implemented for adolescent girls in schools and at mother-and-child health centres.

REFERENCES

AAOS. 2000. *Osteoporosis: your osteoporotic connection.* American Academy of Osteopedic Surgeons (AAOS).

Abd El-Aziz, F., Habib, M., Mohamed, M., Abd El-Hamid, M., Gamil, F., Madkour, S., Mikhail, N., Thomas, D., Fix, A., Strickland, T., Anwar, W. & Sallam, I. 2000. Hepatitis C in a community in the Nile Delta: population description and HCV prevalence. *Hepatology,* 32(1): 111–115.

Abdel Aziz, O. 2000. Lipid profile among Egyptians (LPE) and its impact on ischemic heart disease. A national project. On behalf of the Egyptian Atherosclerosis Investigation Team. *Egypt Heart J.,* 52(1): 1–6.

Abdel Fattah, H.E., Abd-Alla, M.A. & Al-Saeid, H.M. 2000. *Prevention of hypertension in adolescents.* Ain Shams University, Egypt. (M.D. thesis)

Aly, H., Dakroury, A., Said, A., Moussa, W., Shaheen, F., Ghoneme, F., Hassein, M., Hathout, M., Shehata, M. & Gomaa, H. 1981. *National food consumption study, final report.* Cairo, NNI, Ministry of Health.

ARC. 2001/2002. *Final report of the effect of agricultural improvement programmes on the food consumption pattern of the Egyptian family 1999.* Cairo, Agricultural Research Centre (ARC). (in Arabic)

CAPMAS. 2004. *Statistical Year Book.* Cairo. Central Agency for Public Mobilization and Statistics (CAPMAS).

EDHS. 1988. *Egypt Demographic and Health Survey.* Cairo, National Population Council.

EDHS. 1992. *Egypt Demographic and Health Survey.* Cairo, National Population Council.

EDHS. 1995. *Egypt Demographic and Health Survey.* Cairo, National Population Council.

EDHS. 2000. *Egypt Demographic and Health Survey.* Cairo, National Population Council.

EHDR. 2004. *Egypt Human Development Report.* United Nations Development Programme (UNDP) and Institute of National Planning, Egypt.

EIDHS. 2003. *Egypt Interim Demographic and Health Survey.* Cairo, National Population Council.

El Attar. In press. *Cancer Statistics.* Cairo University, National Cancer Institute.

El-Bolkiny, M.N., Nouh, M.A. & El-Bolkiny, T.N. 2005. *Topographic pathology of cancer.* Third edition. Cairo University, National Cancer Institute.

El-Sahn, F. 2004. *Maternal nutrition in Egypt. A critical review.* Cairo, NNI.

El-Sayed, N. 2002. *Profile of micronutrient status in Egypt: compilation of studies and programs.* Cairo, MOHP, Primary Health Care Department.

El-Sayed, N., Nofal, L., El-Sahn, F., Farahat, M., Noweir, A. & El-Sayed, A. 2002. *A national survey to assess the current status of anemia and vitamin A deficiency in Egypt.* Cairo, High Institute of Public Health, MOHP, Primary Health Care Department, in collaboration with UNICEF.

El-Tawela, S. 1997. *Child well-being in Egypt. Results of Egypt multiple indicator cluster survey, final report.* American University in Cairo, Social Research Report Center.

FAO/WHO. 1975. *Recommended dietary allowances.* Rome and Geneva.

FAO/WHO. 2002. *Human vitamin and mineral requirements.* Report of a Joint FAO/WHO Expert Consultation. Rome.

FAO/WHO/UNU. 1985. *Energy and protein requirements.* Report of a Joint FAO/WHO/UNU Expert Consultation. Geneva.

Frank, C., Mohamed, M., Strickland, T., Lavanchy, D., Arthur, R., Magder, L., El-Khoby, T., Abdel-Wahab, Y., Ohn, E., Anwar, W. & Sallam, I. 2000. The role of parenteral antischistosomal therapy in the spread of hepatitis C virus in Egypt. *The Lancet,* 355: 887–891.

Galal, O. 1987. *The Collaborative Research Support Program (CRSP) on Food Intake and Human Function. Final Report.* Grant No. Dan – 1309-G-SS-1070-00. Washington, DC, United States Agency for International Development.

Galal, O. 2002. The nutrition transition in Egypt: obesity undernutrition and the food consumption context. *Public Health Nutrition,* 5(1A): 141–148

GPCR Board. 2002. *Cancer profile in Garbia, Egypt,* by A.S. Ibrahim, I.K. Hussein, A. Hablas, I. Abdel Bar and M. Ramadan. Garbia, Egypt, Garbia Population-Based Cancer Registry (GPCR), MECC, MOHP.

Harrison, G.G. 1998. Experience with dietary assessment in the Middle East. *Public Health Reviews,* 26: 55–63.

Harrison, G.G. 2000. Monitoring micronutrient deficiency conditions. *Public Health Reviews,* 28: 105–115.

Harrison, G.G., Galal, O., Ibrahim, N., Stormer, A., Khorshid, A. & Leslie, J. 2000. Underreporting of food intake by dietary recall is not universal: a comparison of data from Egyptian and American women. *J. Nutrition,* 130: 2049–2054.

Hassan, H.A., Abdel Galil, A. & Moussa, W. 2004. *National survey for the determination of BMD among adolescents and adults,* Cairo, NNI.

Hassan, H.A., Shaheen, F., El Nahry, F., Hussein, M.A., Abdel Galil, A. & Hegazy, I. 1998. *Nutritional deficiencies among primary school children in Egypt.* Cairo, NNI/WHO.

Hassan, H.A., Gargas, S.M., Abdel Galil, A. & Darwish, A.H. 2001. *Focusing on the health requirements and style of living to improve the health of elderly people in different cultural sectors in Egypt.* Final Report. Cairo, NNI.

Hassan, H.A., Moussa, W.A., Tawfik, A.A., Ghobrial, M.A., Youssef, A.N. Abd El-Hady, A.A. 2003. *Nutrition country profile.* Rome, FAO.

Hassanyn, S.A. 2000. *Food consumption pattern and nutrients intake among different population groups in Egypt.* Final Report (part 1). Cairo, NNI, WHO/EMRO.

Herman, W.H., Ali, M.A., Aubert, W.H., Engelgau, M.M., Kenny, S.J., Gunter, E.W., Malarcher, A.M. Brechner, R.J., Wetterhall, S.F., De Stefano, F., Thompson, T.J., Smith, P.J., Badran, A., Sous, E.S., Habib, M., Hegazy, M., Abdel Shakour, S., Ibrahim, A.S. & El-Behairy, A. 1995. Diabetes mellitus in Egypt: risk factors and prevalence. *International Science Diabetic Medicine,* 12: 1126–1131.

Hussein, M.A., Moussa, W.A. & Shaheen, F.M. 1993. *Socio-cultural and dietary determinants of obesity in privileged and underprivileged areas.* Final Report. Cairo, NNI/WHO.

Hussein, M.A., Hassan, H.A., Moustafa, S., Rondos, A.G. & El Ghorab, M. 1989. *The effect of increasing food cost on the behavior of families towards feeding their members.* Final Report. Cairo, NNI/Catholic Relief Services.

Hussein, M.A., Awadalla, M.Z., Shaheen, F.M., Hassan, H.A. & Ismail, M. 1992. *Report on prevalence of iodine deficiency disorders in Egypt.* Cairo, NNI/WHO.

Ibrahim, S. & Eid, N. 1996. Impact of Egyptian socio-economic environment on dietary pattern and adequacy. *Bull. Inst. Cairo, Egypt,* 16(1): 11–33.

Ibrahim, N., Youssef, I.A. & Galal, O. 2002. *Food consumption pattern in Egypt.* Final Report. Cairo. (in Arabic)

Ibrahim, M.M., Rizk, H., Apple, L.J., El-Aroussy, W., Helmy, S., Sharaf, Y,, Ashour, Z., Kandil, H., Rocella, E. & Whelton, P.K. 1995. *Hypertension, prevalence awareness, treatment, and control in Egypt. Results from the Egyptian National Hypertension Project (NHP).* Cairo, for the NHP Investigation Team.

Ismail, M. 2005. *Diet, Nutrition and Prevention of Chronic Non-Communicable Diseases Survey*, phase 1. For the Diet, Nutrition and Prevention of Chronic Non-Communicable Diseases (DNPCNCD) investigation team. Cairo, NNI.

Joint National Committee on Detection, Evaluation and Treatment of High Blood Pressure. 1993. Fifth report. *Arch. Inter. Med.,* 153: 154.

Khorshed, A., Ibrahim, N. & Galal, O. 1995. *Development of food consumption monitoring system in Egypt.* Final Report. Cairo, Ministry of Agriculture, FTRI/ARC.

Khorshed, A., Ibrahim, N., Galal, O. & Harrison, G. 1998. Development of food consumption monitoring system in Egypt. *Adv. Agric. Res. Egypt,* 1(3): 163–217.

Medhat, A., Nafeh, M., Shehata, M., Mikhail, N., Swifee, Y., Abdel-Hamid, M., Watts, S., Strickland, T., Anwar, W. & Sallam, I. 2000. Hepatitis C in a community in upper Egypt: Cross-sectional survey. *Am. J. Trop. Med. Hyg.,* 63(5/6): 236–241.

Ministry of Agriculture/FTRI. 1995. *Egypt Food Consumption Survey.* Cairo

Mokhtar, N. 1991. *Cancer pathology registry (1985–1989).* University of Cairo, Department of Pathology. National Cancer Institute.

Moursi, A. 1992. *Diabetes mellitus* in Egypt. *World Health Statistics Quarterly,* 45: 334–337.

Moussa, W.A. 1989. *Nutritional status in Egypt. Health Profile of Egypt, Health Examination Survey (HPE–HES).* Final Report. Publication No. 38/1. Cairo, MOHP.

Moussa, W.A., El-Nehry, F. & Abdel Galil, A. 1995. *National survey for assessment of vitamin A status in Egypt.* Final report. Cairo, NNI/UNICEF.

Moussa, W.A., Aly, H.E., Goma, H., Michael, K.G. & Said, A.K. 1983. The role of infection in causation of malnutrition in urban areas of Egypt with special reference to diarrheal disease. *Urban Health Policy,* 44: 7.

Moussa, W.A., Shaheen, F.M., El–Nehry, F. & Abdel Galil, A. 1997. Vitamin A status in Egypt. In *Proceedings of the XVIII IVACG meeting,* Cairo.

Nassar, H., Moussa, W., Kamel, A. & Miniawi, A. 1992. *Review of trends, policies and programmes affecting nutrition and health in Egypt* (1970–1990). Cairo, MOHP.

National Centre of Health and Population Information. 2005. Statistics. Cairo, MOHP.

Said, A.K. 1987. Personal habits, health, status and medical care, Final Report, Health Profile of Egypt, Health Interview Survey (HPE, HIS). *In* M.R. Biswas and M. Gabr, eds. *Nutrition in the nineties.* Publication N36/3. Cairo, MOHP.

Shaheen, F.M., Hathout, M. & Tawfik, A.A. 2004. *National Survey of Obesity in Egypt.* Final report. Cairo, NNI.

Shaheen, F.M. & Tawfik, A.A. 2000. Intrahousehold food distribution among Egyptian families. Paper presented to the 17th International Conference on Nutrition. Vienna.

Shaheen, F.M., Tawfik, A.A., Samy, A. & Moussa, W. 2000. *Intrahousehold food distribution among Egyptian families.* Final Report. Cairo, NNI/WHO.

Sherif, M. & Ibrahim, A.S. 1987. *The profile of cancer in Egypt.* Cairo, National Cancer Institute.

UNICEF. 2003. *The state of the world's children 2004. Girls' education and development.* New York.

WHO. 1983. *Measuring changes. Nutritional status guidelines for assessing the nutritional impact of supplementary feeding programmes for vulnerable groups.* Geneva.

WHO. 1989. *Preventing and controlling iron-deficiency anaemia through primary health care. A guide for health administrators and programme managers.* Geneva.

WHO. 1990. *Diet, nutrition and the prevention of chronic diseases.* Report of WHO Study Group. Technical Report Series No. 797. Geneva.

WHO. 1993. *Diabetes prevention and control. a call for action.* Alexandria, Egypt, WHO Regional Office for the Eastern Mediterranean. WHO/EM/3/E/G.

WHO. 1994. *WHO Study Group – Assessment of fracture risk and its application to screening for post-menopausal osteoporosis.* WHO Technical Report Series No. 843. Geneva. 129 pp.

WHO. 1995. *Physical status. The use and interpretation of anthropometry*, pp. 268–369. Report of a WHO Expert Committee. Technical Report Series No. 854. Geneva.

WHO. 2000. *Obesity. Preventing and managing the global epidemic.* Report of a WHO consultation WHO Technical Report Series No. 894. Geneva.

WHO. 2003. *Global strategy on diet, physical activity and health.* Available at: www.who.int/dietphysicalactivity/en/.

WHO. 2004. *Report on the workshop on the WHO STEPwise surveillance system (for Egypt, the Sudan and the Republic of Yemen).* Cairo, 4 to 6 September 2003. WHO EM/NCD/040/E.

WHO. 2005. Administration centre data. Cairo, WHO Eastern Mediterranean Regional Office.

WHO/FAO. 2003. *Diet, nutrition and the prevention of chronic diseases.* Report of a Joint WHO/FAO Expert Consultation. WHO Technical Report Series No. 916. Geneva.

ANNEXES

The NNI and FTRI/ARC surveys used different methods for analysing food intake data. In NNI surveys, data were converted into nutrient intakes using the Food Composition Table of Egypt, which is maintained by NNI and dates from 1996. To analyse the adequacy of nutrient intake, the NNI surveys used the RDAs from FAO/WHO/UNU (1985) for protein and energy, WHO (1989) for iron and FAO/WHO (1975) for vitamins A and C, except in the 2004 survey, for which FAO/WHO (2002) recommendations for vitamins and minerals were used.

The food intake data of ARC/FTRI surveys were converted into nutrient intakes using a modification of the USDA standard reference database (the Food Intake and Analysis System, Version 2.3, University of Texas), which was adjusted to remove the influence of enrichment/fortification and to include more than 1 000 Egypt-specific recipes (Khorshed *et al.,* 1998). Nutrient intake adequacy was expressed using current versions of the United States RDAs (published by the National Academy Press from 1989 onwards).

Because of these important methodological differences between the surveys conducted by NNI and FTRI/ARC, each set is presented separately in these annexes. However, both used internally consistent methodology, so trends over time in the data are reliable.

ANNEX 1:FOOD INTAKE AND NUTRITIONAL STATUS

Survey name	Year	Sample size	Age range	Representation	Method of analysis	Institution	Source
National Food Consumption Survey	1981	6 300 households	2–6 years 10–19 years Adults ≥ 20 years	National	Dietary[1] Anthropometry[2]	NNI	Aly *et al.*, 1981
Effect of increasing food cost on families' behaviour regarding feeding their members	1989	2 022 363	Individuals Households	Regional (Cairo – Assuit, El-Behera)	Dietary[1]	NNI	Hussein, *et al.*, 1989
Household food budget survey	1990/ 1991	1 500 82 109	Households Individuals	National	Questionnaire	CAPMAS	
Assessment of IDD status among schoolchildren	1992	9 538 11 466 9 854	6–11 years 12–14 years 15–18 years	National (22 governorates)	Total goitre rate Lab[3] - urinary iodine	NNI	Hussein *et al.*, 1992
Assessment of vitamin A status in Egypt	1995	1 628 855 M 775 F 1 629 F	0.5–5.99 years	National (five governorates representing different regions of urban and rural Egypt)	Dietary[1] Anthropometry[2] Lab[3] - haemoglobin - plasma retinol	NNI	Moussa, El-Nehry and Abdel Galil, 1995

Survey name	Year	Sample size	Age range	Representation	Method of analysis	Institution	Source
EDHS	1995	9 766 M/F 265 F 6 314 F	0–5 years 15–19 years 15–49 years	National (26 governorates)	Anthropometry[2]	National Population Council	EDHS, 1995
Development of food consumption monitoring system	1995	3 186 households	2–6 years Mothers	National (five governorates representing urban and rural areas: Cairo, Ismalia, Dhakahlia, Aswan, New Valley)	Anthropometry[2] Dietary[1]	Food Technology Research Institute	Khorshed, Ibrahim and Galal, 1995
Household food budget survey	1995/ 1996	14 805 73 939	Households Individuals	National	Questionnaire	CAPMAS	
Child well-being in Egypt	1997	814 M 815 F	0–5 years	National (six governorates: Alexandria, Assuit, Aswan, Great Cairo, Quena, Sohag)	Anthropometry[2]	American University in Cairo, Social Research Center	El-Tawela, 1997

ANNEX 1: FOOD INTAKE AND NUTRITIONAL STATUS (CONTINUED)

Survey name	Year	Sample size	Age range	Representation	Method of analysis	Institution	Source
EDHS	1997	3 328	6–60 months	National (26 governorates)	Anthropometry[2]	National Population Council	EDHS, 1997
Assessment of protein energy malnutrition, iron deficiency anaemia and vitamin A deficiency in Menia, Assuit and Sohag governorates	1997	2 700 2 700	Mothers Children 6–71 months	Regional (Menia Sohag, Assuit)	Anthropometry[2] Dietary[1] Laboratory[3] - haemoglobin - plasma retinol - stool analysis	High Institute of Public Health Alexandria	El-Sayed, 2002

Survey name	Year	Sample size	Age range	Representation	Method of analysis	Institution	Source
Nutritional deficiencies among primary schoolchildren	1998	3 000	6–12 years	Regional (three governorates: Cairo, Quena, Sherkia)	Anthropometry[2] Dietary[1] Laboratory[3] - haemoglobin - serum ferritin - serum zinc - serum retinol - serum selenium - urinary iodine - stool analysis	NNI	Hassan *et al.*, 1998
Transition to adulthood: national survey of Egyptian adolescents	1999	9 128 13 271	10–19 years Households	National (21 governorates)	Anthropometry[2] Dietary[1] Laboratory[3] - haemoglobin	Agriculture Research Centre	ARC, 2001/2002
Household food budget survey	1999/2000	47 949 226 107	Households Individuals	National	Questionnaire	CAPMAS	
Egyptian adolescent anaemia prevention programme	1992/2000	700	Schoolchildren	Regional (Aswan)	Questionnaire	Ministry of Health, health insurance organization	

ANNEX 1: FOOD INTAKE AND NUTRITIONAL STATUS (CONTINUED)

Survey name	Year	Sample size	Age range	Representation	Method of analysis	Institution	Source
Intra-household food distribution among Egyptian families	2000	720 885 532 M 554 F 1 270 M 1 470 F	2–6 years 6–12 years 12–19 years 20–65 years 20–48 years	Subnational: Cairo, Kalyobia and Beheira	Dietary[1] Anthropometry[2]	NNI	Shaheen and Tawfik, 2000
Food consumption pattern and nutrition intake among different population groups	2000	9 134 M/F 384 M/F 1 151 M/F 942 M/F 3 047 M/F 4 562 M/F	< 24 years 2–6 years 6–10 years 10–18 years ≥ 18 years	National (six governorates representing urban and rural areas: Cairo, Alexandria, Sharkia, Beheria, Fayoum, Sohag)	Anthropometric measurement[2] Dietary assessment[1]	NNI	Hassanyn, 2000
EDHS	2000	15 573 M/F	0–5 years 5–10 years 10–20 years 20–65 years ≥ 65 years	National (26 governorates)	Anthropometry[2] Laboratory[3] - haemoglobin	National Population Council	EDHS, 2000

Survey name	Year	Sample size	Age range	Representation	Method of analysis	Institution	Source
Iron supplement distribution system: A trial for primary schoolchildren	2000	1 950 girls 1 250 boys	11–14 years	Regional (Giza)	Laboratory[3] -haemoglobin Focus group discussions	NNI/MOHP	Shaheen *et al.*, 2000
School-based delivery system for iron supplement programme in Egyptian primary schools	2000	7 256	Schoolchildren (11–14 years)	Regional (Sharkia, Kafr El sheikh)	Focus group Laboratory[3] - haemoglobin	NNI/MOHP	Shaheen *et al.*, 2000
Health and nutritional status of the elderly	2001	4 876	≥ 65 years	National (six governorates representing urban and rural areas: Cairo, Alexandria, Port Said, Garbia, Fayoum, Aswan)	Anthropometry[2] Dietary[1] Laboratory[3] - haemoglobin - fasting blood sugar - serum retinol - total cholesterol - liver enzymes - renal function Tests - plasma oestrogen - urinary calcium	NNI	Hassan *et al.*, 2001

ANNEX 1: FOOD INTAKE AND NUTRITIONAL STATUS (CONTINUED)

Survey name	Year	Sample size	Age range	Representation	Method of analysis	Institution	Source
Survey to assess current status of anaemia and vitamin A deficiency	2002	3 000 3 000	F adults 2–6 years	National (Alexandria, Beheria, Garbia, Assuit)	Anthropometry[2] Laboratory[3] - haemoglobin - plasma retinol	High Institute of Public Health/MOHP/ Health Care Department/ UNICEF	El Sayed *et al.*, 2002
EDHS	2003	5 761 3 014 M 2 748 F 8 078 F	< 5 years 15–49 years	National (26 governorates)	Anthropometry[2] Laboratory[3] - haemoglobin	National Population Council	EDHS, 2003
Social marketing campaign for iodized salt	2003/ 2004	1 208 3 114	Market Household	Regional (Quena)	Focus group discussion	NNI	Hassan, Abdel Galil and Moussa, 2004

Survey name	Year	Sample size	Age range	Representation	Method of analysis	Institution	Source
Prevalence of obesity in Egypt	2004	31 798 4 154 2 433 6 190 19 021	Individual 2–6 years 6–12 years 12–19 years ≥ 20 years	National (eight governorates representing urban and rural areas: Cairo, Gharbia, Quena, Beniswef, Marsa Matrouh, El wadi El Gadid, Swey)	Anthropometric measurement[2]	NNI	Shaheen, Hathout and Tawfik, 2004
Determination of bone mass density among adolescents and adults in Egypt	2004	2 520 2 446 2 028 2 039 2 021	Households 20–60 years F adults 20–60 years M adults 20–60 years M adolescents 10–19 years F adolescents 10–19 years	National (Cairo, Red Sea, Sohag, Sharkia)	Dietary[1] Anthropometry[2] - BMD (DXA densitometry) Laboratory[3] - haemoglobin - calcium - phosphorus - alkaline phosphates - osteocalcin - oestrogen - testosterone - cholesterol - retinol - vitamin D - zinc/selenium - TSH	NNI	Hassan, Abdel Galil and Moussa, 2004

[1] Method used for dietary analysis was 24-hour recall, comparing the raw composition of the diet in the analysis with the NNI food composition tables.

[2] Anthropometry analysis was according to age: for two to 12 years – weight, height z-score (weight-for-age, weight-for-height, height-for-age); for 12 to 19 years – BMI for age, height for age; ≥ 20 years – BMI.

[3] The laboratory method used was selected according to the objectives of the study.

ANNEX 2: DIETARY ASSESSMENT

The methods used to measure the food consumption of the families surveyed can be classified into two major categories: dietary pattern methods, for example, those that use food frequency questionnaires; and quantitative daily consumption methods, which are based on recall or records of the quantities of foods and beverages consumed over a one-day period – the 24-hour recall method.

Dietary pattern: food frequency questionnaire

This method obtained qualitative descriptive information about the usual frequency of food and beverage consumption for the whole family per day or per week; food items were categorized according to whether they were consumed – for example – fewer than three times a week, or at least three times a week.

The food groups included in this questionnaire were:

- cereals and starchy roots;
- legumes and pulses;
- oils and fats;
- meat, fish and poultry;
- milk and dairy products;
- vegetables and fruits;
- sugar.

24-hour recall method

In this method, every surveyed person was asked to recall his or her exact food and beverage intake for the previous 24-hour period. Quantities of foods and beverages consumed were estimated in household measures and grams.

The information obtained covered all eating events, in sequence, beginning with the first of the day; each event was classified as major or minor and all the food items consumed were recorded.

Each food and beverage consumed was described in detail, including cooking methods and the amounts of each ingredient used. Household measures were converted into grams by referring to a list of weights of commonly used household measures in Egypt, which was developed by NNI. NNI's food composition tables were used to determine the energy and nutrient intakes of each individual.

Adequacy of the diet consumed was assessed by comparing the energy and nutrient intakes of each person with his or her RDAs (FAO/WHO/UNU, 1985; WHO, 1989).

A food coding system was used, in which the first two digits denoted the food group, the second two digits denoted the food item, and the third two digits denoted the preparation method.

Weights of foods and beverages were converted into energy and nutrient intakes by a computer program developed from an energy and nutrient database.

Analysis was based on:

- energy and nutrients as percentages of RDAs (< 50 percent, 50 to 75 percent, 75 to 100 percent, and ≥ 100 percent);
- iron bioavailability was assessed according to the daily quantity of haem iron sources consumed – meat, poultry and fish – in grams, or of ascorbic acid in milligrams:
  - low bioavailability: < 30 g of haem iron sources, or < 25 mg of ascorbic acid;

      – intermediate bioavailability: 30 to 90 g of haem iron sources, or 25 to 75 mg of ascorbic acid;

      – high bioavailability: ≥ 90 g of haem iron sources, or > 75 mg of ascorbic acid;

• the vitamin A content of the diet was based on the retinol activity equivalent, which is equivalent to 1 µg of all trans retinol, to 6 µg of all trans betacarotene, and to 12 µg of other provitamin A carotenes.

ANNEX 3: DIET-RELATED CHRONIC DISEASES, DATA SETS

Survey name and source	Year	Sample size	Age range	Representation	Method of analysis used
Health Profile of Egypt–Health Examination Survey (HPE–HES) Said, 1987	1987	14 151 48.0% F 52.0% M	> 6 years	National 33.7% urban areas 66.3% rural areas	Measurement of blood pressure Questionnaire, self-reported treatment with antihypertensive medication
National Hypertension Project (NHP) Ibrahim *et al.*, 1995	1991	6 733	25–95 years	National (six governorates: Cairo, Bani Sweif, Aswan, Sharkia, Port Said, El Wadi El Gedid)	Measurements of blood pressure (average of four) Hypertension defined as average systolic blood pressure ≥ 140 mmHg, and/or diastolic ≥ 90 mmHg, and/or self-reported treatment with antihypertensive medication
Prevalence of Hypertension in Adolescents Abdel Fattah, Abd-Alla and Al-Saeid, 2000	2000	5 133 2 660 M 2 473 F Most primary and secondary schools	14–20 years	Regional (Qalyubia governorate)	Measurements of blood pressure (average of three) Blood pressure classified according to Fifth Joint National Committee on Detection, Evaluation and Treatment of High Blood Pressure (JNCV) (1993) for the young age group, as a percentile correlated with height
Diet, Nutrition and Prevention of Chronic Non-Communicable Diseases Ismail, 2005	2003/ 2004	6 000	12–18 years	National, urban and rural areas (seven governorates: Giza, Kalyubia, Kafr al Shekh, Al Sharkia, Aswan, Suhag, Al Menia)	Full medical history Dietary history Anthropometric measurement (weight and height) for BMI Blood pressure measurement Blood pressure classified according to Fifth Joint National Committee on Detection, Evaluation and Treatment of High Blood Pressure (JNCV) (1993) for the young age group, as a percentile correlated with height Blood sugar: fasting and post-prandial Serum lipids: cholesterol, LDL-ch, HDL-ch and triglycerides

ANNEX 3: DIET-RELATED CHRONIC DISEASES, DATA SETS (CONTINUED)

Survey name and source	Year	Sample size	Age range	Representation	Method of analysis used
Diabetes Mellitus in Egypt Hermann *et al.*, 1995	1991–1994	4 620	≥ 20 years	Regional (Cairo, Giza, Kaliubia)	Height, weight, WHR Random capillary glucose For individuals at risk: - fasting blood glucose - glucose 2 hours after 75 g glucose load - diabetes and impaired glucose tolerance (IGT) classified according to WHO (1993) criteria
Focusing on the Health Requirements and Style of Living to Improve the Health of Elderly People in Different Cultural Sectors in Egypt Hassan *et al.*, 2001	2001	4 876	≥ 65 yrs	National, rural and urban areas (six governorates: Cairo, Alexandria, Port-Said, El Garbia, El Fayoum, Aswan)	Full medical history BMD measured by DXA densitometer acting peripherally on calcaneous site Assessment of BMD status based on WHO (1994) diagnostic categories Anthropometric measurements (weight and height) for BMI Dietary history (24-hour recall) Laboratory measurement: liver function, kidney function and heartbeat
National Survey for the Determination of Bone Mass Density (BMD) among Adolescents and Adults in Egypt. Hassan, Abdel Galil and Moussa, 2004	2004	2 520 families	10–19 years 20–60 years	National, rural and urban (six governorates: Cairo, Sohag, Red Sea, Sharkia, Dhakahlia, Beheira)	Full medical history BMD measured by DXA densitometer acting peripherally on calcaneous site Anthropometric measurements (weight and height) for BMI Dietary history (24-hour recall) Laboratory measurement of haemoglobin, calcium, phosphorus, alkaline phosphates, osteocalcin, oestrogen, testosterone, cholesterol, retinol, vitamin D, zinc, TSH, and selenium Assessment of BMD status based on WHO (1994) diagnostic categories

The double burden of malnutrition in India

P. Ramachandran, Director, Nutrition Foundation of India, New Delhi

INTRODUCTION

India is a vast and varied subcontinent. Covering 2.4 percent of the global landmass, it supports more than one-sixth of the world's population. In 2001, India's population had reached 1 028 million people, living in 220 million households in 35 states and union territories (Map). As a developing country with high population density, ever since Indian independence, planners in India have recognized the importance of planned growth of the economy with emphasis on human resource development. Policy-makers recognize that optimal nutrition and health are prerequisites for human development. Article 47 of the Constitution of India states that "the State shall regard raising the level of nutrition and standard of living of its people and improvement in public health among its primary duties". Over the last five decades, successive five-year plans have lain down policies and multisectoral strategies to combat nutrition-related public health problems and improve the nutritional and health status of the population.

Currently, the country is undergoing a rapid socio-economic, demographic, nutritional and health transition. Although India has not yet overcome the problems of poverty, undernutrition and communicable diseases, it is increasingly facing additional challenges related to the affluence that results from industrialization, urbanization and economic betterment. Over the last two decades, overnutrition and obesity have emerged as public health problems; there have been increases in the prevalence of diabetes and cardiovascular disease (CVD), especially in urban areas. The magnitude of these problems varies among states and socio-economic strata and between urban and rural areas, and it is a matter of concern that these diseases occur a decade earlier in India than elsewhere and that they affect poor segments of the population and those in rural areas. Case fatality rates are reported to be higher in poor and rural populations, probably because of poor access to health care and consequent delayed diagnosis and treatment. This case study reviews the impact of ongoing socio-economic, demographic and life style transitions on nutritional status, and the health implications of the ongoing nutrition transition.

Demographic transition

Demographic transition is a global phenomenon. Technological advances and improved quality and coverage of health care have resulted in a rapid fall in India's crude death rate, from 25.1 per 10 000 population in 1951 to 9.8 in 1991. The reduction in crude birth rate has been less steep, falling from 40.8 per thousand in 1951 to 29.5 in 1991 (RGI, 1951 to 2001). As a result, the annual exponential population growth rate was more than 2 percent from 1971 to 1991. The census of 2001 confirmed that the pace of demographic transition in India has been steady, albeit slow, and that India has joined China in having a population of more than 1 billion (Figure 1).

FIGURE 1
Population and birth and death rates in India, 1951 to 2001

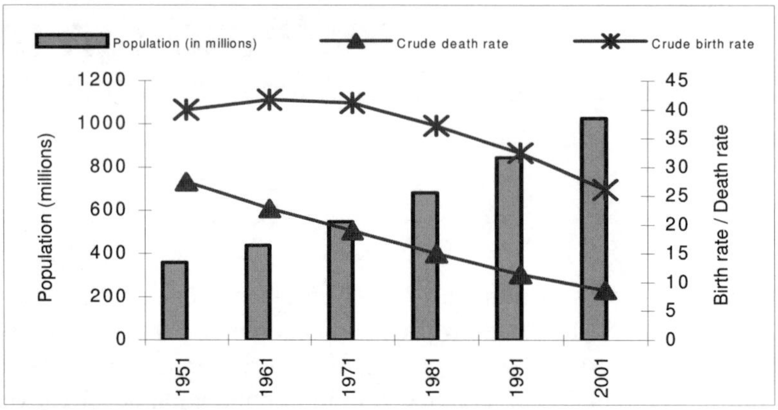

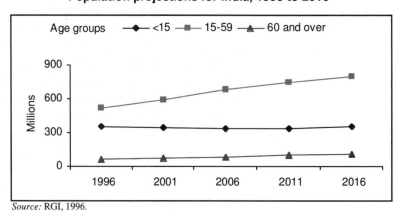

Source: RGI, 1951 to 2001.

Box 1. Population projections 1996 to 2016

The population is projected to increase from 934 million in 1996 to 1 264 million in 2016.
Between 1996 to 2001 and 2011 to 2016 there will be declines of:

- crude birth rate, from 24.10 to 21.41;
- crude death rate, from 8.99 to 7.48;
- natural growth rate, from 1.51 to 1.39 percent;
- infant mortality rate, from 63 to 38 per 1 000 live births for males; and from 64 to 39 for females.

Source: RGI, 1996.

Population projections for the period 1996 to 2016, carried out by the Registrar General of India (RGI, 1996) are given in Box 1. Although there has been a substantial reduction in birth rates, population growth will continue for the next three decades because of:

- the large proportion of the population in the reproductive age group (contributing about 60 percent of total population growth);
- high fertility caused by a lack of contraception (contributing about 20 percent of total population growth);
- high desired fertility resulting from the prevailing high infant mortality rate (contributing about 20 percent of total population growth).

FIGURE 2
Population projections for India, 1996 to 2016

Source: RGI, 1996.

Most of India's population growth between 1996 and 2016 will be caused by increased numbers of people in the 15 to 59 years age group – the working age (Figure 2). The Malthusian assumption that population growth leads to overcrowding, poverty, undernutrition, environmental deterioration, poor quality of life and increase in disease burden has been challenged in the last few decades; population growth can also be a major resource for economic growth, as outlined in Box 2. If India successfully faces the challenge of providing its younger, better-educated, skilled, well-nourished and healthy workforce with appropriate employment and adequate remuneration, the economic status of both the people and the country can improve rapidly.

Box 2. Economic implications of demographic transition

The next two decades will witness:
- increase in the 15 to 59 years age group, from 519 to 800 million;
- low dependency ratios.

The challenge is to ensure:
- adequate investment in human resources development;
- appropriate employment and adequate remuneration for the workforce.

The opportunity is to:
- utilize the abundant human resources available to accelerate economic development.

The current phase of demographic transition also represents a major opportunity for improving the health and nutritional status of the population. The under 15 years age group will not increase in numbers. The health and nutrition infrastructure will therefore not have to cope with ever-increasing numbers of children needing health and nutrition care, leaving it free to concentrate on the quality and coverage of health and nutrition services needed to improve health and nutritional status. If the health and nutrition needs of the literate and aware 15 to 59 years age group are met, massive improvement in nutrition and health status can be made. Appropriate counselling will enable people to adopt life styles and diets that prevent the escalation of overnutrition and the attendant non-communicable disease (NCD) risk. For the increasing numbers of people over 60 years of age, provisions for managing their nutritional and health problems would have to be made.

Economic transition

Since the 1950s, India has adopted the concept of a mixed economy for overall agricultural and industrial development. In the last decade, the service sector has become the high-growth sector. Over the last three decades, there has been a steady increase in gross domestic product (GDP) and per capita net national income; per capita net national product reached US$237 in 2000 (Government of India, 2003). Agriculture remains a major determinant of GDP growth, and is the most important sector for rural employment. Over the years there has been slow but steady reduction in poverty (Table 1), which had declined to 26.2 percent in 2000 (Planning Commission, 2004). Rises in per capita income (Figure 3) have not been matched by increased energy consumption (NNMB, 1979 to 2002), and there are large inter-state differences in per capita income and poverty ratios.

FIGURE 3
Trends in per capita income and energy intake, 1974 to 2002

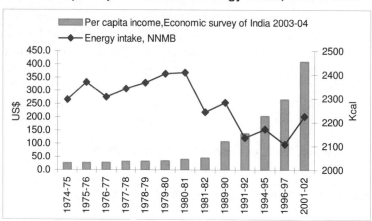

TABLE 1
Economic indicators, 1950 to 2001

	1950/1951	1960/1961	1970/1971	1980/1981	1990/1991	2000/2001
GDP at current prices (million US$)	2 195	3 729	9 706	29 926	117 461	440 856
Per capita net national product (1993/1994 prices, US$)	85	102	115	123	168	237
Poverty (%)*			54.9	44.5	36	26.1

US$1 = RS 43.5.
Sources: Government of India, 2003; * Planning Commission, 2003.

Social transition

Improvement in the quality of life is the central pillar of India's planned development. The adult literacy rate improved from 18.3 percent in 1951 to 65.4 percent in 2001 (Table 2). India now has the world's largest trained workforce in science, administration and technology. Attempts are under way to ensure universal primary education and to improve secondary and vocational education (Government of India, 2003). Efforts are also being made to ensure that higher and technical education gets due attention (Table 3) (Department of Education, 2002). The urban population has continued to grow because of rural–urban migration; in 2001, 30 percent of Indians lived in urban areas. Of the 26 megacities (each housing more than 10 million people) that are forecast worldwide by 2015, five will be in India.

Although urban amenities have failed to cope with the increase in population, cities and towns have become the engines of social change, rapid economic development and improved access to education, employment and health care. Rural and urban populations continue to lack access to safe drinking-water (38 percent in 1981 and 68 percent in 2001) and good environmental sanitation (less than 30 percent) (RGI, 1951 to 2001). With better communication and transportation, urban and rural areas can be linked, both economically and socially, to create an urban–rural continuum of communities and to achieve sustained, rapid improvement in quality of life in both.

TABLE 2
Social indicators, 1950 to 2001

	1950/1951	1960/1961	1970/1971	1980/1981	1990/1991	2000/2001
Population (millions)	359	434	541	679	839	1 019
Urban population (%)	17.3	18.0	19.8	23.1	25.5	27.7
Male literacy rate (%)	27.16	40.40	45.96	56.38	64.10	75.85
Female literacy rate (%)	8.86	15.35	21.97	29.76	39.30	54.16
Overall literacy rate (%)	18.33	28.30	34.45	43.57	52.20	65.38

Source: Government of India, 2003.

TABLE 3
School enrolment by gender (millions), 1970 to 2001

Year	Primary (I–V)			Middle/upper primary (VI–VIII)			Higher/secondary (IX–XII)		
	Boys	Girls	Total	Boys	Girls	Total	Boys	Girls	Total
1970/1971	35.7	21.3	57.0	9.4	3.9	13.3	5.7	1.9	7.6
1980/1981	45.3	28.5	73.8	13.9	6.8	20.7	7.6	3.4	11.0
1990/1991	57.0	40.4	97.4	21.5	12.5	34.0	12.8	6.3	19.1
2000/2001	64.0	49.8	113.8	25.3	22.0	42.8	16.9	10.7	27.6

Source: Department of Education, 2002.

Health transition

Over the last five decades, there have been steady but slow reductions in the rates of births, deaths, infant mortality and under-five mortality (RGI, 1971 to 2000) (Table 4). India still has high infant, perinatal and neonatal mortality (Figure 4), but there has been a steady reduction in the death rate and an improvement in longevity.

FIGURE 4
Child mortality indicators, 1971 to 1997

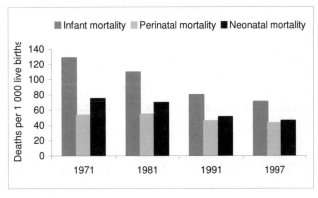

Source: RGI, 2000.

TABLE 4
Health indicators, 1950 to 2001

	1950/1951	1960/1961	1970/1971	1980/1981	1990/1991	2000/2001
Birth rate (per 1 000)	39.9	41.7	41.2	37.2	33.9	25.8
Death rate (per 10 000)	27.4	22.8	19	15	12.5	8.5
Male life expectancy at birth (years)	32.5	41.9	46.4	50.9	58.6	63.8
Female life expectancy at birth (years)	31.7	40.6	44.7	50	59	66.9
Overall life expectancy at birth (years)	32.1	41.3	45.6	50.4	58.7	

Source: Government of India, 2003; RGI, 2000; UNDP, 2003.

Access to health services is still sub-optimal, especially in remote areas with high morbidity. Immunization coverage is low (complete immunization coverage at 12 months was 35.4 percent in 1992/1993 and 42.0 in 1998/1999), and child morbidity and mortality rates are high (IIPS, 1992/1993; 1998/1999). India's shares of global communicable disease and maternal and perinatal problems are high and have not shown substantial reduction in the last two decades (Box 3) (Planning Commission, 2002). The estimated disease burden to communicable diseases and ischaemic heart disease (IHD) is shown in Table 5. Diabetes and CVD have shown sharp rises in the last two decades; India faces the dual burden of high communicable and rising non-communicable disease prevalence (World Bank, 1993).

Box 3. India's share of global health problems

India accounts for:

- 26 percent of the world's childhood vaccine-preventable deaths;
- 20 percent of maternal deaths;
- 68 percent of leprosy cases;
- 30 percent of tuberculosis cases;
- 10 percent of HIV-infected people.

Source: Planning Commission, 2002.

TABLE 5
Burden of five major diseases (million DALYs)[1]

Disease	Age (years)					
	0-4	5-14	15-44	45-59	60+	Total
Diarrhoea						
Male	42.1	4.6	2.8	0.4	0.2	50.2
Female	40.7	4.8	2.8	0.4	0.3	48.9
Worm infection						
Male	0.2	10.6	1.6	0.5	0.1	13.1
Female	0.1	9.2	0.9	0.5	0.1	10.9
Tuberculosis						
Male	1.2	3.1	13.4	6.2	2.6	26.5
Female	1.3	3.8	10.9	2.8	1.2	3120
IHD						
Male	0.1	0.1	3.6	8.1	13.1	25
Female	-	-	1.2	3.2	13	17.5

[1] DALY = disability-adjusted life year.
- = less than 0.05 million.
Source: World Bank, 1993.

SUSTAINABLE FOOD PRODUCTION TO MEET NUTRITIONAL NEEDS
Nutritionists view agriculture as an input for dietary intake, while farmers look for returns on their investments. The green revolution showed that food grain production can be increased fourfold when farmers are assured of returns on investment (Figure 5). However pulse and coarse grain production has stagnated (Ministry of Agriculture, 2002a).

Cereals and pulses
Over the last five decades, the per capita net availability of cereals has been improving, and by 1991 it was sufficient to meet the recommended dietary allowance (RDA) (Figure 6). However, per capita pulse availability and consumption have declined. Pulses are a major source of protein among poorer segments of the population, so this trend must be reversed (Ministry of Agriculture, 2002b).

FIGURE 5
Trends in production of important food items, 1950 to 2001

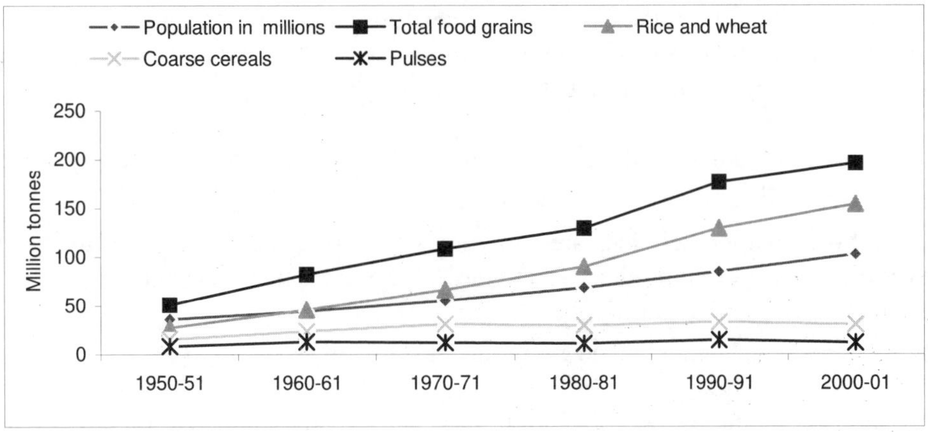

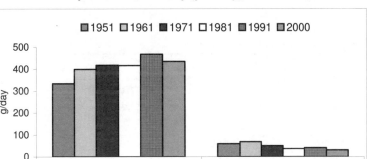

Source: Ministry of Agriculture, 2002a.

FIGURE 6
Per capita net availability (per day), 1950 to 2001

Source: Ministry of Agriculture, 2002b.

Horticulture

Vast areas of India are subtropical, and agroclimatic conditions are well suited to the cultivation of vegetables, fruits and plantation crops. Horticultural products provide higher yields per hectare, obtain higher sale prices and sustain agro-industries. As a result, greater areas are being brought under horticulture, and the production of fruits and vegetables is increasing. In 2000, India produced 46.6 million tonnes of fruits and 96.5 million tonnes of vegetables. Less than 1 percent of this production is processed. Losses during packaging and transport are about 30 percent.

Except among affluent urban segments of the population, per capita vegetable and fruit consumption continues to be low because of problems with access and affordability. Investment in infrastructure for preservation, cold storage, refrigerated transportation, rapid transit, grading, processing, packaging and quality control will help the horticultural sector to achieve its full economic potential and to provide vegetables and fruits at affordable cost throughout the year. In this way, the micronutrient needs of the population can be met through a sustainable food-based approach.

National agricultural policy

The National Agricultural Policy (NAP) (Ministry of Agriculture, 2000) emphasizes crop diversification, horticulture and food processing for sustainable agriculture growth. NAP and the Tenth Five-Year Plan (Planning Commission, 2002) have set a target of a 3.97 percent growth for agriculture. This is to be achieved through:

- efficient use of resources and the conservation of soil, water and biodiversity;
- equity across different regions and farmers;
- a demand-driven approach that caters to domestic markets and maximizes the benefits of exporting agricultural products in the face of the challenges of economic liberalization and globalization;
- technological, environmental and economic sustainability.

Increasing economic growth and improved access are expected to lead to dietary diversification and increased consumption of pulses, vegetables, fruits and dairy products. Once dietary diversification at affordable cost is possible and the majority of the population have a balanced diet, it will be possible to achieve nutrition security.

MAP: INDIA'S STATES (CENSUS INDIA)

CONSUMPTION EXPENDITURE ON FOOD

The National Sample Survey Organization (NSSO) is a permanent survey organization that was set up in the Department of Statistics of the Government of India in 1950. NSSO has been carrying out five-yearly consumer expenditure surveys since 1972/1973, providing time series data in rural and urban areas of all India's states. Household food consumption at the national and state levels is computed on the basis of data on household monthly per capita consumption expenditure (MPCE) in 12 MPCE classes (with expenditure ranging from less than US$5 to $30). NSSO surveys have excellent sampling design, large sample sizes, clearly stated estimation procedures and national coverage, but do not provide insight into the actual dietary intake of households or individuals or into the intra-family distribution of food.

FIGURE 7
Expenditure on cereals (percentages), 1972 to 2001

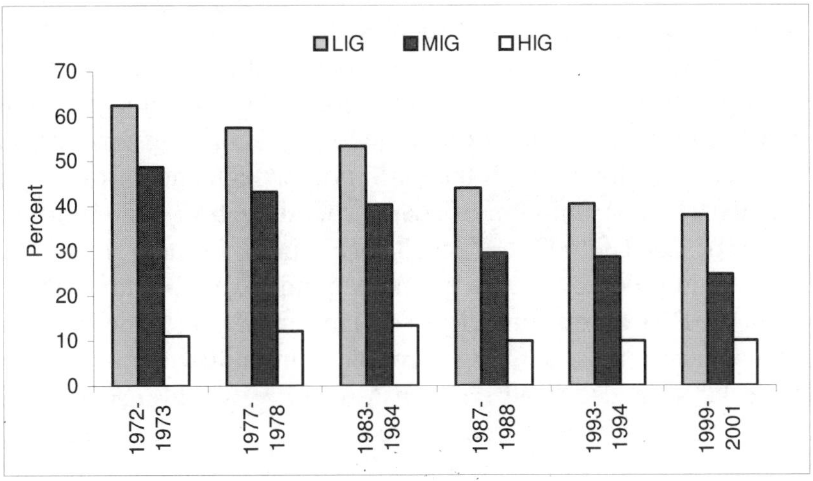

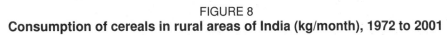

Source: NSSO, 2001.

FIGURE 8
Consumption of cereals in rural areas of India (kg/month), 1972 to 2001

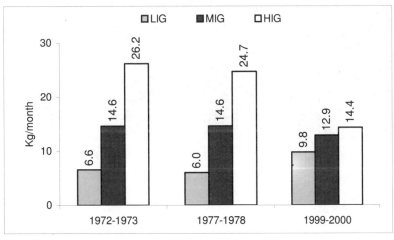

Source: NSSO, 2001.

Cereals

Data from NSSO surveys from 1972 to 2000 show that expenditures on cereal in the lowest (LIG) and middle-income groups (MIG) declined. Among the highest income group (HIG), cereals accounted for a fairly low proportion of total expenditure, which has remained essentially unchanged over the last three decades (Figure 7). People in the lowest income group were consuming greater quantities of cereals, even though they were also spending a reduced proportion of their total expenditure on these (Figure 8). This is because there has been a reduction in the relative cost of cereals, especially those supplied through the public distribution system (PDS). There was a decline in household consumption of cereals in the middle-income group, while monthly cereal consumption in high-income rural households dropped from 26.2 kg in 1972/1973 (about 1kg/day) to 14.4 kg in 1999/2000. Data from diet surveys conducted by the National Nutrition Monitoring Bureau (NNMB, 1979 to 2002) show that the average intake of cereals in even the highest income group has never exceeded 400 g/day. It would therefore seem likely that the high cereal consumption among high-income rural households might be because cooked food is shared with guests, relatives and servants. The sharing of food with guests and servants has declined over the last two decades, which accounts for the steep reduction in cereal consumption in high-income group households. The simultaneous increase in cereal consumption in the lower-income group confirms this.

With wheat and rice available through the PDS, poorer segments of the population now use these as staple cereals. The consumption of coarse cereals rich in micronutrients and minerals has declined (Figure 9). The Tenth Five-Year Plan (Planning Commission, 2002) recommends that locally produced and procured coarse grains be made available through a targeted public distribution system (TPDS) at subsidized rates. This may substantially reduce the cost of subsidies without any decrease in the energy provided; an improved micronutrient intake from coarse cereal would be an added benefit. Such a measure would also improve targeting, as only the most needy are likely to buy these coarse grains.

FIGURE 9
Cereal consumption, 1972 to 2000

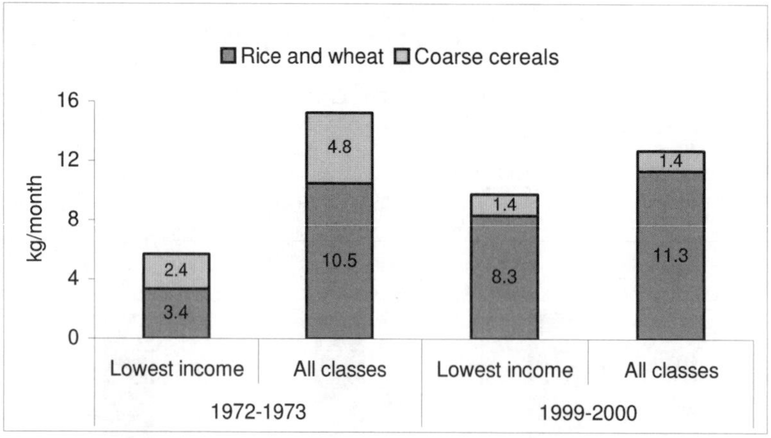

Source: NSSO, 2001.

Pulses

Between 1972 and 2001, there was a substantial increase in the proportion of expenditure spent on pulses in the lowest income group (Figure 10), but expenditure on pulses remained relatively unaltered in the middle and highest income groups. In spite of increased expenditure, household consumption of pulses declined in all income groups and in both urban and rural areas (Figure 11). Data from the NSSO 2000 survey show that middle and upper income groups spent more on milk and animal products, so their protein intakes were not adversely affected by the reduction in pulses. Pulses are still the major source of protein in the lowest income group. In order to ensure adequate protein intake for this group, it is therefore essential to increase the cultivation of a variety of pulses and legumes, so that they can be made available at affordable prices, perhaps through TPDS.

FIGURE 10
Expenditure on pulses (percentages of total), 1972 to 2001

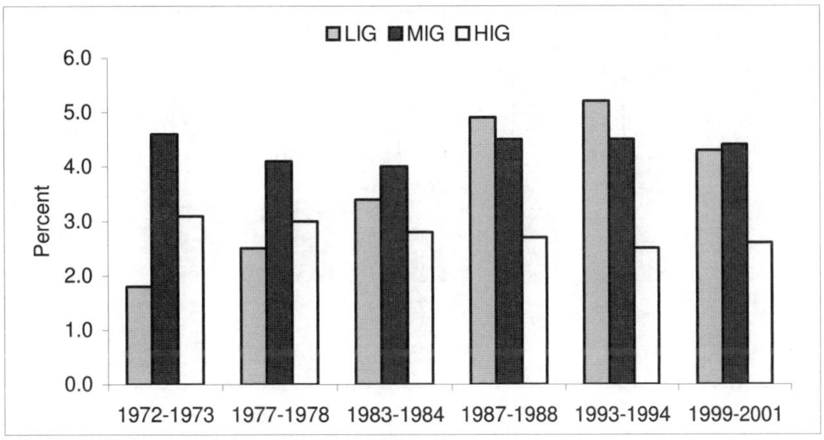

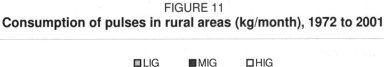

Source: NSSO, 2001.

FIGURE 11
Consumption of pulses in rural areas (kg/month), 1972 to 2001

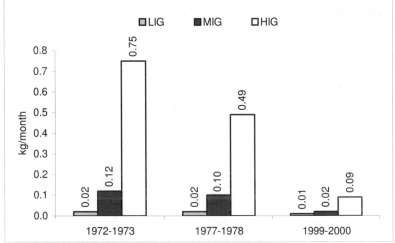

Source: NSSO, 2001.

Time trends in monthly per capita expenditure

MPCE on food and non-food items over the last three decades is shown in Figure 12. The proportion of total expenditure spent on foodstuffs has declined considerably over the last three decades – from 70.6 percent in 1972 to 55.3 percent in 1999/2000 – mainly because of the decline in cereal prices. Expenditures on pulses, vegetables, other foods and beverages increased. However, pulse and vegetable intakes among the poor remain low. There are massive urban–rural and inter-district/state differences in the costs of vegetables, milk, fish and meat. Therefore data on the quantities of these foodstuffs consumed by state or expenditure group are not available from NSSO surveys. India uses diet surveys for such information.

FIGURE 12
Percentage distribution of MPCE in rural areas, 1972 to 2001

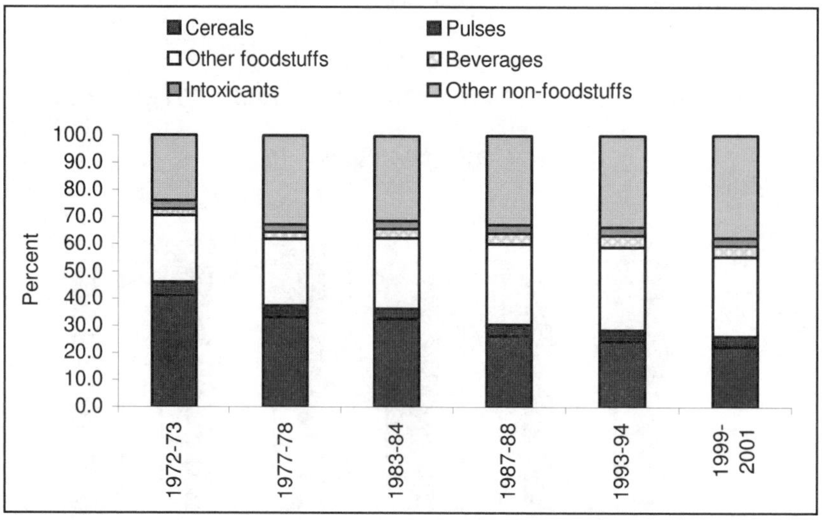

Source: NSSO, 2001.

Nutrient intake computed from NSSO surveys

NSSO uses household expenditures on food to compute the energy, protein and fat intakes of the population. Over the last three decades, overall energy and protein consumption in rural areas has shown a small decline while remaining unaltered in urban areas. There have been increases in fat consumption in both rural and urban areas (Table 6).

TABLE 6
Average daily per capita nutrient intakes, 1972 to 2000

Year	Energy (kcal)		Protein (g/day)		Fat (g/day)	
	Rural	Urban	Rural	Urban	Rural	Urban
1972/1973	2 266	2 107	62	56	24	36
1983	2 221	2 089	62	57	27	37
1993/1994	2 153	2 071	60.2	57.2	31.4	42
1999/2000	2 149	2 156	59.1	58.5	36.1	49.6

Source: NSSO, 2001.

TABLE 7
Average per capita calorie consumption by income group, 1972 to 1994

Expenditure class	Rural			Urban		
	1972/1973	1977/1978	1993/1994	1972/1973	1977/1978	1993/1994
Lowest 30 percent	1 504	1 630	1 678	1 579	1 701	1 682
Middle 40 percent	2 170	2 296	2 119	2 154	2 438	2 111
Top 30 percent	3 161	3 190	2 672	2 572	2 979	2 405

Source: NSSO, 2001.

Changes in energy consumption in different income groups in urban and rural areas are shown in Table 7; energy consumption has shown small increases in both the urban and rural poor and substantial declines among the urban and rural rich. As indicated earlier, data on household consumption expenditure in high-income groups include the food shared with guests and servants, so therefore have to be interpreted with caution. There are massive interstate differences in food expenditures.

Urban–rural differences

Data from the NSSO 55th round (1999/2000) on urban–rural differences in food expenditure are given in Figure 13. Among the urban and rural poor, most food expenditure was on cereals. Dietary diversification is seen mainly among middle- and high-income groups in both urban and rural areas; diversity is greater in urban areas, perhaps because of access to a wider variety of foodstuffs.

FIGURE 13
Expenditure on foodstuffs by income group

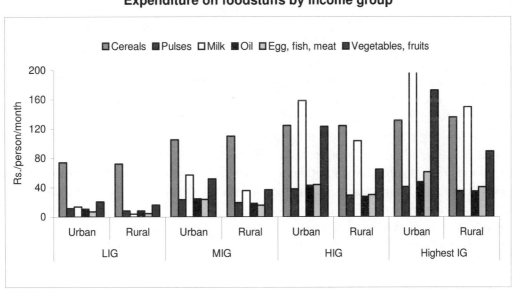

Source: NSSO, 2001.

Summary

Data from NSSO consumption expenditure surveys indicate the following:

- Expenditure on food has declined, mainly because of reductions in the cost of cereals.
- In spite of a steep decline in cost, cereal consumption has not increased, except in the lowest income group. This apparent paradox has been the subject of widespread debate among economists and nutritionists in India, and the consensus view is that it might be because cereal requirements are being met.
- In spite of increased expenditure on pulses, consumption among all segments has declined because of the soaring cost of pulses. Pulse consumption is very low among the poor.
- Rural populations consume more cereals, fewer pulses and less oil and fat compared with urban populations.

- Dietary diversification is seen mainly in middle- and high-income groups in urban and rural areas. Increasing incomes and wider availability of diverse foodstuffs accelerated this trend in the 1990s.
- There has been only a small increase in energy consumption among the poor in spite of steep declines in the cost of cereals. Among the middle- and high-income groups, energy consumption has declined.
- The energy consumption of the urban high-income group is associated with consumption of increased quantities of sugar, oil, milk and milk products and lower quantities of cereals. Changes in the energy density of the diet and sedentary lifestyles appear to be the major factors for the steep increase in obesity among this group.

DIETARY INTAKE DATA FROM NUTRITION SURVEYS

Since 1975, the National Nutrition Monitoring Bureau (NNMB) has been providing data on dietary intake (by 24-hour dietary recall) and nutritional status (by anthropometry and nutritional deficiencies) for ten states of India (Kerala, Karnataka, Andhra, Tamil Nadu, Maharashtra, Orissa, Gujarat, Madhya Pradesh, West Bengal and Uttar Pradesh). NNMB is the only survey that provides data on intra-family food distribution and the dietary intake and nutritional status of all age groups. Proposals to expand the network to cover all states have not yet been implemented. A one-time district nutrition survey was carried out in the mid-1990s in order to obtain data on the dietary intake and nutritional status of individuals in other states. Both the NNMB 1994 survey and this one-time survey used the same methodology of data collection, using representative samples of households in every state. The combined data were reported as the India Nutrition Profile (INP) (DWCD, 1995/1996).

INP provides data on the dietary intake and nutritional status of all age groups, in all states and in both urban and rural areas. Both the NNMB and INP surveys used 24-hour dietary recall to assess food intake. The amounts consumed were compared with the RDAs for India drawn up in 1989 by the Indian Council of Medical Research (ICMR, 1989).

Household food intake obtained by 24-hour dietary recall is used to compute the average intakes of household members expressed as consumption units (CUs) per day (NNMB, 1981). The CUs for different age and gender groups were worked out from the basis of the energy consumption of an average adult male doing sedentary work being 1 CU (Box 4). The reference man is between 20 and 39 years of age, weighs 60 kg and is physically fit and moderately active. The reference woman is between 20 and 39 years of age, weighs 50 kg and is moderately active.

Box 4. Consumption units

Adult male (sedentary worker)	1.0	Child (nine to 12 years)	0.8
Adult male (moderate worker)	1.2	Child (seven to nine years)	0.7
Adult male (heavy worker)	1.6	Child (five to seven years)	0.6
Adult female (sedentary worker)	0.8	Child (three to five years)	0.5
Adult female (moderate worker)	0.9	Child (one to three years)	0.4
Adult female (heavy worker)	1.2		
Adolescent (12 to 21 years)	1.0		

Source: NNMB, 1981.

Nutrient intake is computed using the *Nutritive value of Indian foods* (NIN, 2004), first published by the National Institute of Nutrition (NIN) in 1971 and updated many times since then. Analysis of the iron content of foodstuffs using recent techniques shows that the iron available is only about 50 percent of the values previously reported; hence, values for iron content have been revised in the latest edition.

Food intake in urban and rural areas

Data from the NNMB and INP surveys show that average intakes of cereals in the mid-1990s were near the RDAs, but intakes of pulses, vegetables and fruits were low (Table 8). There are significant differences in food intake among states. Reported intakes of foodstuffs are higher in INP than in NNMB data, probably because there are higher dietary intakes – especially of cereals and pulses – in states not included in the NNMB survey, but covered by INP. Dietary intake was higher in some states with high per capita income (Punjab), but not others (Maharashtra), which suggests that greater per capita income is not always associated with higher dietary intake. Data from both NNMB and INP show that cereal intakes were higher in some of the poor states (Orissa in NNMB, Uttar Pradesh in INP), perhaps because most of the population of these states work as manual labourers and require high cereal intakes. NSSO (1975 to 2001) consumer expenditure surveys show similar interstate differences. Consumption of cereals is higher in rural areas, while that of pulses, milk and milk products, fruits and fat and oils is higher in urban areas.

TABLE 8
Food intakes in rural and urban areas (g/CUs per day)

| | NNMB | | | | | | INP (1995/1996) | | RDA |
| | Rural | | | | Urban slums | | Rural | Urban | |
	1975–1979	1988–1990	1995–1996	2000–2001	1975–1979	1993–1994			
Cereals and millets	505	490	450	457	416	380	488	420	460
Dairy products	116	92	85	85	42	75	126	143	150
Pulses and legumes	34	32	29	34	33	27	33	55	40
Vegetables									
Green leafy	8	9	15	18	11	16	32	23	40
Others (includes tubers)	54	49	47	57	40	47	70	75	60
Fruits	13	23	24	25	26	26	15	37	50
Fats and oil	14	13	12	14	13	17	14	21	20
Sugar and jaggery	23	29	21	23	20	22	20	22	30

Sample sizes: NNMB, rural – 1975–1979, 33 048; 1996–1997, 14 391; 2000–2001, 30 968. Urban slums – 1975–1980, 32 500; 1993–1994, 5 447. INP – 46 457.
Sources: NNMB; INP.

Time trends in food intake

Data on time trends in food intake in rural areas and urban slums in nine states are available from NNMB surveys (Table 8). These data show that there has been some decline in cereal consumption in both urban and rural areas over the last three decades. There has also been a substantial decline in the cost of cereals and an improvement in their availability. The decline is therefore not due to economic constraints. Over the same period, there has also been a decline in the consumption of pulses, which are a major source of protein in Indian diets. This is partly attributable to soaring costs and the inability of poor people to purchase them in adequate quantities, in spite of higher expenditure on pulses.

Although India's milk output has increased massively, there has not been any improvement in the per capita consumption of milk. Consumption of vegetables and fruits also continues to be very low. In rural areas, there has not been any significant increase in the per capita consumption of fats and oils and of sugar and jaggery. However in urban areas – even among slum dwellers – there has been an increase in oil consumption and some increase in sugar consumption. Data from NNMB surveys suggest that dietary intake has not undergone any major shift towards increased consumption of fat and oils, sugar and processed food, and there has been no increase in energy intake. These data are confirmed by the consumer expenditure on food items reported in NSSO.

Nutrient intake

INP provides data on nutrient intake in the urban and rural areas of all states (Table 9). The nutrient intakes reported in INP are higher than those in NNMB because of higher intakes in states not covered by NNMB. At the aggregate national level, total energy intake was less than 2 300 kcal/CUs/day in the mid-1990s. There are substantial interstate differences in energy and other nutrient intakes.

TABLE 9
Nutrient intakes in rural and urban areas (g/CUs/day)

| | RDA (sedentary man) | NNMB | | | | | | | | INP (1995/1996) | |
| | | Rural | | | | | Urban Slums | | | Rural | Urban |
		1975–1979	1988–1990	1996–1997	2000–2001	% Δ¹	1975–1979	1988–1990	% Δ²		
Energy (kcal)	2 425	2 340	2 283	2 108	2 255	-4	2 008	1 896	-6	2 321	2 259
Protein (g)	60	62.9	61.8	53.7	58.7	-7	53.4	46.75	-12	70	70
Calcium (mg)	400	590	556	521	523	-11	492	*		631	673
Iron (mg)	28.0	30.2	28.4	24.9	17.5³	-42	24.9	19.0	-24	23.2	22.3
Vitamin A (mcg)	600	257	294	300	242	-6	248	352	42	355	356
Thiamine (mg)	1.2	1.6	1.5	1.2	1.4	-13	1.3	*		1.9	1.9
Riboflavin (mg)	1.4	0.9	0.9	0.9	0.8	-11	0.8	0.8	-2	1.0	1.0
Niacin (mg)	16.0	15.7	15.5	12.7	17.1	9.0	14.6	*		19.7	18.8
Vitamin C (mg)	40	37	37	40	51	38	40	42	5	55	62
Folic acid (mcg)	100	*	*	153	62		*	*		*	*

Sample sizes: NNMB, rural – 1975–1979, 33 048; 1996–1997, 14 391; 2000–2001, 30 968. Urban slums – 1975–1980, 32 500; 1993–1994, 5 447. INP – 46 457.
¹ Changes in intake from 1975–1979 to 2000–2001.
² Changes in intake from 1975–1979 to 1993–1994.
³ Method of estimation different.
* Data not available.
Sources: NNMB, 1979; 2002; INP, 1996.

Time trends in nutrient intakes

Data on time trends in nutrient intakes are available from NNMB surveys (Table 9). These data show there has been a small decline in energy intake over the last three decades (Figure 14). There has also been some decline in the intakes of most nutrients in both urban and rural areas. The percentage of total energy intake derived from carbohydrates has declined and there has been some increase in the percentage dietary energy from fats (Figure 15). In spite of this, the proportion of dietary energy from fat remains less than 15 percent. These aggregate measures mask large disparities between the intakes of urban and rural populations and among different socio-economic groups. In India, the dietary intake of iron has always been low. The steep decline in iron intake reported in the last NNMB survey can be attributed to different estimation methods, which showed that absorbable iron was 50 percent less than it was in earlier surveys.

FIGURE 14
Time trends in energy intake, 1975 to 2001

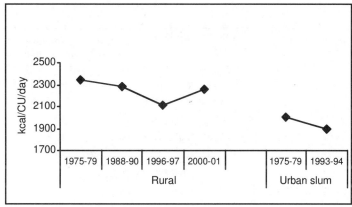

Source: NNMB reports.

FIGURE 15
Macronutrient intake in rural areas as percentage of total energy, 1979 to 2001

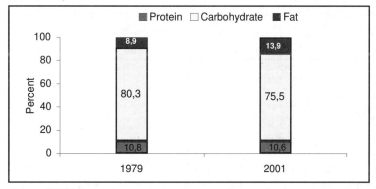

Source: NNMB reports.

Urban–rural differences in nutrient intakes

Energy intake is lower in urban areas (Table 9), in spite of higher intake of fats and oils, because of lower cereal consumption. Data from NNMB surveys suggest that the consumption of all nutrients is lower in urban slums than in rural areas. INP, which covered most states, did not show any significant differences in nutrient intake between urban and rural areas. Interstate differences in nutrient consumption and the fact that NNMB data were available only on urban slums are two of the factors responsible for the apparent differences between NNMB and INP survey data.

Source of dietary energy

Data on total energy intakes and percentages of energy intake from fat, carbohydrate and protein for different age groups, as reported by NNMB and INP, are given in Table 10. Carbohydrates remain the major source of energy in Indian diets. There has been some reduction in the percentage of total energy intake from carbohydrates and some increase in the percentage from fats over the past three decades.

TABLE 10
Sources of dietary energy

Gender and age (years)	Total dietary energy intake (kcal)				Percentage dietary energy from fat				Percentage dietary energy from protein				Percentage dietary energy from carbohydrates			
	NNMB			INP	NNMB			INP	NNMB			INP	NNMB			INP
	1979	1996	2001	1996	1979	1996	2001	1996	1979	1996	2001	1996	1979	1996	2001	1996
Males and females[1]																
1–3	834	807	706	926	14.8	14.3	12.1	15.1	10.9	10.4	10.1	13.2	74.3	75.3	77.7	71.7
4–6	1 118	1 213	1 029	1 299	12.9	13.6	10.8	13.2	10.8	10.3	10.2	12.7	76.3	76.4	79.1	74.1
7–9[2]		1 467	1 251	1 520		12.3	10.1	13.9		10.6	10.1	13.1		77.1	79.8	73.1
Males																
10–12	1 439	1 738	1 524	1 847	8.8	12.7	11.8	12.1	10.9	10.5	10.6	12.3	80.3	76.7	77.6	75.6
13–15	1 618	2 004	1 856	2 185	9.3	12.4	11.9	11.9	10.7	10.5	10.5	12.3	80.0	77.1	77.6	75.8
16–17	1 926	2 369	2 114	2 514	8.0	12.6	11.0	11.3	10.4	10.4	10.4	12.6	81.6	77.0	78.7	76.1
< 18[3]	2 065	2 488	2 225	2 592	8.9	12.4	13.9	12.2	10.8	10.2	10.6	12.3	80.3	74.8	75.5	75.5
Females																
10–12	1 394	1 635	1 500	1 482	9.0	12.2	11.3	12.3	11.2	10.4	10.5	12.3	79.8	77.4	78.1	75.4
13–15	1566	1 848	1 689	2 097	9.1	11.7	11.2	12.2	10.5	10.4	10.3	12.5	80.4	77.9	78.5	75.3
16–17	1 704	2 030	1 856	2 327	8.8	12.9	11.7	12.3	10.3	10.2	10.1	12.8	80.9	76.6	77.7	74.9
<18[3]	1 698	2 106	1 878	2 293	9.1	13.9	13.9	12.6	10.7	9.9	10.6	12.4	80.2	76.2	75.5	75.0

Sample sizes: NNMB – 1975–1979, 33 048; 1996–1997, 14 391; 2000–2001, 22 945. INP – 46 457.
[1] No gender disaggregation of data before ten years of age.
[2] Data not available.
[3] No gender disaggregation of data after 18 years of age.
Sources: NNMB, 1979; 2002; INP, 1996.

Dietary diversity

The second National Family Health Survey (NFHS-2) (IIPS, 1998/1999) collected data on frequency of consumption of various types of foods (daily, weekly or occasionally) to assess dietary diversity among 90 000 married women aged 15 to 49 years living in 26 states. The survey did not include the quantities of intake. Data from the survey are presented in Tables 11 and 12. Adult women in India consume cereals every day; their diets tend to be monotonous and there is very little dietary diversity. Fruits are eaten daily by only 8 percent of women, and once a week by only one-third. Almost one-third of women never eat chicken, meat or fish, and very few (only 6 percent) eat these foods every day. Eggs are consumed even less frequently than chicken, meat or fish.

TABLE 11
Women's frequency of consumption of selected foods

Type of food	Daily	Weekly	Occasionally	Never
Milk or curd	37.5	17.4	34.1	10.9
Pulses or beans	46.9	40.8	11.6	0.6
Green leafy vegetables	41.8	43.4	14.3	0.4
Other vegetables	65.1	28	6.6	0.2
Fruits	8.1	24.9	62.3	4.7
Eggs	2.8	25.0	37.9	34.2
Chicken, meat or fish	5.8	26.1	37.3	30.8

Source: IIPS, 1998/1999.

There were substantial differences in food consumption patterns according to background characteristics (Table 12). Age does not play an important role in women's consumption patterns, but women in urban areas are more likely than those in rural areas to include every type of food in their diet, particularly fruits and milk or curd. Illiterate women have less varied diets than literate women, and seldom eat fruits. Poverty has a strong negative effect on dietary diversity. Women from households in the low socio-economic group are less likely than others to eat items from each type of food group listed, and their diets are particularly deficient in fruits and milk or curd. There are substantial interstate differences in the consumption of different types of food.

TABLE 12
Women's food consumption (percentages of survey population)

	Milk or curd	Pulses or beans	Green leafy vegetables	Other vegetables	Fruits	Eggs	Chicken, meat or fish
			Residence				
Urban	65.3	92.8	88.4	95.0	53.9	39.7	41.7
Rural	51.3	86.0	84.1	92.4	25.6	23.6	28.5
			Economic status				
Low	35.0	81.4	82.1	91.6	17.0	23.8	29.1
Medium	58.1	89.4	85.3	93.1	31.5	28.6	33.1
High	80.0	94.3	90.0	95.7	62.0	32.3	33.6
Total	**55.0**	**87.8**	**85.2**	**93.1**	**33.0**	**27.8**	**31.9**

Source: IIPS, 1998/1999.

Summary
During the past three decades there have been:

- reductions in energy intake from cereals, except among the poor; overall there has been a small decrease in total energy intake in both urban and rural areas;

- some increase in percentage of dietary energy derived from fat, and a reciprocal reduction in that derived from carbohydrate;

- some increase in consumption of fats and oils in urban populations, even in urban slums;

- increasing dietary diversity among upper-income groups in rural and – especially – urban areas;

- cereal-based and monotonous diets for the rural poor, with low micronutrient content;

- low iron intake, which coupled with the poor bioavailability of iron from Indian diets is responsible for a high prevalence of anaemia

DIETARY INTAKE AND NUTRITIONAL STATUS IN DIFFERENT AGE GROUPS

As well as the dietary intake and nutritional status data collected by NNMB and INP, NFHS 1 and 2 (IIPS, 1992/1993; 1998/1999) provide state-level estimates of time trends in the nutritional status of women and preschool children in all major states during the 1990s. The District-Level Household Survey (DLHS) 2002/2003 (Ministry of Family and Health Welfare, 2004) provides district-level estimates on the nutritional status of preschool children. In addition, several smaller studies provide follow-up data on the nutritional status of specific groups over decades. This section reviews these data on time trends in the dietary intake and nutritional status of different age groups.

Time trends in anthropometric indices

Data from NNMB rural surveys of trends in weight, height, mid-arm circumference and triceps fat fold thickness in males and females of all age groups are shown in Figures 16 to 21. Even in the rural population, adult height has increased by about 4 cm. Increases in body weight have been greater, mainly due to fat deposition, as shown by rising fat fold thickness over this period. These affected all age groups, and especially women.

FIGURE 16
Trends in mean weights in rural males, 1975 to 2001

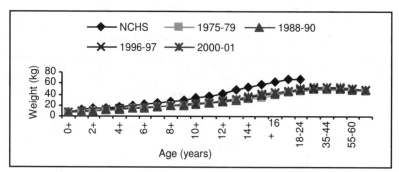

Source: NNMB reports.

FIGURE 17
Trends in mean heights in rural males, 1975 to 2001

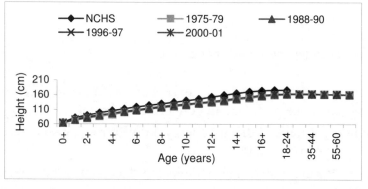

Source: NNMB reports.

FIGURE 18
Trends in mean tricep fat fold thickness in rural males, 1975 to 2001

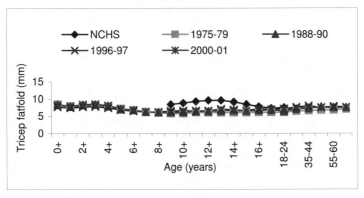

Source: NNMB reports.

FIGURE 19
Trends in mean weights in rural females, 1975 to 2001

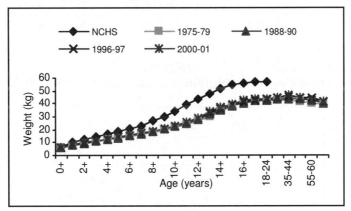

Source: NNMB reports.

FIGURE 20
Trends in mean heights in rural females, 1975 to 2001

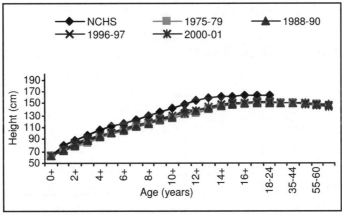

Source: NNMB reports.

FIGURE 21
Trends in mean tricep fat fold thickness in rural females, 1975 to 2001

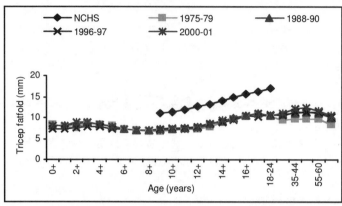

Source: NNMB reports.

Data from NNMB surveys in urban slums are shown in Figures 22 to 25. Mean body weight, mid-upper arm circumference and fat fold thickness at triceps have increased in all age groups. Most of the body weight increase is due to increased fat, as shown by rising fat fold thickness.

FIGURE 22
Trends in mean weights in urban males, 1975 to 1994

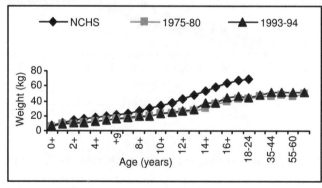

Source: NNMB reports.

FIGURE 23
Trends in mean tricep fat fold thickness in urban males, 1975 to 1994

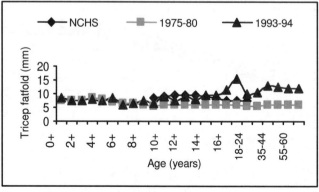

Source: NNMB reports.

FIGURE 24
Trends in mean weights in urban females, 1975 to 1994

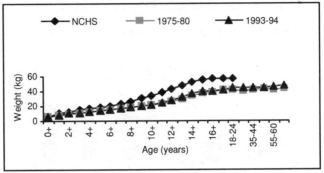

Source: NNMB reports.

FIGURE 25
Trends in mean tricep fat fold thickness in urban females, 1975 to 1994

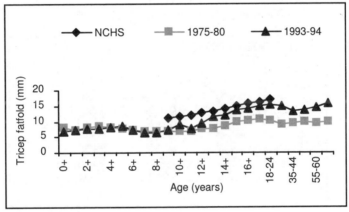

Source: NNMB reports.

Low birth weight

Nearly one-third of Indian infants weigh less than 2.5 kg at birth. Incidence of low birth weight (LBW) is highest among low-income groups (Table 13). There is clear correlation between birth weight and maternal body weight (Figure 26); low birth weight rate doubles when Hb levels fall below 8 gm/dl. Low birth weight incidence has remained unaltered over the last three decades (Figure 27) (NFI, 2004).

TABLE 13
Birth weight and socio-economic status

	Low-income	Middle-income	High-income
Age (years)	24.1	24.3	27.8
Parity	2.41	1.96	1.61
Height (cm)	151.5	154.2	156.3
Weight (kg)	45.7	49.9	56.2
Hb (g/dl)	10.9	11.1	12.4
Birth weight (kg)	2.70	2.90	3.13

Source: Ramachandran, 1989.

FIGURE 26
Birth weight in relation to maternal body mass index

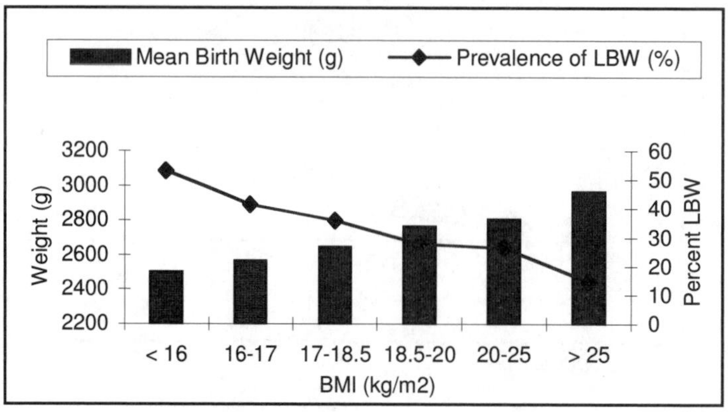

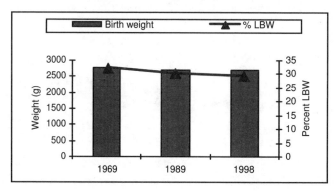

Source: Planning Commission, 2002.

FIGURE 27
Trends in birth weight, 1969 to 1998

Source: NFI, 2004.

Although there has been no decline in the prevalence of low birth weight, India has achieved a substantial decline in infant mortality (RGI, 2002). As more low-birth-weight newborns survive, there is growing concern regarding the relationship between low birth weight and poor growth during childhood and adolescence, as well as increased risk of chronic degenerative diseases in later life.

Under the Reproductive and Child Health Programme 1 and 2 (Ministry of Family and Health Welfare, 1998/1999; 2002), efforts are under way to provide effective antenatal care and reduce rates of low birth weight. Factors such as maternal height, which has a significant influence on birth weight, cannot be improved with short-term corrective interventions, but anaemia, pregnancy-induced hypertension and low maternal weight gain during pregnancy can be detected and treated. Effective management of these could result in substantial reductions in both pre-term births and the birth of small-for-date infants.

Growth during infancy and early childhood
Growth during infancy and childhood depends on birth weight, adequacy of infant feeding and absence of infection. Available data clearly indicate that exclusively breastfed infants thrive better during the first six months of life and have lower morbidity episodes (diarrhoea,

respiratory tract infection and fever) than those receiving supplements in addition to breastmilk. In India, steps taken to protect and promote the practice of breastfeeding have been effective, and breastfeeding is now almost universal (Planning Commission, 2002). However, the message that exclusive breastfeeding up to six months followed by the gradual introduction of semi-solids is critical for the prevention of undernutrition in infancy has not been as effectively communicated. Data from NFHS 2 (IIPS, 1998/1998) indicate that although breastfeeding is nearly universal and the mean duration of lactation is more than two years, only 55.2 percent of infants up to three months of age receive exclusive breastfeeding. In spite of the emphasis on the need to introduce complementary food gradually, only 33.5 percent of infants in the six to nine months age group receive breastmilk and semi-solid food.

There are substantial interstate differences in exclusive breastfeeding and the timely introduction of semi-solid food (Figure 28). Early introduction of supplements is a major problem in states such as Delhi, Himachal Pradesh and Punjab, while late introduction is a problem in Bihar, Uttar Pradesh, Madhya Pradesh, Rajasthan and Orissa. Kerala fares well in terms of appropriate infant feeding practices, and this might be one of the reasons for the relatively low undernutrition rates in this state (IIPS, 1998/1999).

Early introduction of milk substitutes and late introduction of complementary food are associated with increased risk of undernutrition and infection. Faulty infant feeding practices are causing the prevalence of undernutrition to increase steeply with age, from 11.9 percent at less than six months to 58.5 percent in the 12 to 23 months age group (Figure 29). A major thrust of the Tenth Five-Year Plan is to prevent the onset of undernutrition in infancy and early childhood through nutrition education, so that by 2007 more than 80 percent of women breastfeed exclusively up to six months and the complementary feeding rate at six months goes up to 75 percent (IIPS, 1998/1999).

FIGURE 28
Infant feeding practices by state

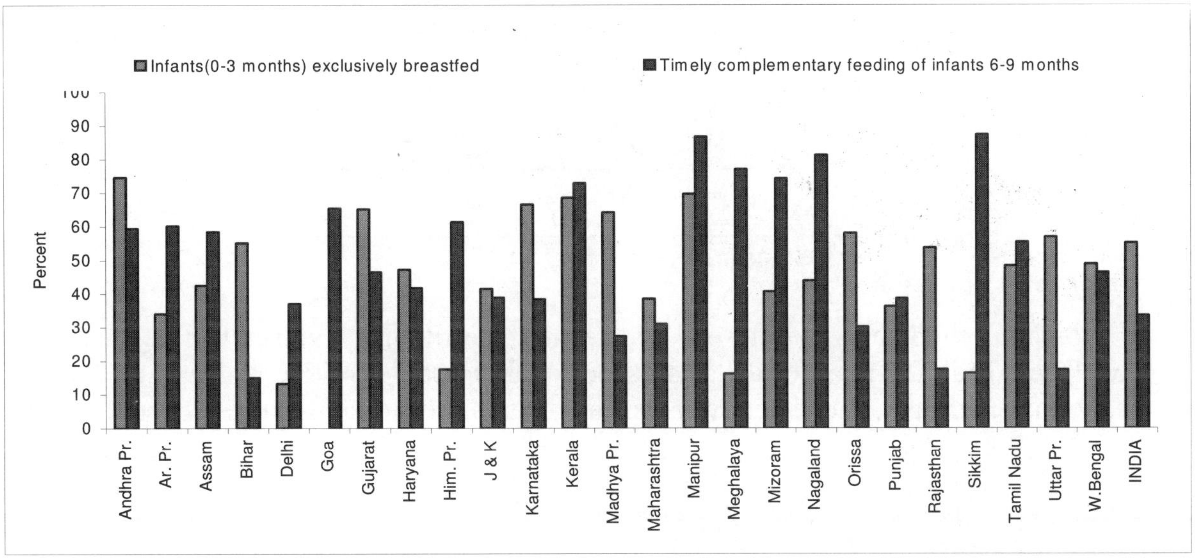

FIGURE 29
Prevalence of undernutrition (weight for age less than –2 SD)

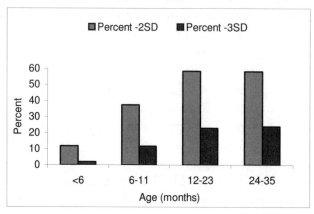

Source: IIPS, 1998/1999.

Time trends in the dietary intake and nutritional status of preschool children

Data from NNMB on energy intake and the prevalence of undernutrition in children under three years of age are shown in Figure 30. There has been a steady decline in undernutrition in children, even though the dietary intake has not shown a major change. The decline in undernutrition is most probably attributable to better access to health care and the effective management of infections.

FIGURE 30
Energy intake and undernutrition in children aged one to three years, 1979 to 2002

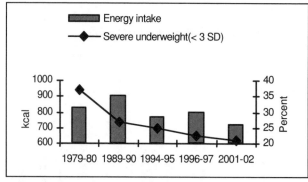

Source: NNMB reports.

Preschool children constitute one of the most nutritionally vulnerable segments of the population, and their nutritional status is considered to be a sensitive indicator of community health and nutrition. Their dietary intake has not improved substantially over the last two decades (Table 14).

TABLE 14
Average nutrient intakes among preschool children, 1975 to 1997

	1–3 years			4–6 years		
	1975–1979	1988–1990	1996–1997	1975–1979	1988–1990	1996–1997
Protein (g)	22.8	23.7	20.9	30.2	33.9	31.2
Energy (kcal)	834	908	807	1 118	1 260	1 213
Vitamin A (µg)	136	117	133	159	153	205
Thiamine (mg)	0.50	0.52	0.40	0.76	0.83	0.70
Riboflavin (mg)	0.38	0.37	0.40	0.48	0.52	0.60
Niacin (mg)	5.08	5.56	4.60	7.09	8.40	7.40

Source: NNMB, 2000.

Data on energy intake in children, adolescents and adults from NNMB 2000 are shown in Table 15. Mean energy consumption as a percentage of RDA is lowest among preschool children. Time trends in the intra-family distribution of food (Figure 31) indicate that although the proportion of families in which both adults and preschool children have adequate food has remained at about 30 percent over the last 20 years, the proportion of families with inadequate intake has decreased substantially. However, the proportion of families in which preschool children receive inadequate and adults adequate intakes has nearly doubled, even though the RDA for preschool children forms only a very small proportion (an average of 1 300 kcal/day) of the family's total intake of about 11 000 kcal/day (assuming a family size of five). It therefore appears that poor young child feeding and care practices – and not poverty – is the factor responsible for inadequate dietary intake. The Tenth Five-Year Plan (Planning Commission, 2002) emphasizes the importance of health and nutrition education to ensure proper intra-family distribution of food, based on needs.

TABLE 15
Average energy intakes for children, adolescents and adults

Age group	Males			Females		
	kcals	RDA	% RDA	kcals	RDA	% RDA
Preschool	889	1 357	65.5	897	1 351	66.4
School age	1 464	1 929	75.9	1 409	1 876	75.1
Adolescents	2 065	2 441	84.6	1 670	1 823	91.6
Adults	2 226	2 425	91.8	1 923	1 874	102.6

Source: NNMB, 2000.

FIGURE 31
Comparison of adequate energy status of preschool children and adults, 1975 to 1997

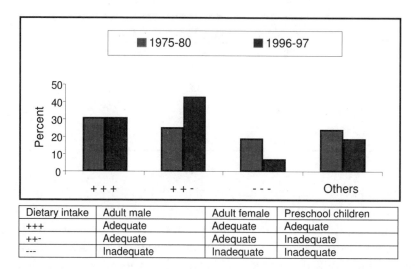

Dietary intake	Adult male	Adult female	Preschool children
+++	Adequate	Adequate	Adequate
++-	Adequate	Adequate	Inadequate
---	Inadequate	Inadequate	Inadequate

Time trends in prevalence of undernutrition in preschool children

Over the last three decades, there has been a steep decline in the prevalence of moderate and severe undernutrition as assessed by weight-for-age and height-for-age (Figures 32 and 33), but very little change in the prevalence of wasting. In spite of the steep decline in the prevalence of stunting, the mean height of children has changed only very slightly. The increase in adult height has also been a modest 2 to 4 cm in three decades.

FIGURE 32
Trends in prevalence of undernutrition in children (percentages), 1975 to 1999

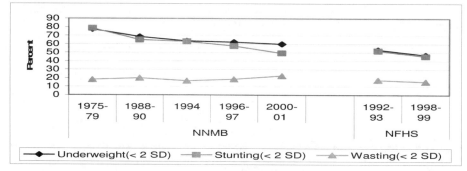

Sample sizes: NNBB – 1975–1980, 6 428; 1988–1990, 13 432; 1996–1997, 8 654; 2000–2001, 6 646. INP – 46 457. NFHS – 1992–1993, 25 584; 1998–1999, 24 600.
Sources: NNMB; INP; IIPS.

FIGURE 33
Prevalence of severe undernutrition in children (percentages), 1975 to 1999

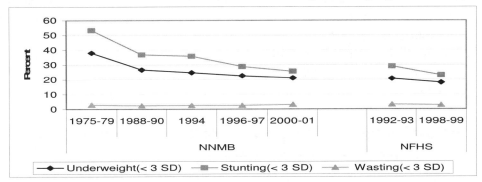

Sample sizes: NNBB – 1975–1980, 6 428; 1988–1990, 13 432; 1996–1997, 8 654; 2000–2001, 6 646. INP – 46 457. NFHS – 1992–1993, 25 584; 1998–1999, 24 600.
Sources: NNMB; INP; IIPS.

Indian children are short compared with the National Center for Health Statistics (NCHS) norms; even when they have appropriate weight for height they are classified as undernourished according to these norms. The so-called South Asian paradox (high undernutrition rates but comparatively good health status) disappears when the body mass index (BMI)-for-age is the criterion for defining undernutrition. Early detection and correction are needed if wasting is to be reduced so that Indian children can achieve their growth potential. There are considerable interstate differences in the dietary intake and nutritional status of children (Figure 34). Although dietary intake is a major determinant of nutritional status in children, it is not the only one. Energy intake is low and undernutrition high in Uttar Pradesh, Bihar and Rajasthan. However, in spite of low energy intakes, the prevalence of undernutrition in Kerala and Tamil Nadu is low, probably because there is more equitable intra-family distribution of food based on needs, and better access to health care. The combination of high energy intakes and high undernutrition prevalence in Madhya Pradesh and Orissa is probably due to inequitable food distribution and poor access to health care (IIPS, 1998/1999).

FIGURE 34
Energy intake and undernutrition among children, by state

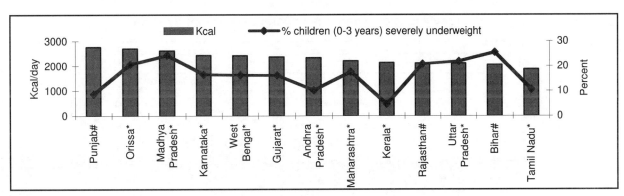

Sources: INP; IIPS, 1998/1999.

The nutritional status of poor children in Kerala is similar to that of rich children in Uttar Pradesh and Orissa (Figure 35). This is probably attributable to better access to health care and more equitable intra-family food distribution in Kerala than in Uttar Pradesh. These data clearly indicate that lack of access to health care is a major factor in undernutrition among preschool children. The decline in fertility and the reduction in family size may also have contributed to this because the prevalence of severe forms of undernutrition is higher in large families (IIPS, 1998/1988).

FIGURE 35
Nutritional status of children (weight-for-age) by income group and state

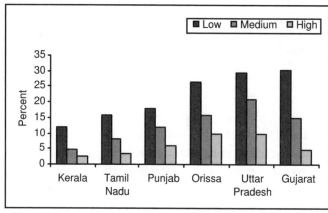

Sources: IIPS, 1992-93.

Poor dietary intake, poor care practices and poor access to health care are some of the major factors responsible for undernutrition and a high under-five mortality rate (U5MR). In most of the states where undernutrition is high (e.g., Orissa), U5MR is also high; in states where undernutrition is low (e.g., Kerala), U5MR is also low (Figure 36). There are exceptions to this, however; in Maharashtra U5MR is relatively low, in spite of relatively high undernutrition rates – this might be because access to health care is relatively good. In Punjab, in spite of high per capita income and dietary intake and good access to health care, both undernutrition and U5MR are relatively high. These data indicate the importance of health care in reducing both undernutrition and U5MR (IIPS, 1992/1993).

FIGURE 36
Prevalence of severe underweight and U5MR by state

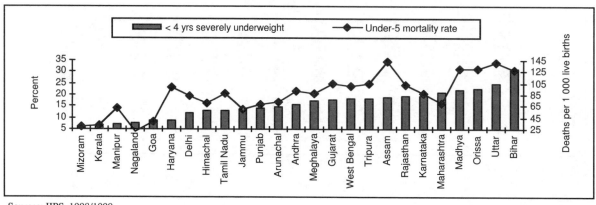

Sources: IIPS, 1998/1999.

Nutritional status of affluent schoolchildren

Studies carried out by NFI in 1991 (NFI, 2004) show that the growth of affluent children up to six years of age is similar to the NCHS and WHO norm. Data from NFI studies in Delhi between 2000 and 2004 (NFI, 2004) show that while undernutrition is a problem among children from low-income groups (LIG) who are studying in government schools, overnutrition is the cause for concern among high-income-group (HIG) schoolchildren from six years of age (Figure 37).

FIGURE 37
Comparison of weight-for-age in Delhi schoolboys

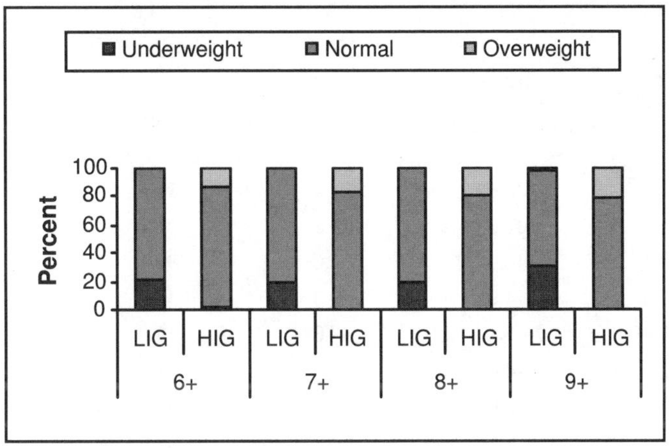

Source: NFI, 2004.

Growth of adolescents from affluent urban families

The heights and weights of adolescent girls and boys from affluent income groups are comparable to NCHS norms (Table 16), and higher than those of adolescents surveyed by NNMB. NFI data on height and weight distribution (compared with NCHS norms) in Delhi schoolchildren from affluent families are shown in Figures 38 and 39. Even in these affluent segments of the population, some children are stunted (-2 SD height for age). There are overweight children in all classes and age groups. Among children over ten years of age there is a reduction in overweight because children of this age try to lose weight through exercise or skipping meals (NFI, 2004). However, the adolescents have inconsistent eating and exercise habits and tend therefore to have cyclical weight gain and loss, thereby incurring the health hazards associated with this pattern.

FIGURE 38
Height-for-age

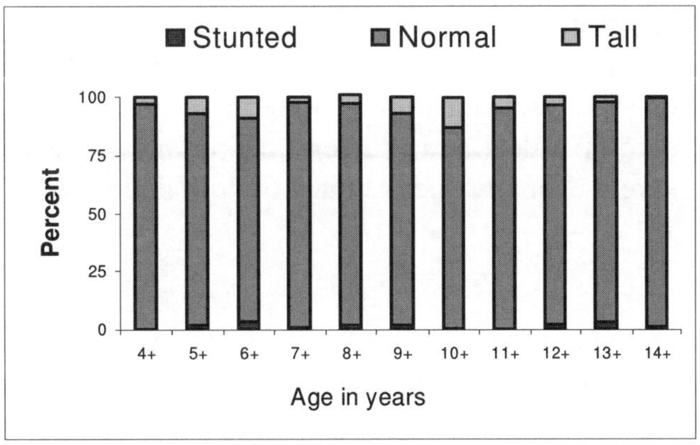

TABLE 16
Growth of adolescents from urban affluent families

Age (years)	Well-to-do		NCHS		Average Indian	
	Boys	**Girls**	**Boys**	**Girls**	**Boys**	**Girls**
Height (cm)						
10+	138.5	138.9	137.5	138.3	128.1	128.1
11+	143.4	145.0	140.0	142.0	133.1	133.1
12+	148.9	151.0	147.0	148.0	137.4	138.4
13+	154.9	153.4	153.0	155.0	143.0	144.1
14+	161.7	155.0	160.0	159.0	148.6	147.9
15+	165.3	156.0	166.0	161.0	153.0	149.8
16+	168.4	156.0	171.0	162.0	158.0	151.2
17+	173.0		175.0	163.0	161.2	152.1
Weight (kg)						
10+	32.3	33.6	31.4	32.5	23.1	23.1
11+	35.3	37.2	32.2	33.7	25.1	25.7
12+	38.8	43.0	37.0	38.7	27.3	28.7
13+	42.9	44.5	40.9	44.0	30.8	32.6
14+	48.3	46.7	47.0	48.0	34.8	36.0
15+	52.2	48.8	52.6	51.4	38.6	38.9
16+	55.5	49.8	58.0	53.0	42.3	41.3
17+	57.9		62.7	54.0	46.0	42.8

FIGURE 39
Weight-for-age

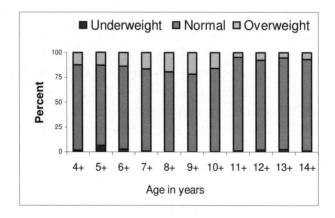

Nutritional status of adults

NNMB and INP data show that the prevalence of undernutrition in adults is higher in rural than urban areas (Table 17). Overnutrition is higher in urban areas. Over the last three decades there has been a progressive decline in undernutrition and some increase in overnutrition in both urban and rural areas. The prevalence rates of both under- and overnutrition are higher in women than men.

TABLE 17
Prevalence of under- and overnutrition among adults, 1975 to 2001

	Underweight						Overweight					
	NNMB				INP		NNMB				INP	
	1975–1979	1989–1990	1996–1997	2000–2001	1993–1994	1995–1996	1975–1979	1989–1990	1996–1997	2000–2001	1993–1994	1995–1996
Rural	53.2	49.0	48.5	38.6		34.6	2.9	3.1	46.5	6.6		4.1
Urban					20.3	27.7						6.0
Male	55.6	49.0	45.5	37.4	22.2	28.6	2.3	2.6	4.1	5.7	5.0	4.3
Female	51.8	49.3	47.7	39.3	19.4	36.3	3.4	4.1	6.0	8.2	10.6	4.6

Sample sizes: NNMB – 1975–1979, 11 973; 1989–1990, 21 398; 1993-1994, 2 772; 1996–1997, 30 773; 2000–2001, 11 074. INP – 17 7841.
Sources: NNMB; INP.

Nutritional status of women

Data from NFHS-2 (IIPS, 1998/1999) indicate that the prevalence of undernutrition among women in urban areas is half that of rural areas (Table 18). Overnutrition is four times higher in urban than in rural areas. In women, as age increases, the prevalence of undernutrition declines while that of overnutrition increases.

TABLE 18
Prevalence of under- and overnutrition among women (15 to 45 years)

Characteristic	Mean BMI	BMI < 18.5	BMI ≥ 25
Rural	19.6	40.6	5.9
Urban	21.1	22.6	23.5
Age (years)			
15–19	19.3	38.8	1.7
20–24	19.3	41.8	3.6
25–29	19.8	39.1	7.3
30–34	20.4	35.0	11.7
35–49	21.1	31.1	16.8
Overall	**20.3**	**35.8**	**10.6**

Sample size: 77 119.
Source: IIPS, 1998/1999.

Data from NFHS-2 show that although undernutrition continues to be high among women in poorer segments of the population, overnutrition and obesity are emerging as major problems in all states of India. There are substantial differences in the prevalence of under- and overnutrition among states, but all states have to prepare to detect and manage this dual nutrition problem in women (Figure 40).

FIGURE 40
Comparison of BMI in women, by state

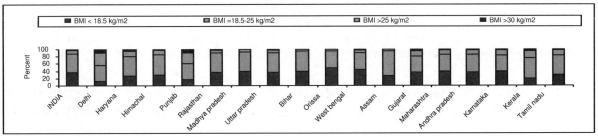

Source: IIPS 1998/1999.

Summary

Over the past three decades there have been:

- a very small (2 to 4 cm) increase in adult height;
- a significant increase in mean body weights, mostly owing to increased body fat as shown by increased fat fold thickness, which is greater in urban than rural areas.

In the absence of increased energy consumption, increased fat deposition is attributed to reduced physical activity. Very few studies have documented changes in physical activity patterns over the last three decades, but it is documented that over this period there have been:

- reduction in the number of people engaged in manual work;
- substantial improvement of mechanical aids in agriculture, industry and allied activities;
- improved access to water and fuel near households, in both urban and rural areas;
- improved availability of urban transport at affordable costs, resulting in fewer people walking or cycling to work, school or market;
- more mechanical aids that reduce physical activity during cooking and household tasks;
- TVs and computers in affluent urban households, which contribute to steep reductions in physical activity.

These lifestyle changes have led to reductions in energy requirements. Unchanged energy intakes combined with reduced energy requirements are associated with a positive energy balance and fat deposition.

MICRONUTRIENT DEFICIENCIES

Goitre caused by iodine deficiency, blindness by vitamin A deficiency (VAD) and anaemia by iron and folate deficiency are major public health problems in India. Over the last three decades, there has been a steep decline in keratomalacia caused by severe VAD, but no decline in the prevalence of anaemia caused by iron and folic acid deficiency; the declines in VAD and iodine deficiency disorders (IDDs) have been very slow. Data from NNMB surveys, IIPS and DLHS provide valuable insights for assessing the progress achieved in combating these deficiencies, help to formulate future interventions and provide baseline information for assessing the impacts of future interventions.

Anaemia

In India, the prevalence of anaemia is high because of:

- low dietary intake of iron (less than 20 mg/day, according to NNMB 2000) and folate (less than 70 mg/day);
- poor bioavailability of iron (only 3 to 4 percent) in the phytate fibre-rich Indian diet;
- chronic blood loss caused by infections such as malaria and hookworm infestations.

Data from DLHS (all states 1 100 households/district; Ministry of Family and Health Welfare, 2002/2003) and the NNMB survey (from eight states, NNMB, 2002) show that prevalence of anaemia is very high (ranging from 80 to more than 90 percent) in preschool children, pregnant and lactating women and adolescent girls (Figure 41). Criteria used for assessing anaemia in DLHS are given in Table 19.

FIGURE 41
Prevalence of anaemia (percentage)

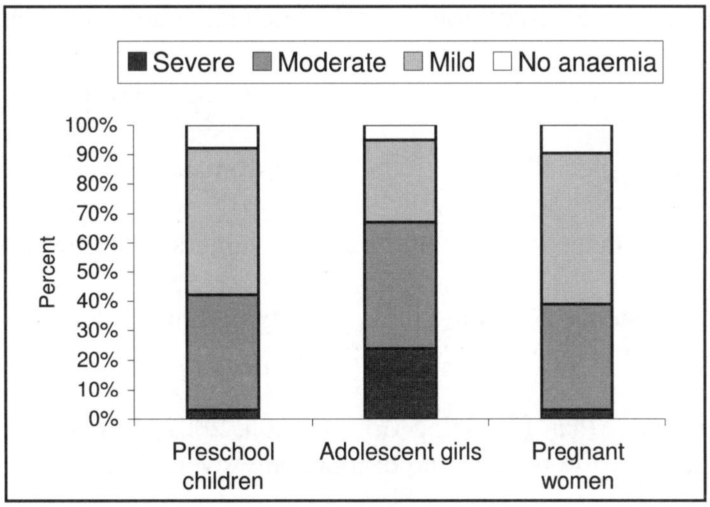

Source: Ministry of Family and Health Welfare, 2002/2003.

TABLE 19
Anaemia measurement criteria used in DLHS (g/dl)

	Normal	Mild	Moderate	Severe
Pregnant women and preschool children	≥ 11	8.0–10.9	5.0–7.9	≤ 5
Adolescent girls	≥ 12	10.0–11.9	8.0–9.9	≤ 8

Source: Ministry of Family and Health Welfare, 2002/2003.

Moderate and severe anaemia is seen even among upper-income group families. There are interstate differences in prevalence, which are probably attributable to differences in dietary intake and access to health care.

Anaemia is associated with increased susceptibility to infections, reduced work capacity and poor concentration. Anaemia remains a major cause of maternal mortality in India, accounting for more than 20 percent of all maternal deaths. In response to the low dietary intake of iron and folate, the high prevalence of anaemia and its adverse health consequences, India was the first developing country to adopt a National Nutritional Anaemia Prophylaxis Programme to prevent anaemia among pregnant women and children. Screening for anaemia and iron–folate therapy in appropriate doses have been essential components of antenatal and paediatric care for the last three decades, but coverage of these programmes is very low. As a result, very high rates of anaemia in pregnant women persist, and the impacts of severe anaemia on birth weight and maternal mortality remain unaltered. Anaemia continues to be a major problem affecting all segments of the population, and there has been no substantial decline in the adverse health consequences associated with it.

Strategies for the prevention, detection and management of anaemia in the Tenth Five-Year Plan

The total Indian population of more than 1 billion people will have to double their iron and folate intakes and sustain these new levels life long. The major intervention strategies required for the prevention and management of anaemia are:

- dietary diversification to include iron- and folate-rich foods and food items that promote iron absorption;
- health and nutrition education to improve the consumption of iron- and folate-rich foodstuffs;
- food fortification, especially the introduction of iron and iodine-fortified salt at affordable costs;
- screening for early detection of anaemia among vulnerable groups (such as children and pregnant women);
- management of anaemia according to its severity/chronicity, the physiological status of the individual and the time available for treatment.

The Tenth Five-Year Plan (Planning Commission, 2002) has set the goal of reducing the prevalence of anaemia by 25 percent and of moderate/severe anaemia by 50 percent, by 2007.

Vitamin A deficiency

Vitamin A is an important micronutrient for maintaining normal growth, regulating cellular proliferation and differentiation, controlling development, and maintaining visual and reproductive functions. Diet surveys show that intakes of vitamin A are significantly lower than the recommended daily allowance in all groups, and that they have not increased over the decades (NNMB, 1979 to 2002). IIPS, Ministry of Family and Health Welfare (1998/1999) and DLHS surveys show that coverage of the Massive Dose Vitamin A Programme has been poor (Figure 42). However, over the years there has been a steep decline in severe forms of VAD in children; blindness caused by VAD is now very rare. All the large national surveys (NNMB, 2002; ICMR, 2004a; NNMB, 2001) have clearly shown that the prevalence of clinical VAD in children under five years of age in India is currently less than 1 percent (Figure 43). The decline in VAD in children appears to be caused by better access to health care and a consequent reduction in the severity and duration of common childhood morbidity to infections, especially measles.

FIGURE 42
Coverage of the Massive Dose Vitamin A Programme by state

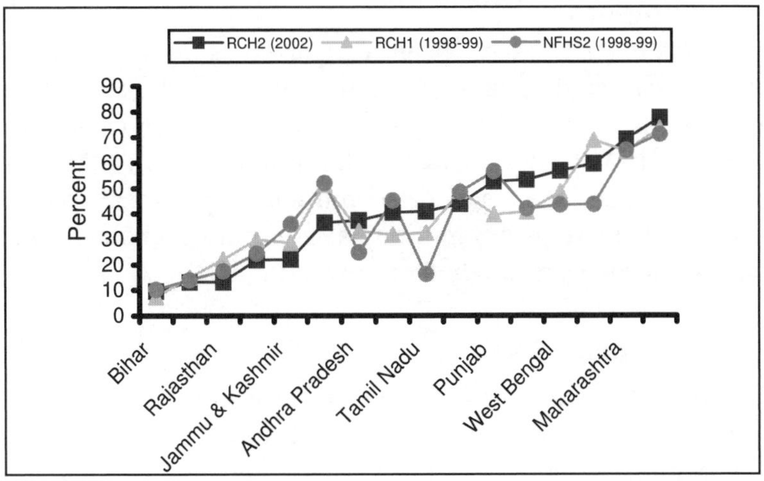

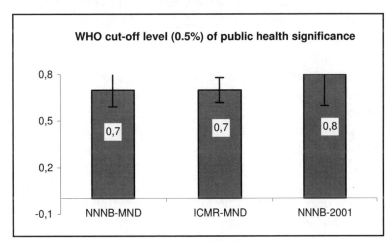

Sources: Ministry of Family and Health Welfare, 1998/1999; 2002/2003; IIPS, 1998/1999.

FIGURE 43
Prevalence of Bitot's spots among children aged one to five years (percentages)

Sources: NNMB, 2002; ICMR, 2004a; NNMB, 2001.

Strategies for managing VAD in the Tenth Five-Year Plan

Clinical VAD often coexists with other micronutrient deficiencies; hence there is a need for broad-based dietary diversification programmes aimed at improving the overall micronutrient status of the population. In addition, the ongoing Massive Dose Vitamin A Programme in children aged nine to 36 months will be continued and its implementation strengthened.

Goals for the Tenth Plan

- Achieve universal coverage for each of the five doses of vitamin A.
- Reduce prevalence of night blindness to less than 1 percent, and that of Bitot's spots to less than 0.5 percent, in children between six months and six years of age.

- Eliminate VAD as a public health problem.

Iodine deficiency disorders

Iodine deficiency disorders (IDDs) have been recognized as a public health problem in India since the 1920s. IDD is caused by a lack of iodine in water, soil and foodstuffs, and it affects all socio-economic groups in defined geographic areas. Surveys carried out by central and state health directorates, ICMR and medical colleges have shown that no Indian territory is free from the problem of IDD. An estimated 167 million people are at risk of IDD – 54 million of whom have goitre while more than 8 million have neurological handicaps. Universal use of iodized salt is a simple, inexpensive method of preventing IDD.

Ongoing interventions to reduce IDD

The Government of India launched the National Goitre Control Programme (NGCP) in 1962. Initially, the programme aimed to provide iodized salt to the well-recognized sub-Himalayan "goitre belt". However, the erratic availability of the salt, the availability of cheaper non-iodized salt and a lack of awareness regarding the need to use iodized salt meant that there was no substantial reduction in IDD. It was then decided to introduce universal iodization of all the salt used for human consumption. This was implemented in a phased manner from 1986, and major efforts were made to increase the production of and access to iodized salt (Salt Department, 2003/2004). In August 1992, the NGCP was renamed the National Iodine Deficiency Disorders Control Programme (NIDDCP) and took into its ambit control of the entire spectrum of IDD. India became the second largest producer of iodized salt in the world, after China. In 1997, the central government banned the storage and sale of non-iodized salt, but lifted the ban in October 2000 because "matters of public health should be left to informed choice and not enforced".

NNMB 2002 data on prevalence rates of goitre in six- to 12-year-old children are shown in Figure 44. The relatively high prevalence of goitre in these non-endemic states is a source of concern. Data from DLHS (Ministry of Family and Health Welfare, 2002/2003), which undertook spot tests of iodization in the salt consumed in 3 05 106 households, are presented in Figure 45. There has been some decline in the consumption of iodized salt since the ban on using non-iodized salt was lifted.

FIGURE 44
Prevalence of goitre in children aged six to 12 years, by state

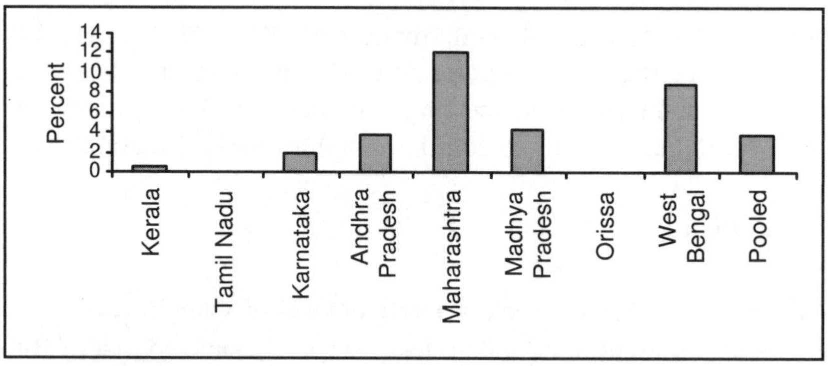

Source: NNMB, 2002.

FIGURE 45
Percentages of households consuming iodized salt, by state

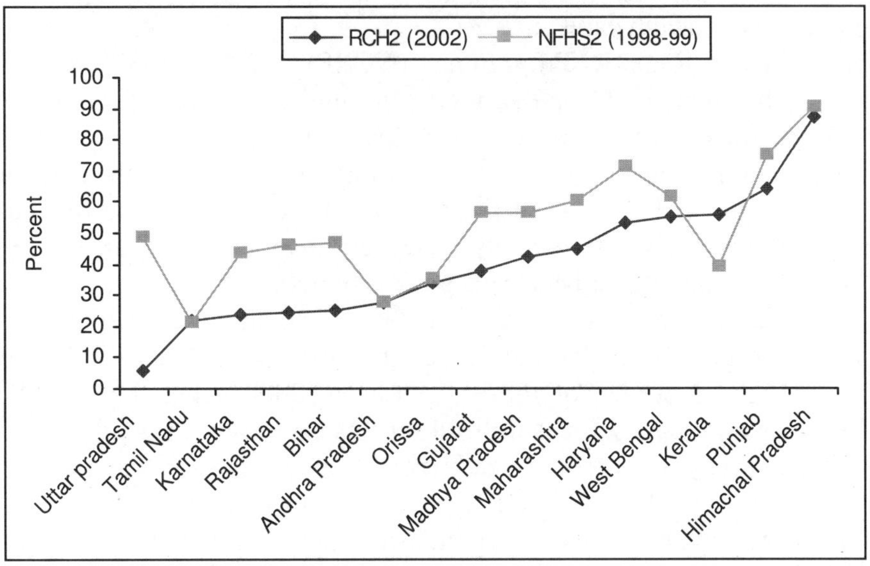

Source: Ministry of Family and Health Welfare, 2002/2003.

Strategies for the prevention of IDDs in the Tenth Five-Year Plan

On 25 June 2005, the Union Minister for Health and Family Welfare announced the decision of the Government of India to reimpose the ban on sales of non-iodized salt for human consumption. It is expected that this announcement will ensure universal access to iodized salt, such that the goals set in the Tenth Five-Year Plan can be achieved.

Goals for the Tenth Plan

- Achieve universal access to iodized salt.
- Generate data on iodized salt consumption by district.
- Reduce the prevalence of IDD in India to less than 10 percent by 2010.

PREVALENCE OF NON-COMMUNICABLE DISEASES

Soon after independence, India established systems for assessing per capita income, purchasing power, poverty, undernutrition and micronutrient deficiencies. Data from these surveys were used to assess interstate differences and time trends. A similar system for tracking overnutrition and the risk of non-communicable diseases (NCDs) was not established until the 1990s, and even now the coverage of this is not as extensive as that of other surveys. In view of this, for documenting time trends in prevalence of NCDs related to overnutrition, India has to depend on research studies carried out in different parts of the country. The differences in methodology of data collection, criteria used for case definition and parameters reported make it difficult to make comparisons among studies and to draw conclusions regarding time trends. However, from the existing data, it is clear that there has been an increase in prevalence rates of diabetes, hypertension and CVD over the last two decades, especially in affluent urban segments of the population. Prevalence of these diseases is lower in poorer segments and in rural areas, but case fatality rates may be higher in these areas because of poor access to health care.

The National Cancer Registry Programme (NCRP) (ICMR, 1983) established cancer registries based on hospitals and populations in the mid-1980s, and generates data on time trends and regional differences in cancer incidence, prevalence and mortality. Data from NCRP show that India has the lowest cancer rates in the world, although it also has relatively high rates of tobacco use (nearly half of the cancers in men are tobacco-related). In spite of increasing longevity, there has not been any increase in overall cancer incidence over the last two decades. However, there have been changes in the incidences of cancer in specific sites, for example, a decrease in prevalence of cervical cancer and an increase in breast cancer.

As NCDs are emerging as major public health problems in India, ICMR undertook an assessment of the disease burden of these diseases in 2004 using the DISMOD II model (ICMR, 2004b). The major data sources utilized for this exercise were medical certifications of causes of disease, a survey of causes of death (rural), cancer registry data, and review of 180 published articles, ten published reports, five unpublished reports and one personal communication dealing with diabetes, hypertension, IHD, stroke and cancers. The ICMR assessment provides national-level estimates of the disease burden of NCDs in the first five years of the new millennium.

This section of the case study reviews the available data on time trends in prevalence of hypertension, diabetes, IHD, stroke and cancers over the last two decades; ICMR estimates of the disease burdens of NCDs; and the relationship between nutritional status and NCD.

Diabetes and impaired glucose tolerance

Community-based studies on prevalence of diabetes in urban and rural areas have been conducted in all regions of the country (Figure 46); all these studies show that there has been progressive increase in prevalence of diabetes in both urban and rural areas over the last three decades.

Data from the Chennai on time trends in prevalence of diabetes and impaired glucose tolerance (IGT) in urban and rural urban populations (Figures 47 and 48) show that both have increased at escalating rates in urban and rural areas (A. Ramachandran, 2005). Potential factors associated with the higher prevalence of diabetes in urban areas are shown in Figure 49.

FIGURE 46
Prevalence of diabetes, 1971 to 1998

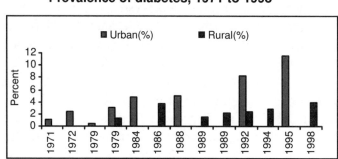

FIGURE 47
Increasing prevalence of diabetes and IGT in urban southern India, 1989 and 2003

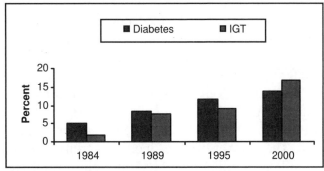

Source: A. Ramachandran, 2005.

FIGURE 48
Temporal changes in prevalence of diabetes and IGT in urban southern India

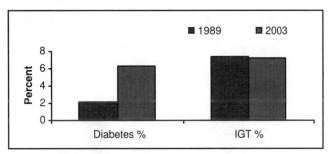

Source: A. Ramachandran, 2005.

FIGURE 49
Factors associated with the prevalence of diabetes and IGT in urban areas

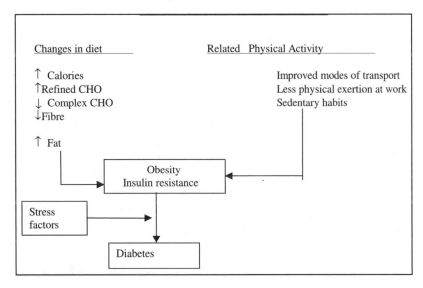

In 2000, the Diabetes Epidemiology Study group initiated a multicentre community-based study using the stratified random sampling method to assess the prevalence of diabetes and IGT in Bangalore, Chennai, Mumbai, Delhi, Kolkata and Hyderabad. The oral glucose tolerance test was carried out on 11 216 people (5 288 men and 5 928 women) aged 20 years and over in a representative sample drawn from all socio-economic strata. Information on socio-economic status, physical activity and anthropometric data were collected (National Urban Diabetes Survey, 2001). Age-standardized prevalence rates of diabetes and IGT are shown in Figure 50. Diabetes and IGT increase progressively with age (Figure 51), and subjects under 40 years of age have higher prevalence of IGT than diabetes (12.8 percent versus 4.6 percent, p < 0.0001). Diabetes is not usually listed as a predisposing cause of death in death certificates in India; data from hospital-based studies suggest that major causes of death in patients with diabetes are infections, renal failure, IHD and stroke.

Summary results of ICMR's estimates of the disease burden of diabetes in 1998 and 2004 are presented in Table 20. The number of cases increased from 58.35 million in 1998 to 66.58 million in 2004 (37.73 million in urban and 28.85 million in rural areas). By 2004, diabetes accounted for 100 000 deaths a year, and is responsible for 1.15 million years of life lost (YLLs) to disease and 2.26 million disability-adjusted life years (DALYs) (ICMR, 2004b)

FIGURE 50
Prevalence rates of diabetes and IGT in India's urban population

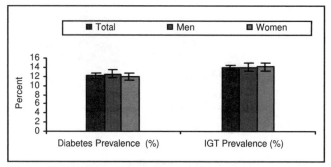

Source: National Urban Diabetes Survey, 2001.

FIGURE 51
Prevalence rates of type-2 diabetes and IGT in India's urban population

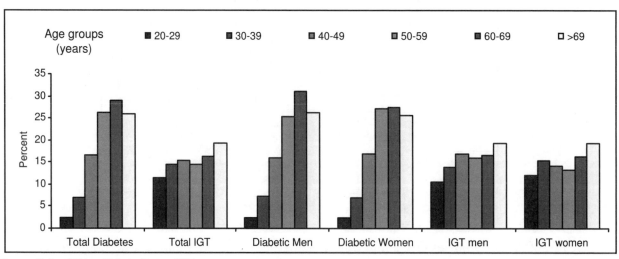

Source: National Urban Diabetes Survey, 2001.

TABLE 20
Projections of disease burden of diabetes, 1998 and 2004

	1998			2004		
	Urban	Rural	Total	Rural	Urban	Total
Population (thousands)	262 152	708 781	970 933	319 727	746 031	1 065 758
No. of cases of diabetes (thousands)	30 939	27 409	58 348	37 734	28 849	66 583
No. of deaths due to diabetes	51 251	44 299	95 550	62 506	46 627	109 133
No. of YLLs	529 959	484 983	1 014 942	646 351	510 471	1 156 822
No. of DALYs	1 016 866	971 890	1 988 756	1 240 195	1 022 968	2 263 163

Source: ICMR, 2004b.

A WHO burden of disease study carried out in 2000 estimated that 2.7 million DALYs are attributable to diabetes; ICMR estimates for 2004 correspond closely to this estimate (ICMR, 2004).

Hypertension

Hypertension is probably the most common NCD, and is the most common factor responsible for IHD and cerebrovascular accidents. In the early 1970s, the reported prevalence of hypertension was low, ranging from 2 to 5 percent of the adult population. However, over the years rates have increased and currently range from 5 to 15 percent in urban adults. Yagnik (1998) showed that some Indian people are prone to developing hypertension from early childhood. Gopinath *et al.* (1994) investigated 10 200 Delhi schoolchildren (5 709 males and 4 506 females) aged five to 14 years and showed that hypertension existed even among this age category. Prevalence of hypertension increases with age, BMI, parental history of hypertension, and diabetes. A community-based study of hypertension (systolic BP > 140 and diastolic BP more than 85) in 6 543 people aged 15 to 25 years in Delhi in 1985 to 1987 showed overall prevalence of hypertension was 3.9 per 1 000 population (Reddy, 1998; Table 21).

TABLE 21
Hypertension rates by age and gender (thousands)

Age (years)	Male			Female			Total		
	No. examined	Hyper-tensive	PR ± SE	No. examined	Hyper-tensive	PR ± SE	No. examined	Hyper-tensive	PR ± SE
15–19	1 744	47	26.9 ± 4.0	1 874	27	14.4 ± 3.7	3 618	74	20.5 ± 2.0
20–24	1 342	80	59.6 ± 8.2	1 583	48	30.3 ± 6.7	2 925	128	43.8 ± 6.6
Total	**3 086**	**127**	**41.2 ± 5.0**	**3 457**	**75**	**21.7 ± 4.0**	**6 543**	**202**	**30.9 ± 3.6**

Sample size: 6 543.
PR = prevalence rate per 1 000, SE = standard error.
Source: Gopinath *et al.,* 1994.

Results from some of the major community-based studies on hypertension over the last two decades are shown in Figures 52 and 53. There have been clear increases in prevalence of hypertension among men and women living in urban and rural areas. Prevalence is lower in rural than in urban areas.

ICMR undertook an assessment of the burden of disease of hypertension (systolic BP > 140 mmHg and/or diastolic BP > 90 mmHg), based on studies carried out between 1995 and 2002 in the urban and rural areas of different regions. Meta-analysis of the data indicated that prevalence of hypertension was 157.4 per thousand at the national level (ICMR, 2004b).

FIGURE 52
Prevalence of hypertension (SBP > 140/DBP > 90), 1959 to 2005

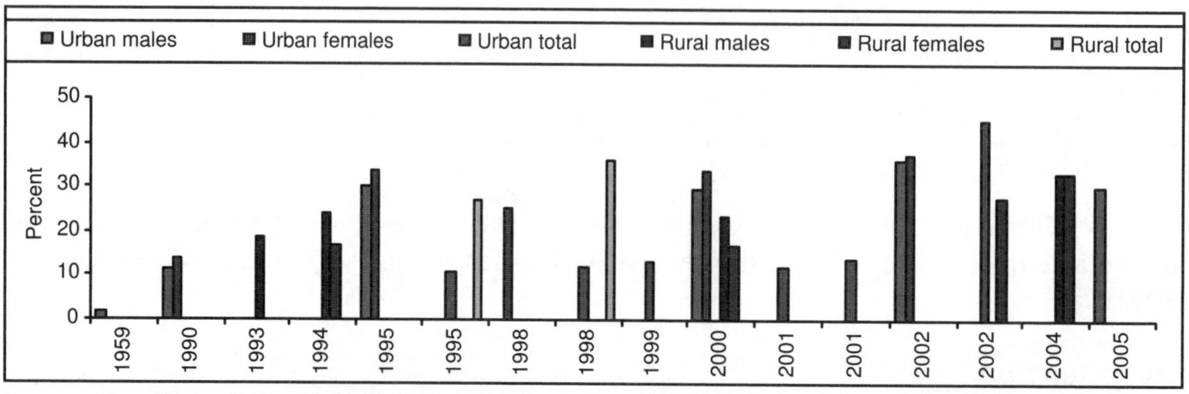

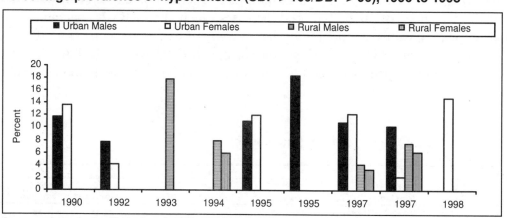

Sources and sample size: Padmavathy et al, 1959: 1642;Gopinath et al, 1990: 6372(Males), 7351 (Females); Kutty et al, 1993: 1130; (Females); Gupta et al., 1994: 1982 (rural males), 1166(rural females); Gupta et al, 1995: 1415 (males) 797(females); Gopinath etal.5998 (Urban males), 7136 (Urban females), 616 (Rural males), 1116 (Rural females), Singh et al, 1998: 3714; Chadha et al., 1998: 13134 (urban), 1982 (rural); Gupta et al.,2000: 1415(urban males), 797 (urban females), 1982 (rural males), 1166(rural females); Misra et al., 2001: 532; Mohan et al., 2001: 1175; Gupta et al., 2002: 550 (urban males), 573 (urban females); Ahlawat et al, 2002: 937; Reddy et al, 2002: 3307; Hazarika et al, 2004: 3180; Prabhakaran et al., 2005: 2122.

FIGURE 53
Percentage prevalence of hypertension (SBP > 160/DBP > 90), 1990 to 1998

Sources and sample size: Gopinath et al, 1990: 6372(Males), 7351 (Females); Kutty et al, 1993: 1130; (Females); Gupta et al., 1994: 1982 (rural males), 1166(rural females); Gupta et al, 1995: 1415 (males) 797(females); Gopinath etal.5998 (Urban males), 7136 (Urban females), 616 (Rural males), 1116 (Rural females), Singh et al, 1998: 3714.

Health consequences of hypertension

ICMR estimated the risk ratios for NCD that are associated with hypertension; 16 percent of IHD, 21 percent of peripheral vascular disease, 24 percent of acute myocardial infarctions and 29 percent of strokes can be attributed to hypertension (ICMR, 2004b). ICMR also computed the risks of NCDs that are attributable to diabetes and hypertension (Figure 54). Because hypertension and diabetes often coexist, the actual risk of various NCDs when both are present may be higher than the risk for either individually.

FIGURE 54
Risks of NCD that are attributable to diabetes and hypertension

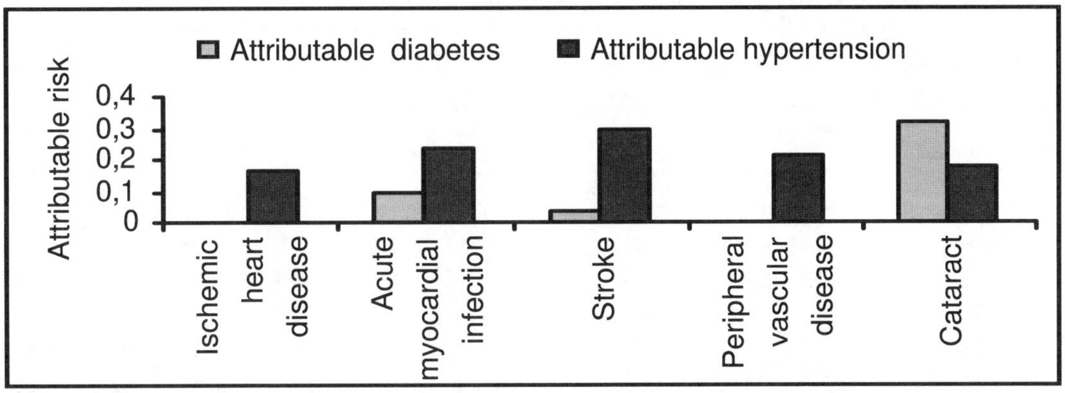

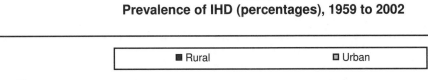

Source: ICMR, 2004b.

Ischaemic heart disease

IHD, also known as coronary artery disease, is becoming an important cause of death in India. The findings of some of the major studies on prevalence of IHD in urban and rural areas in different parts of India are shown in Figure 55. Over the last three decades, there has been a progressive increase in prevalence of IHD, particularly during the last decade, especially in urban areas. Most of this increase is attributed to lifestyle changes, which have affected people in urban areas more than rural ones (ICMR, 2004b). For the purpose of ICMR's meta-analysis of these studies, which were carried out during the 1990s, IHD was diagnosed on the basis of:

- history of documented angina or infarction and previously diagnosed CHD;
- affirmative response to the Rose questionnaire;
- electrocardiogram changes: Minnesota codes 1-1, 4-1, 5-9, 5-2 or 9-2.

FIGURE 55
Prevalence of IHD (percentages), 1959 to 2002

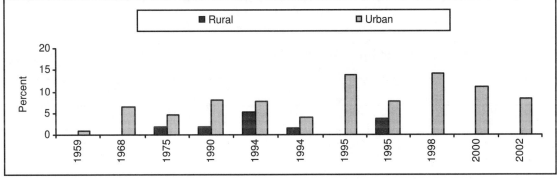

Age-specific prevalence rates of IHD among males and females were obtained by pooling the data of these five studies (separately for urban and rural areas), the results of which are given in Table 22. There is a steep increase in IHD prevalence in both sexes in the 40 to 50 years age group. Prevalence rates in women are similar to or higher than those in men.

TABLE 22
Age-specific prevalence derived from selected studies of IHD

Age group	Urban						Rural					
	Male			Female			Male			Female		
	Sample size	No. of cases	PR	Sample size	No. of cases	PR	Sample size	No. of cases	PR	Sample size	No. of cases	PR
20–24	125	1	8.0	147	1	6.8	285	5	17.5	191	2	10.5
25–29	1 374	27	19.6	1 677	44	26.2	512	7	13.7	624	9	14.4
30–34	1 584	27	17.1	2 091	48	22.9	888	11	12.4	1 302	14	10.8
35–39	1 459	63	43.2	1 796	87	48.4	1 011	19	18.8	1 376	22	15.9
40–44	1 418	67	47.3	1 549	102	65.8	836	15	17.9	1 033	24	23.2
45–49	1 093	91	83.2	1 234	130	105.4	724	15	20.7	954	37	38.8
50–54	1 053	98	93.1	1 162	130	111.9	675	21	31.11	722	36	49.9
55–59	985	160	162.4	1 054	161	152.8	937	25	26.7	825	42	50.9
60 +	835	145	173.6	941	165	175.4	591	42	71.1	519	35	67.4

PR = prevalence rate per thousand.
Source: ICMR, 2004b.

Indices of the burden of disease of IHD in India are presented in Table 23. Estimated prevalence rates are 64.4 per thousand in urban and 25.3 per thousand in rural populations. Projections of the burden of disease of IHD in India from 1998 to 2004 are given in Table 24. The number of IHD cases is estimated to have increased from 34.78 million in 1998 to about 39.43 million in 2004 (20.58 million in urban and 18.85 million in rural areas). In 2004 , the total number of DALYs attributable to IHD was estimated to be 16 million (ICMR, 2004b).

TABLE 23
Indices of disease burden of IHD

	Urban	Rural
Prevalence rate/1 000	64.4	25.3
Death rate/1 000	0.8	0.4
YLLs/100 000	728.7	351.5
DALYs/100 000	2 703.4	986.2

Source: ICMR, 2004b.

TABLE 24
Projections of disease burden of IHD, 1998 and 2004

	1998			2004		
	Urban	Rural	Total	Rural	Urban	Total
Population (thousands)	262 152	708 781	970 933	319 727	746 031	1 065 758
No. of cases of IHD	16 874 724	17 910 896	34 785 620	20 580 827	18 852 203	39 433 030
No. of deaths to IHD	207 548	256 014	463 562	255 782	298 412	554 194
No. of YLLs	1 991 451	2 470 149	4 461 600	2 329 851	2 622 299	4 952 150
No. of DALYs	7 388 453	6 930 974	14 319 427	8 643 450	7 357 358	16 000 808

Source: ICMR, 2004b.

It is often assumed that IHD affects mainly the well-to-do. However, several studies suggest that poor people are vulnerable to IHD. A community-based cross-sectional survey looked at the prevalence of CHD and coronary risk factors in Rajasthan by educational level in 3 148 residents over 20 years of age (1 982 men and 1 166 women) in three villages (Gupta, Gupta and Ahluwalia, 1994). The prevalence of CHD (diagnosed by electocardiography) showed an inverse relation with education in both sexes; prevalence of coronary risk factors such as smoking and hypertension were higher among the uneducated. NSSO (1975 to 2000) surveys have documented higher prevalence of tobacco use among the poorer segments of the population (Figure 56). Lack of physical exercise and stress are common among the urban poor in sedentary jobs. It is therefore not surprising that there is high prevalence of hypertension and IHD among this segment. Results of some of the studies carried out in Delhi show that prevalence of hypertension and IHD is high among poorer segments of the population in urban areas. Some data indicate that untreated/poorly controlled severe hypertension and IHD were higher among low-income groups, perhaps because of poor access to health care; data also indicate that mortality rates associated with IHD are higher among the poor (Srinath Reddy, personal communication). It is therefore important to recognize that not only the urban affluent are at risk of hypertension and IHD in India. Programmes aimed at lifestyle modifications for all segments of the population are of critical importance for preventing IHD. Facilities for screening to detect IHD and for managing those with the disease also have to be built up.

FIGURE 56
Prevalence of alcohol and tobacco use in India, by income quintale

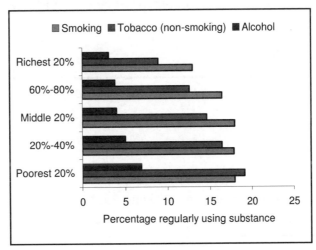

Source: NSSO, 1995/1996.

Stroke

WHO defines stroke as "rapidly developed clinical signs of focal disturbances of cerebral function, lasting more than 24 hours or leading to death, with no apparent cause other than vascular origin". The 24-hour threshold in the definition excludes transient ischaemic attacks. Stroke is the acute severe manifestation of cerebrovascular disease, and is one of the leading causes of mortality and morbidity in developed countries.

ICMR undertook a meta-analysis of stroke from well-designed studies with adequate sample sizes (Figure 57). The weighted average of stroke prevalence was 1.54 per thousand. Estimated prevalence of stroke is lower in India than in developed countries. However, it may increase proportionally with increasing longevity. The prevalence rates, stroke-specific mortality rates, case fatality rates, all-cause mortality rates and age distribution of population (1998) were inputs for a DISMOD analysis of stroke data.

FIGURE 57
Prevalence of stroke, 1985 to 2001

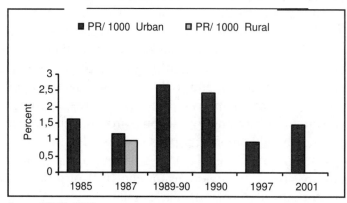

Source: ICMR, 2004b.

The YLLs to stroke are 496.3 per 100 000, and the DALYs 597.6 per 100 000 (Table 25).Projections of the burden of disease of stroke in India for 1998 to 2004 are given in Table 26. In 2004, the total number of stroke cases in India was expected to be 1.64 million and the total number of DALYs attributable to stroke 6.37 million.

TABLE 25
Indices of disease burden of stroke

Prevalence rate/1 000	**1.54**
Death rate/1 000	0.6
YLLs/100 000	496.3
DALYs/100 000	597.6

Source: ICMR, 2004b.

TABLE 26
Projections of disease burden of stroke, 1998 and 2004

	1998	**2004**
Population (thousands)	970 933	1 065 758
No. of cases of stroke	14 95 237	16 41 267
No. of deaths due to stroke	5 93 362	6 39 455
No. of YLLs	48 18 740	52 89 357
No. of DALYs	58 02 295	63 68 970

Source: ICMR, 2004b.

Cancers

NCRP estimates that there are about 700 000 new cases of cancer a year and about 2 million cases of cancer in the country (ICMR, 1990 to 2005). Age-adjusted cancer incidence in India varies from 91.9 to 120.9 per 100 000 in urban males and from 108.7 to 134.8 per 100 000 in urban females. The cumulative incidence rates in selected population-based cancer registries in India are given in Table 27. Over all, cancer incidence in India is among the lowest in the world. Incidences of cancers reported in the urban cancer registries are similar to cancer incidences among Indians in Singapore and are substantially lower than cancer rates reported in other countries. Cancer epidemiologists have been exploring the protective role of the Indian diet – with its high fibre, phytate and spices, including turmeric – in the observed low prevalence of malignancies in India. Cancers associated with tobacco use account for 36 to 55 percent of all of cancers in men and for 10 to 16 percent of those in women. Anti-tobacco education and reduction of tobacco use can result in further substantial reductions in cancer rates in India. Data on time trends in prevalence of cancers (all sites) from the six population-based cancer registries are shown in Figure 58. It is obvious that, unlike CVD and diabetes, there has not been any increase in overall cancer prevalence over time.

TABLE 27
Cumulative incidence rate, cumulative risk and possibility of developing cancer at all sites

Registry	Cumulative rate (%)		Cumulative risk (%)		Possibility of one in no. of persons developing cancer	
	Males	Females	Males	Rural	Males	Females
			0 to 64 years			
Bangalore	8.06	10.80	7.75	10.24	13	10
Barshi	4.05	5.04	3.97	4.91	25	20
Bhopal	10.49	10.80	9.96	10.24	10	10
Chennai	10.11	11.69	9.62	11.03	10	9
Delhi	10.45	12.21	9.92	11.49	10	9
Mumbai	9.37	11.17	8.94	10.57	11	9
			0 to 74 years			
Bangalore	11.08	13.39	10.49	12.53	10	8
Barshi	5.10	5.86	4.97	5.69	20	18
Bhopal	15.34	12.50	14.22	11.75	7	9
Chennai	13.19	14.35	12.35	13.37	8	7
Delhi	13.97	15.23	13.04	14.13	8	7
Mumbai	13.98	14.82	13.04	13.77	8	7

Source: ICMR, 1990 to 2005.

FIGURE 58
Trends in prevalence of cancer rates (per 100 000 population), 1990 to 1998

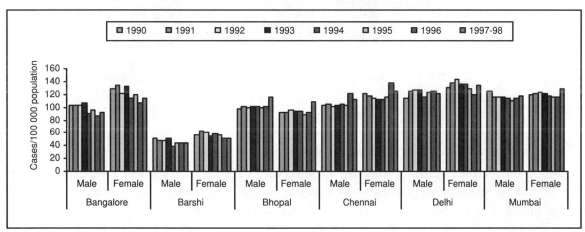

Source: ICMR, 1990 to 2005.

The Bombay cancer registry has population-based data on incidence of cancer from the 1960s to the present (Yeole, 2001). Analysis of time trends from the 1960s until 1999 confirms that although there have been massive changes in prevalence of some cancers (reductions in cervical cancer and increases in breast cancer) there has been no increase in overall prevalence of cancers over the last five decades.

ICMR estimates of the burden of disease of cancer (all sites), based on data from NCRP's population-based cancer registries, are given in Table 28. The number of cases of cancer in 2004 is expected to be 820 000, and the total number of DALYs due to cancer in India is estimated at 5.9 million. This estimate is low compared with the 8.6 million DALYs estimated in the WHO burden of disease study (2000) (Figure 59). To obtain cancer disease burden estimates, ICMR used mortality rates obtained by pooling the data of all six population-based registries. However, if the cancer mortality rates reported in the Chennai registry (which are the highest reported) are used, the figures become comparable to those in the WHO study.

TABLE 28
Projections of disease burden of cancer

	Male	Female
Population (thousands)	550 404	515 354
No. of cases	390 809	428 545
No. of deaths	138 622	121 192
No. of YLLs	13 96 508	16 17 787
No. of DALYs	25 48 392	33 48 444

Source: ICMR, 2004b.

FIGURE 59
WHO and ICMR estimates/projections of disease burden of cancer, 1990 to 2004

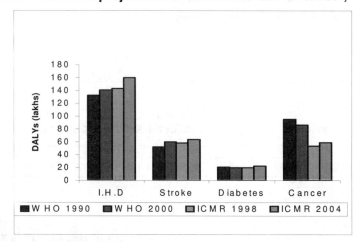

Source: ICMR, 2004b.

Tobacco as a risk factor for NCDs in India

Data on tobacco use in India from the fiftieth NSSO survey (NSSO, 1975 to 2000) are shown in Figure 60. Prevalence rates of tobacco use are highest among urban males, followed by rural males. The countrywide prevalence of tobacco use (rural and urban) is 35.5 percent.

The risk ratios associated with tobacco use in NCDs are presented in Figure 61; 15 percent of IHD cases, 48 percent of acute myocardial infarction (AMI) and 22 percent of strokes are attributable to tobacco use, which is also the major factor responsible for cancers of the lung, mouth and oesophagus. A strategy for controlling the use of tobacco would therefore result in significant reductions of these NCDs.

FIGURE 60
Use of tobacco in various forms

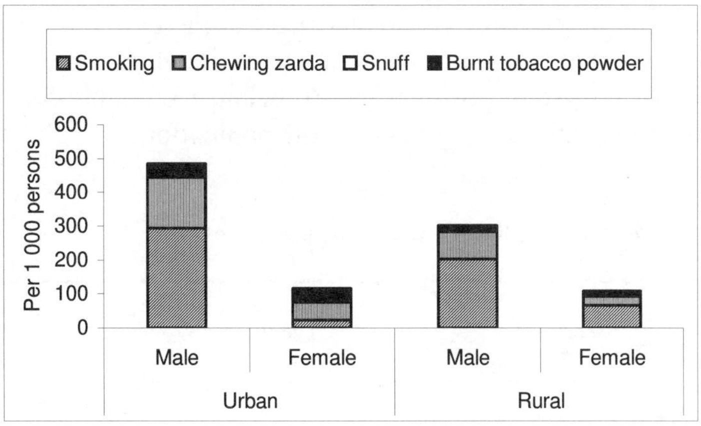

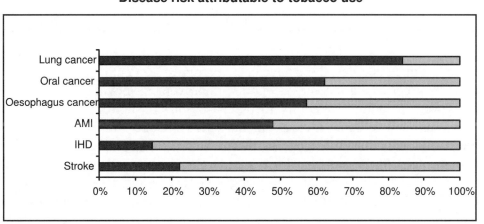

Source: ICMR, 2004b.

FIGURE 61
Disease risk attributable to tobacco use

Source: ICMR, 2004b.

FACTORS RESPONSIBLE FOR THE EMERGING PROBLEM OF OVERNUTRITION

Data presented in the section on food and nutrient intake indicate that over the last three decades there has not been any significant change in the energy intake of the Indian population, except in affluent families, especially in urban areas; even in this segment, however, most of the increase in consumption of energy-dense fast foods is among adolescents and youth. It is therefore obvious that increase in dietary intakes of fats, oils and sugar is not a major factor in overnutrition in India. Over this period, there has been a progressive reduction in physical activity in all segments of population. Reduction in energy expenditure and unchanged dietary intake results in a positive energy balance, and could be a major factor responsible for the rising prevalence of overnutrition in adults in India. Available evidence to support this is reviewed in this section.

Cross-sectional studies undertaken among affluent housewives aged 30 to 60 years in Delhi show that their dietary intake remained unaltered, at between 2 100 and 2 300 kcal/day (Wasuja and Siddhu, 2003). In each age group, energy expenditure is lower than intake by about 50 to 75 kcal/day. This is associated with a weight gain of about 5 kg per decade (Table 29). The women were not making any conscious effort to increase physical activity or take up regular exercise. It is possible that a similar situation exists among men in these segments of population. A small but persistent positive energy balance accounts for the slow but steady weight gain in adults among affluent segments of the population.

TABLE 29
Energy intake and expenditure in affluent urban housewives

Group	Weight (kg)	BMI (kg/m2)	% body fat	Total daily energy intake (kcal/day)	Total daily energy expenditure (kcal/day)	Energy balance (kcal)	Measured RMR (kcal/day)	PAR$_{RMR}$ (TDEE/ measured RMR)
D3 (30–39 yrs) [n = 22]	59	24.8	32.8	2 134	2 056 ± 238.7 (1 724.5 - 2 665.5)	+ 78	1 562 ± 260 (1 166 - 2 059)	1.33 ± 0.14 (1.12 - 1.59)
D4 (40–49 yrs) [n = 20]	64	26.4	36.5	2 264	2 191 ± 306.6 (1 785.4 - 2 817.3)	+ 73	1 779 ± 273 (1 267 - 2 304)	1.24 ± 0.10 (1.10 - 1.49)
D5 (50–59 yrs) [n = 20]	69	28.6	40.3	2 195	2 146 ± 173.1 (1 849.4 - 2 494.0)	+ 49	1752 ± 274 (1224 - 2203)	1.24 ± 0.12 (1.06 - 1.51)

Source: Wasuja and Siddhu, 2003.

During the last three decades, there have been a progressive decline in the poverty ratio and a steep increase in per capita income. Economic improvement inevitably results in improved purchasing power, including the ability to purchase and consume higher-value food items. This, in turn, can lead to some increase in the energy intake from fats, sugar and refined carbohydrates, and reductions in the energy intake from complex carbohydrates and in dietary fibre. Simultaneously, there has also been a reduction in physical activity and perhaps an increase in work-related stress because of changes in occupation. This combination of factors might be responsible for some of the rapid increase in overnutrition and hypertension in segments of the population that are emerging from poverty. It would also apply to rural migrants who settle in urban areas.

It is well documented that Indians have higher body fat per BMI compared with Caucasians. Prevalence of abdominal obesity is higher in India. Both overnutrition and abdominal obesity are associated with increased risks of hypertension, diabetes and CVD.

It is however important to remember that the seeds of obesity in adult life are often sown decades earlier. The thrifty gene hypothesis proposes that populations who have faced energy scarcity over millennia may have evolved so that the majority have the thrifty gene, which conserves energy. If energy intake of people with this gene obtain adequate or excess energy intake, they lay down fat, develop abdominal obesity and insulin resistance – which may progress to diabetes – and incur risk of hypertension and CVD. Barker's thrifty phenotype hypothesis puts the evolution of thriftiness into the intrauterine period; Indians with one-third low birth weight rate can be deemed to have acquired the risk of this metabolic syndrome before birth.

Yagnik and colleagues in Pune explored the relationship between low birth weight and glucose and insulin metabolism using the oral glucose tolerance test on 477 children born in KEM hospital, Pune (Yagnik, 1998). They found that Indian newborns weighed less because they had low muscle mass and small abdominal viscera. However, they also conserved their subcutaneous fat. At four years of age, plasma glucose and insulin concentrations 30 minutes after glucose administration were inversely related to birth weight (Table 30), and directly related to current weight and skin fold thickness. The relationship between glucose/insulin and birth weight was independent of current weight. Thus, poor intrauterine growth with relatively excess growth later was associated with metabolic endocrine abnormalities, which could lead to diabetes in adult life. Adolescent obesity is well-documented in both urban and rural areas and may be the stepping-stone to adult obesity.

TABLE 30
Birth weight, plasma glucose and insulin concentrations in four-year-old urban children

Birth weight (kg)	Number	Plasma glucose (mmol/l) at 30 min	Plasma insulin (pmol/l) at 30 min
=< 2.4	36	8.1	321
-2.6	36	8.3	337
-2.8	44	7.8	309
-3.0	42	7.9	298
=>3.0	43	7.5	289
All	201	7.9	310
P for trend		0.01	0.04

Source: Yagnik, 1998.

In a study in urban Delhi, Bhargava and colleagues found that low- and middle-income adults who were undernourished in infancy, childhood and adolescence were prone to develop overweight, abdominal obesity, hypertension and diabetes by the time they were 30 years of age (Bhargava *et al.,* 2004) (Tables 31 and 32).

TABLE 31
Trends in nutritional status of the Delhi cohort

	Male		Female	
Age	Number	Weight (kg)	Number	Weight (kg)
At birth	803	2.89 ± 0.44	561	2.79 ± 0.38
2 yrs	834	10.3 ± 1.3	609	9.8 ± 1.2
12 yrs	867	30.9 ± 5.9	625	32.2 ± 6.7
30 yrs	886	71.8 ± 14.0	640	59.2 ± 13.4

Source: Bhargava *et al.*, 2004.

TABLE 32
Current status of the Delhi cohort

Characteristic	Men		Women	
	Number	**Value**	**Number**	**Value**
Weight (kg)	886	71.8 ± 14.0	640	59.2 ± 13.4
Height (m)	886	1.70 ± 0.06	638	1.55 ± 0.06
BMI	886	24.9 ± 4.3	638	24.6 ± 5.1
Waist: hip ratio	886	0.92 ± 0.06	639	0.82 ± 0.07
BMI >= 25	886	47.4	638	45.5
BMI >= 23	886	66.0	638	61.8
Central obesity (%)	886	65.5	639	31
IGT test	849	16	539	14

Source: Bhargava *et al.*, 2004.

The lesson to be learned from these data is that it is never too early for Indians to start practising healthy lifestyle and dietary habits. Early detection and correction of undernutrition, until children attain appropriate weight-for-height is essential to promote linear growth. Adolescents and adults should ensure a balanced diet with no more than adequate energy intake. Exercise has to become part of the daily routine in order to promote muscle and bone health, as well as to prevent the development of adiposity in all age groups.

LINKAGES BETWEEN OVERNUTRITION AND NCDS
Overnutrition and diabetes
Studies from Chennai (Ramachandran, 2005) show that increasing BMI brings an increased risk of diabetes in both men and women, and a steep increase when BMI rises beyond 23 (Figure 62). There is a progressive increase in prevalence of diabetes with increasing waist-to-hip ratio (WHR) in both men and women (Figure 63). Indians have higher body fat per BMI than Caucasians (Figure 64). The associations between abdominal obesity and the metabolic syndrome of hypertension, dyslipedaemia, insulin resistance and diabetes have been well documented. Comparison of the insulin resistance and insulin response of Indians and United Kingdom citizens showed that both fasting and two-hour insulin levels are lower in Indians in rural areas and in Caucasians in the United Kingdom; urban Indians and Indians residing in the United Kingdom have substantially higher fasting and two-hour insulin levels, indicating insulin resistance (Figure 65). Data from the affluent urban population show that the prevalence of insulin resistance is high in children and young adults, as well as adults (Yagnik, 1998).

FIGURE 62
Risk for diabetes associated with increasing BMI

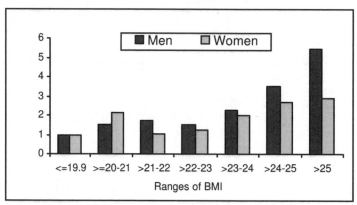

FIGURE 63
Diabetes and WHRs

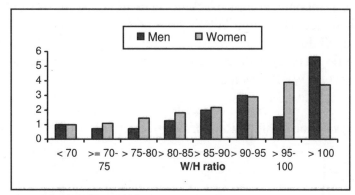

Source: Ramachandran, 2005.

FIGURE 64
Comparison of body fat (percentage) and BMI in Indians and Caucasians

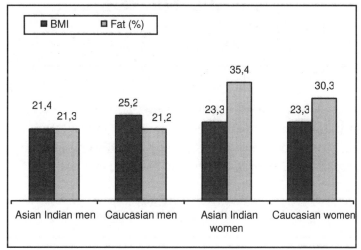

Source: Ramachandran, 2005.

FIGURE 65
Insulin resistance/serum insulin responses in Indians and Caucasians

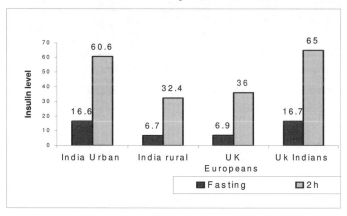

Source: Ramachandran, 2005.

Overnutrition and hypertension

NFI carried out studies to explore the relationships between overnutrition and hypertension in people from different income groups working at a government institution (NFI, 2004). A larger proportion of subjects had high WHR (50.3 percent) than BMI > 25 (30.8 percent). The higher the BMI and WHR, the higher were the prevalence rates of hypertension in both men and women (Figure 66). The prevalence of high blood pressure in the normal and overweight subjects was higher when WHR was high.

FIGURE 66
Prevalence of high blood pressure by income group and BMI

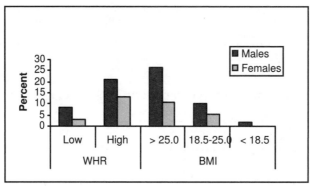

Source: NFI, 2004.

Serum cholesterol and triglycerides in men were significantly higher in subjects with BMI > 25, and increased significantly with increasing BMI and WHR in both men and women (Figures 67 and 68). Most cholesterol levels greater than 180 mg percent and most blood sugar levels of 140 mg percent were seen in subjects with high BMI and WHR.

FIGURE 67
Effect of BMI on biochemical parameters

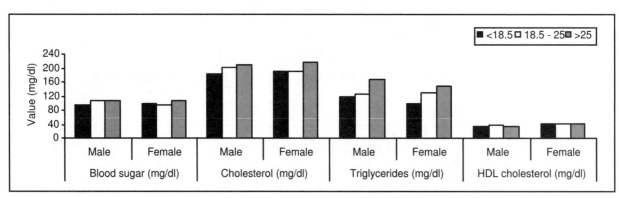

Source: NFI, 2004.

FIGURE 68
Effect of WHR on biochemical parameters

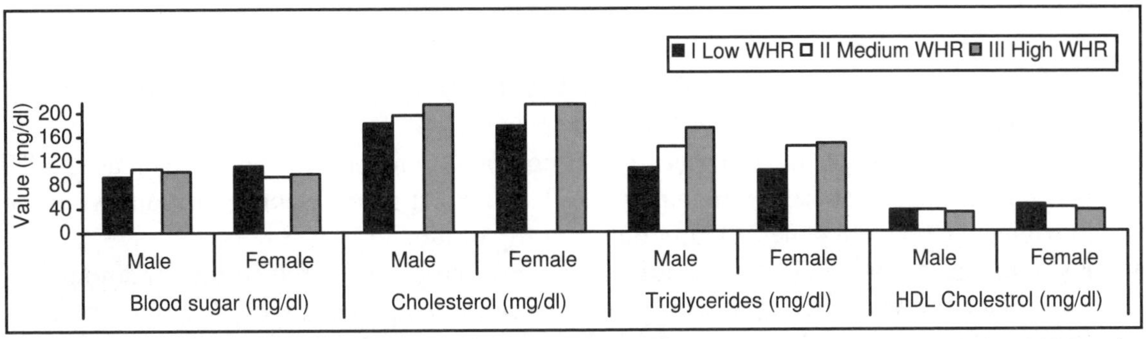

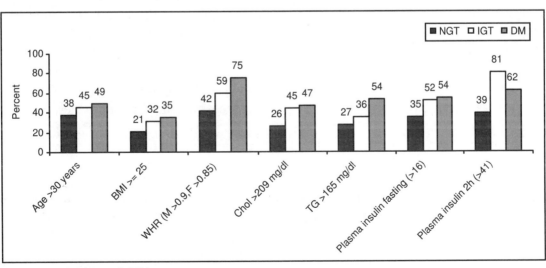

Source: NFI, 2004. WHR I Males < 0.93, Females < 0.81; WHR II Males 0.93-1.00, Females 0.81-0.89; WHR III Males >1.00, Females >0.89.

Linkages between obesity and diabetes and CVD

The susceptibility of urban Indians to central adiposity has been highlighted in all studies. All studies in India show that central obesity is more strongly associated with glucose intolerance than generalized obesity is. A cluster of risk factors have been demonstrated to be associated with central obesity. These include glucose intolerance, general obesity, hyperinsulinaemia, hypertriglyceridaemia and hypertension, all of which are important risk factors for IHD. Recent studies comparing body fat topography in migrant Asians with that of Caucasians have also reported a higher WHR, with hyperglycaemia, elevated plasma insulin concentrations, altered blood lipids and increased risk of coronary heart disease in Indians.

Indians are at higher risk of metabolic syndrome, with type-2, diabetes, dyslipedaemia, hypertension and CVD (Ramachandran, Snehlata and Vijay, 2004). Data from Chennai provide information on glucose tolerance and different CVD risk factors (Figure 69). These data indicate that the risk of glucose intolerance and diabetes increases with age, BMI, WHR, blood cholesterol (> 209 mg/dl) and triglyceride level (> 165 mg/dl). Cardiovascular risk is lowest in people with normal glucose tolerance and highest in those with diabetes.

FIGURE 69
Glucose intolerance and CVD risk factors

Source: Ramachandran *et al.*, 2004.

Comparison of newly diagnosed non-insulin-dependent diabetes mellitus patients at KEM hospital, Pune with migrant Indian and Caucasian patients in the United Kingdom showed the following:

- Diabetic patients in India are about a decade younger at diagnosis (20 percent are under 35 and 50 percent under 40 years of age).
- Obesity (using BMI as the criterion) is less common, but central obesity (increased WHR) is a very striking feature in Indian patients. The highest glucose concentrations were found in subjects who were generally thin but centrally obese.
- Hypercholesterolaemia is uncommon (5 percent), but plasma triglycerides and non-esterified fatty acids are significantly elevated in Indian patients with IGT or diabetes compared with those who have normal glucose tolerance (NGT).
- Both IGT and diabetic patients show higher fasting hyperinsulinaemia than NGT subjects do, but post-glucose plasma immunoreactive insulin (IRI) concentrations are diminished in diabetic patients. Plasma IRI concentrations show an inverted U-shaped distribution in relation to plasma glucose concentration, suggesting that insulin resistance and compensatory hyperinsulinaemia precede diabetes. Even NGT Indians are substantially more hyperinsulinaemic and insulin-resistant than Caucasians.

In Indians the cardiovascular risk factors (obesity, central obesity, hypertension, high plasma triglycerides and elevated non-esterified fatty acids) are increased in diabetic patients and also in those with IGT, a condition that precedes diabetes by many years. Electrocardiographic changes suggestive of IHD were associated with older age, higher blood pressure, higher plasma triglycerides and immunoreactive insulin concentrations. Cardiovascular risk factors were all related to plasma insulin levels and seem to occur as part of the complex metabolic profile called the insulin resistance syndrome, the metabolic syndrome or Syndrome X.

NATIONAL NUTRITION POLICY AND PLAN OF ACTION: THE RESPONSE TO NUTRITION TRANSITION

In 1950, India faced two major nutritional problems. One was the threat of famine and the resultant acute starvation caused by low agricultural production and the lack of an appropriate food distribution system. The other was chronic energy deficiency caused by:

- low dietary intake because of poverty and low purchasing power;
- high prevalence of infection because of poor access to safe drinking-water, sanitation and health care;
- poor utilization of available facilities because of low literacy and lack of awareness.

The country adopted a multisectoral, multipronged strategy to combat these problems and improve the nutritional status of the population (Box 5). Successive five-year plans laid down the policies and strategies for achieving these goals.

Box 5. Initiatives to improve the nutritional status of the population, 1950 to 1990

- Increasing food production: building buffer stocks.
- Improving food distribution: building up the public distribution system (PDS).
- Improving household food security through:
- improving purchasing power;
- food-for-work programmes;
- direct or indirect food subsidies.
- Food supplementation to address the special needs of vulnerable groups, the Integrated Child Development Services (ICDS) and midday meals.
- Nutrition education, especially through the Food and Nutrition Board (FNB) and ICDS.
- Efforts of the health sector to tackle:
- adverse health consequences of undernutrition;
- adverse effects of infection and unwanted fertility on nutritional status;
- micronutrient deficiencies and their health consequences.

Source: Planning Commission, 2002.

Progress achieved in seven five-year plans was reviewed in 1991/1992. It was obvious that the threat of famine has disappeared and there has been a significant decline in severe forms of undernutrition. However, mild and moderate undernutrition and micronutrient deficiencies were widespread. India prepared and adopted the National Nutrition Policy in 1993 (DWCD, · 1993). This policy advocated a comprehensive intersectoral strategy involving 14 sectors (which directly or indirectly affect the dietary intake and nutritional status of the population) in combating the multifaceted problem of undernutrition and improving the nutritional status of all sections of society. The policy sought to strike a balance between short-term direct nutrition interventions and long-term institutional/structural changes to create an enabling environment and the necessary conditions for improving nutritional and health status. It also set goals to be achieved in each sector by 2000. A National Plan of Action (DWDC, 1995) was drawn up and approved in 1995. In order to achieve intersectoral coordination at the highest level, a National Nutrition Council was formed with the Prime Minister as chairperson and the Planning Commission as the Secretariat. The council was to act as the national forum for policy and strategy formulation, review performance and suggest mid-course corrections. A similar set-up was envisaged for the state level. An interdepartmental coordination committee under the Department of Women and Child Development (DWCD) was to coordinate and review the implementation of nutrition programmes.

Review of the situation in 2000/2001 prior to formulation of the Tenth Five-Year Plan (Planning Commission, 2002) showed that although undernutrition and micronutrient deficiencies continue to be major public health problems, overnutrition and obesity are also emerging as a major problem in many states. In response to this, the Tenth Five-Year Plan envisaged a paradigm shift:

- from household food security and freedom from hunger to nutrition security for the family and the individual;
- from untargeted food supplementation to screening of all the people in vulnerable groups, identification of those with various grades of undernutrition and appropriate management;
- from ad hoc unfocused interventions addressing the prevention of overnutrition to the promotion of appropriate lifestyles and dietary intakes for the prevention and management of overnutrition and obesity.

The plan gave high priority to the effective implementation of focused and comprehensive interventions aimed at improving the nutritional and health status of individuals. It was emphasized that the increased outlays to combat the dual nutrition burden should result in improved outcomes and outputs in terms of reducing both under- and overnutrition. In view of the massive interstate differences, the Tenth Five-Year Plan laid down state-specific goals based on the current nutritional status and investment provided for the sector in the state plan. The national goals conform to the Millennium Development Goals and, although ambitious, may be achievable through improved coverage, quality and content of nutrition-related services.

SUMMARY AND CONCLUSIONS

Data suggest that there has not been much change in the predominantly cereal-based dietary intake in India over the last three decades, except among affluent segments of the population. In spite of increasing per capita income and reduced poverty, dietary diversity is seen mainly among the affluent. Undernutrition rates remain high; starting before birth, they are aggravated throughout infancy by poor infant feeding practices and perpetuated in childhood by poor intra-family distribution of food and poor access to health care. There has been a substantial reduction in severe undernutrition, most of which is due to improved access to health care. India can achieve substantial improvement in nutritional status through health and nutrition education and improved access to health and nutrition services.

Prevention of intrauterine growth retardation through antenatal care, and early detection and correction of undernutrition so that children attain appropriate weight for height are essential to promoting linear growth; they can be achieved through the effective implementation of ongoing intervention programmes utilizing the available infrastructure.

Low intakes of vegetables and fruit, poor bioavailability of iron and limited use of iodized salt are responsible for micronutrient deficiencies' being major public health problems even today. Dietary diversification, better coverage under the national anaemia control programme, massive-dose vitamin A administration and universal access to iodized, and later iron and iodine-fortified, salt are some of the interventions that could help the country to achieve rapid reductions in micronutrient deficiencies.

Over the last decade, there has been a progressive increase in overnutrition. Reduced physical activity is the major factor behind this. In affluent urban segments, increased energy intake from fats, refined cereals and sugar, combined with simultaneous reductions in physical activity have contributed to steep increases in overnutrition in all age groups. Nutrition education on healthy dietary patterns containing plenty of fruit and vegetables, maintenance of energy balance through regulation of dietary intake, and increasing energy expenditure through physical activity as part of the daily routine will promote muscle and bone health and prevent the development of adiposity in all age groups. Such information can be passed on to large segments of the urban upper- and middle-income groups through the media (television, Internet) that this segment has access to.

Indians appear to have a predisposition for adiposity – especially abdominal – insulin resistance and diabetes, hyper-triglyceridaemia and CVD. This predisposition could be genetic or environmental, and can manifest itself at birth, in childhood, during adolescence and in adult life. It is never too early for Indians to start practising healthy lifestyle and dietary habits.

It therefore seems that India could combat the dual nutrition burden through efficient implementation of time-tested, effective and inexpensive interventions to achieve significant reductions in both over- and undernutrition and their adverse health consequences within the next two decades.

REFERENCES

Bhargava, S.K., Sachdev, H.P., Fall, H.D., Osmond, C., Lakshmy, R., Barker, D.J.P., Biswas, S.K.D., Ramji, S., Prabhakaran, D. & Reddy, K.S. 2004. Relation of serial changes in childhood body mass index to impaired glucose tolerance in young adulthood. *New Eng. J. Med.,* 350: 865–875.

Department of Education. 2002. *Selected educational statistics 2000–01.* New Delhi, Government of India.

DWCD. 1993. *National Nutritional Policy.* Government of India, New Delhi, Department of Women and Child Development (DWCD).

DWCD. 1995/1996. *Indian Nutrition Profile.* Government of India, New Delhi.

Gopinath, N., Chadha, S.L., Sood, A.K., Shekhawat, S., Bindra, S.P.S. & Tandon, R. 1994. Epidemiological study of hypertension in young (15 to 24 years) Delhi urban population. *Ind. J. Med. Res.,* 99: 32–37.

Government of India. 2003. *Economic Survey of India 2003–04.* New Delhi.

Gupta, R., Gupta, V.P. & Ahluwalia, N.S. 1994. Educational status, coronary heart disease, and coronary risk factor prevalence in a rural population of India. *Br. Med. J.,* 309: 1332–1336.

ICMR. 1989. *Nutrient requirements and recommended dietary allowances for Indians.* New Delhi.

ICMR. 1990 to 2005. *Reports of the National Cancer Registry Programme 1990 to 2005.* New Delhi, Indian Council of Medical Research (ICMR).

ICMR. 2004a. *Micronutrient profile of Indian population.* New Delhi.

ICMR. 2004b. *Assessment of burden of non-communicable diseases.* New Delhi.

IIPS. 1992/1993. *National Family Health Survey 1.* International Institute of Population Sciences (IIPS). Mumbai.

IIPS. 1998/1999. *National Family Health Survey 2.* Mumbai.

Ministry of Agriculture. 2000. *National Agriculture Policy.* New Delhi, Government of India.

Ministry of Agriculture. 2002a. *Agriculture statistics at a glance 2002.* New Delhi, Government of India.

Ministry of Agriculture. 2002b. *Report of Department of Economics and Statistics 2002.* New Delhi, Government of India.

Ministry of Family and Health Welfare. 1998/1999. *Reproductive and Child Health 1.* New Delhi, Government of India.

Ministry of Family and Health Welfare. 2002. *Reproductive and Child Health 2.* New Delhi, Government of India.

Ministry of Family and Health Welfare. 2002/2003. *District-Level Household Survey.* New Delhi, Government of India.

Ministry of Family and Health Welfare. 2004. *District-Level Household Survey 2002–03.* New Delhi, Government of India.

National Urban Diabetes Survey. 2001. *Diabetologia.,* 44(9): 1094–1101.

NFI. 2004. *Twenty-Five Years Report 1980 to 2005.* New Delhi, Nutrition Foundation of India (NFI).

NIN. 2004. *Nutritive value of Indian foods.* Hyderabad, National Institute of Nutrition (NIN).

NNMB. 1979 to 2002. *NNMB reports.* Hyderabad, National Nutrition Monitoring Bureau (NNMB), National Institute of Nutrition.

NNMB. 2000. *NNMB report.* Hyderabad, National Institute of Nutrition.

NNMB. 2001. *NNMB report.* Hyderabad, National Institute of Nutrition.

NNMB. 2002. *NNMB micronutrient survey.* Hyderabad, National Institute of Nutrition.

NSSO. 1975 to 2000. *Reports of NSSO.* New Delhi, National Sample Survey Organization (NSSO), Department of Statistics, Government of India.

Planning Commission. 2002. *Tenth Five-Year Plan.* New Delhi, Government of India.

Planning Commission. 2004. *Annual Plan 2003–04.* New Delhi, Government of India.

Ramachandran, A. 2005. Epidemiology of diabetes in India – three decades of research. *J. Assoc. Phy. India,* 53: 34–38.

Ramachandran, A., Snehlata, C. & Vijay, V. 2004. Low risk threshold for acquired diabetogenic factors in Asian Indians. *Diab. Res. Clin. Prac.,* 65: 189–195.

Ramachandran, P. 1989. Nutrition in pregnancy. *In* C. Gopalan and Suminder Kaur, eds. *Women and nutrition in India.* Special Publication No. 5. New Delhi, NFI.

Reddy, K.S. 1998. The emerging epidemiology of cardiovascular diseases in India. *In* P. Shetty and C. Gopalan, eds. *Diet, nutrition and chronic disease: An Asian perspective,* pp. 50–54. London, Smith-Gordon and Co.

RGI. 1951 to 2001. *Report of census 1951–2001.* New Delhi, Registrar General of India (RGI).

RGI. 1971 to 2000. *Reports of sample registration system.* New Delhi.

RGI. 1996. *Population projections 1996–2016.* New Delhi.

RGI. 2002. *Bulletin of sample registration system.* New Delhi.

Salt Department. 2003/2004. *Annual Reports – 2003–04.* New Delhi, Government of India.

UNDP. 2003. *Human Development Report.* New York, United Nations Development Programme (UNDP).

Wasuja, M. & Siddhu, A. 2003. *Decade-wise alterations in energy expenditure and energy status of affluent women (30 to 88 years) – A cross-sectional study.* New Delhi, Delhi University. (Ph.D. thesis)

World Bank. 1993. *World Development Report.* New York.

Yagnik, C.S. 1998. Diabetes in Indians: small at birth or big as adults or both? *In* P. Shetty and C. Gopalan, eds. *Diet, nutrition and chronic disease: An Asian perspective,* pp. 43–46. London, Smith-Gordon and Co.

Yeole. 2001. *Cancer in India in 2001.* (Ph.D. thesis)

Food consumption, food expenditure, anthropometric status and nutrition-related diseases in Mexico

S. Barquera, C. Hotz, J. Rivera, L. Tolentino, J. Espinoza, I.Campos and T. Shamah, National Institute of Public Health, Cuernavaca, Mexico

INTRODUCTION

Mexico, as are other Latin American countries, is experiencing an epidemiological and nutrition transition characterized by a rapid rise in the prevalence of obesity and chronic diseases such as diabetes mellitus, high blood pressure and cardiovascular diseases (CVDs) (Flores *et al.,* 1998; Rivera-Dommarco *et al.,* 2001). Although the morbidity and mortality related to acute communicable diseases, such as diarrhoeas and respiratory infections, undernutrition and some micronutrient deficiencies, have shown important reductions during the last three decades, different forms of undernutrition, such as child stunting and anaemia, remain relevant public health problems.

Mexico's gross national product (GNP) per capita increased by 62 percent between 1970 and 2003. This change is greater than that observed for the Latin America and the Caribbean (LAC) region as a whole (43 percent) (Figure 1a). Currently, 75 percent of the population live in urban locations. The percentage of population living in rural locations decreased by 39 percent in the 1970 to 2003 period (Figure 1b). During recent decades, health status has been affected by environmental and economic conditions. Child mortality has decreased by 74.5 percent in 33 years, which is similar to the LAC regional average (Figure 1c) but three times greater than the rate observed for other Organisation for Economic Co-operation and Development (OECD) countries during the same period. In Mexico, health expenditure as a percentage of GNP was lower than the average for Latin American countries during the 1998 to 2002 period.

Currently, Mexico has more than 100 million inhabitants. As one of the world's mega-countries, implementation of social policies is complex, and the expected impact difficult to measure (Barquera, Rivera-Dommarco and Gasca-Garcia, 2001). Although Mexico has been developing food and nutrition programmes since the early twentieth century and has devoted more resources to these programmes than any other Latin American country (Rivera-Dommarco *et al.,* 2001; Rivera *et al.,* 2004b), until recently social policies were not evaluated (Barquera, Rivera-Dommarco and Gasca-Garcia, 2001; Ministry of Social Development, 2000). Food and nutrition programmes in the last eight years have improved their targeting and have incorporated objectives related to improving nutritional status and education. It is expected that these improved programmes will have positive impacts on nutrition and health. Conversely, consumer access to industrialized foods has increased in recent years owing to technological developments and economic growth.

FIGURE 1
Development indicators in Mexico, Latin America and the Caribbean

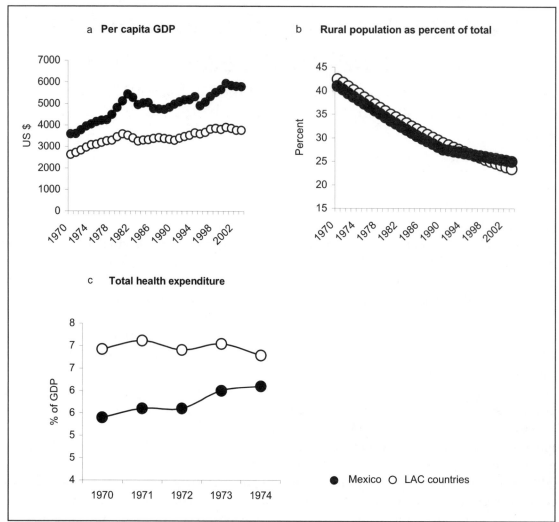

Mexico is also characterized by major epidemiological differences across country regions, urban/rural residence and socio-economic status. Imbedded in these differences is the *polarization* of the transition, which means that different subpopulations within the country are undergoing different stages of transition. In Mexico, polarization has been described across four regions (Bobadilla *et al.,* 1993; Hernandez-Diaz *et al.,* 1999; Rivera-Dommarco *et al.,* 2001). The *North region* is the most industrialized. It has a higher per capita income and infrastructure level than the rest of the country, close cultural and economic relations with the border states of the United States and adequate access to basic and health services. The *Central region* is less developed than the North, but still contains large developed cities such as Guadalajara and many rural towns that live from agriculture. *Mexico City* is the third most populated city in the world. It has a very developed economy and access to food and basic services, combined with high immigration from the south and poverty pockets. It also receives several subsidies and social programmes targeting the poor. The *South region* is considered the least developed. It has the largest rural and indigenous population in the country, and access to certain basic services and subsidies is limited; in this region health problems such as infectious diseases and undernutrition still represent a relevant public health concern. While the health sector in all of these regions is still facing the challenge of preventing and treating acute diseases (Frenk *et al.,* 1991), non-communicable chronic diseases such as diabetes and hypertension are rapidly increasing.

In order to address this complex situation, it will be important to understand how nutrition and related health conditions have evolved together over the last decades in the context of social, economic and market changes. The following subsections document the main characteristics of the epidemiologic and nutrition transition in Mexico, including nutrient intake, trends in food expenditure, nutritional status, prevalence of obesity and chronic diseases and mortality trends, with emphasis on polarization among the different regions of the country, between urban and rural populations and among socio-economic groups. The information is used to discuss the double burden of disease and the role of current and future national programmes in addressing emerging health challenges.

METHODS

The analysis in this case study is based on diverse nationwide databases generated from surveys collected mostly by the National Institute of Public Health and from other cross-sectional surveys and registries collected by diverse governmental agencies (Table 1). Variables and measurements were stratified by region, urban/rural residence and socio-economic status, when possible. The case study team also analysed trends over time for variables such as nutrient intake in women, household food expenditure, prevalence of chronic diseases and mortality.

TABLE 1
Socio-demographic and health surveys used in this report

Survey name and year	Agency	Description
Mexican Nutrition Survey I (MNS–1), 1988	Ministry of Health	Women 12 to 45 years and children < 5 years Representative of the country, four regions and urban/rural locations n = 7 426 children, and 9 449 women
Mexican Nutrition Survey 2 (MNS–2), 1999	National Institute of Public Health	Children < 12 years, and women 12 to 45 years Representative of the country, four regions and urban/rural locations n = 3 521 children, and 2 596 women
Mexican Chronic Diseases Survey (MCDS), 1994	Ministry of Health	Adults 20 to 69 years Representative of urban locations of the country and four regions n = 2 125
Mexican Health Survey (MHS), 2000	National Institute of Public Health	Adults > 19 years Representative of the country, states, regions and urban/rural locations n = 45 294
Mexican Household Income and Expenditure Surveys (MHIES), 1989 to 2002	National Institute of Informatics, Statistics and Geography (INEGI)	Representative of the country, states, regions and urban/rural locations n = 11 531 in 1989, 10 508 in 1992, 12 815 in 1994, 14 042 in 1996, 10 952 in 1998, 10 089 in 2000, 17 167 in 2002
National Mortality Register, 1980 to 2000	INEGI	All reported mortality from 1980 to 2000

Country regions

The country was divided into four regions with common geographic and socio-economic characteristics: 1) North region, which comprises Baja California, Southern Baja California, Coahuila, Durango, Nuevo Leon, Sonora, Sinaloa, Tamaulipas and Zacatecas; 2) Central region, which comprises Aguascalientes, Colima, Guanajuato, Hidalgo, Jalisco, Mexico, Michoacan, Nayarit, Querétaro, San Luis Potosí and Tlaxcala; 3) Mexico City; and 4) South region, which comprises Campeche, Chiapas, Guerrero, Morelos, Oaxaca, Puebla, Quintana Roo, Tabasco, Veracruz and Yucatan. This regionalization scheme was used in epidemiologic transition analysis for intra-country comparisons (Hernandez-Diaz *et al.,* 1999; Rivera *et al.,* 2002; Sepulveda-Amor *et al.,* 1990).

Place of residence

In addition, subjects were classified as urban or rural according to the population size of their place of residence. For variables obtained from the Mexican Nutrition Survey (MNS), these classifications were ≥ 2 500 inhabitants for urban areas and < 2 500 inhabitants for rural ones, while for variables obtained from the Mexican Health Survey (MHS) and the Mexican Household Income and Expenditure Survey (MHIES) the corresponding figures were ≥ 15 000 inhabitants and < 15 000 inhabitants.

Socio-economic status index

MNS–1 (1988) and MNS–2 (1999) obtained socio-economic information such as household conditions, basic services infrastructure (i.e., water source and disposal) and possession of domestic appliances (i.e., radio, television and refrigerator). A principal components factor analysis was carried out using this information to extract a main factor that explained more than 50 percent of the socio-economic information variability (Flores *et al.,* 1998; Long-Dunlap *et al.* 1995). This factor was divided into quintiles and used as a relative measure of socio-economic status.

Nutrient and dietary information

Nutrient intake information for Mexico was obtained from MNS–1 and MNS–2, which are two nationwide representative surveys with sufficient sampling power to allow data to be disaggregated by region and urban/rural location. Detailed descriptions of the survey sampling procedures and methods have been published elsewhere (Resano-Perez *et al.,* 2003; Rivera-Dommarco *et al.,* 2001; Sepulveda-Amor *et al.,* 1990). Food and nutrient intake information was available for females aged 12 to 49 years and for children aged one to 11 years in 1999. These surveys also had anthropometric information for women aged 12 to 49 years and for children under five years of age.

A 24-hour dietary recall (24HDR) was administered to obtain dietary information for randomly selected sub-samples of 9 449 (MNS–2) and 2 596 (MNS–1) women. Trained and standardized personnel applied the questionnaires and converted consumption into grams or millilitres of food items. For MNS–2, aberrant food consumption was reviewed by hand and updated when a clear mistake was detected, or eliminated if the value was not biologically plausible. Complete food intake data were not available from MNS–1, but a database with estimated nutrient intake generated from 24HDR was obtained and used for the analysis. Nutrient intakes were then estimated for foods, using a comprehensive nutrient composition database compiled from several sources (Muñoz *et al.,* 1996; Souci, Fachmann and Kraut, 2000; USDA/ARS, 1999; Wuleung and Flores, 1962). Nutrient adequacies were calculated relative to the dietary reference intakes (Institute of Medicine, 2000a; 2000b; 2001; 2002; National Research Council, 1989); the estimated average requirement was used for protein, vitamins A and B12, folic acid, iron and zinc; the adequate intake was used for calcium and vitamin D; and the estimated energy requirement was used for energy. A cut-off of 30 percent of total energy intake was considered fat adequacy. Requirements were adjusted for pregnant and lactating women. To estimate intake by food groups, grams consumed were aggregated into selected groups and reported as mean consumption, stratified by region, location and socio-economic index tertile.

Estimation of household adult equivalent

To estimate household food expenditure using MHIES, the individual adult equivalent (AE) was obtained by dividing the recommended dietary allowance (RDA) for energy of each household member – according to age and sex – by the energy RDA for an average adult. The sum of all of the individual AEs within a household was then computed to obtain the number of household AEs. Family members not currently living in the house were excluded from this estimation, but their income contribution was included in the total household income.

Quantity of food purchased per AE

Household food quantities purchased per AE were used as a proxy for food intake. Data from seven MHIES conducted between 1989 and 2002 were used. These surveys were collected by the National Institute of Geography, Informatics and Statistics. They contain nationally representative information on approximately 15 000 households and their members. Information was available for 1989, 1992, 1994, 1996, 1998, 2000 and 2002. A questionnaire based on a seven-day diary record of house purchases and containing about 215 foods was included in each MHIES, with slight variations in some years. A database with the quantities of each food purchased per household was developed. All foods were converted into grams, and food group quantities were estimated for cereals, meats, eggs, milk and dairy products, legumes, fats and oils, vegetables, fruits, and sugars. In addition, soda, alcohol and tobacco were converted into millilitres and grams and included in the final tables. From this database, the following indicators were obtained: 1) percentage of families purchasing each food group during the seven-day survey period; 2) percentage of total food expenditure allocated to each food group; 3) mean g/day per AE in families reporting expenditure on that item; and 4) per capita mean g/day per AE. The data were stratified by region, urban/rural residence and income quintile (only the extreme income quintiles are presented in this case study).

Percentage of food expenditure outside the home

In addition to food expenditure at home, MHIES also reported expenditure on food outside the home. It was therefore possible to calculate food expenditure outside the home as a percentage of total food expenditure per AE. This expenditure was not disaggregated according to food item.

Breastfeeding characteristics in Mexico

The information on breastfeeding practices in Mexico in this case study is based on a previous analysis of MNS–2 (González-Cossío *et al.*, 2003).

Children's nutritional status

Nutritional status derived from anthropometric indicators was available for children under five years of age from MNS–1 and MNS–2. In addition, MNS–2 collected information for children of five to 12 years of age. Using weight, height (or length) and age, the case study team calculated height-for-age, weight-for-height and weight-for-age Z-scores relative to the National Center for Health Statistics/World Health Organization (NCHS/WHO) reference population (HAZ, WAZ and WHZ, respectively) (WHO, 1983; 1995). Underweight was defined as WAZ < -2, stunting as HAZ < -2, wasting as WHZ < -2 and overweight as WAZ > +2. For school-age children, MNS–2 used two different criteria of classification for overweight (Cole *et al.*, 2000; Must, Dallal and Dietz, 1999).

Adult nutritional status and chronic disease prevalence

Adult nutritional status and prevalence rates of chronic diseases were obtained from two representative national surveys: the Mexican Chronic Diseases Survey (MCDS, 1994) and MHS (2000) (Olaiz, Rojas and Barquera, 2003). MCDS was implemented in four urban areas of Mexico and is representative of the country's urban locations. MHS was implemented in urban and rural locations with sample power to be representative of each state. In this survey, the rural population was defined as those living in locations with < 15 000 inhabitants. Prevalence rates of low weight (body mass index [BMI] < 18.5 kg/m^2), normal weight (BMI 18.5 to 24.9 kg/m^2), overweight (BMI > 25 kg/m^2) and obesity (BMI > 30 kg/m^2) were calculated. Diabetes mellitus was defined as a fasting glucose concentration of $\geq$ 126 mg/dl, or a non-fasting concentration of > 200 mg/dl, and/or a previous medical diagnosis of diabetes (Expert Committee on the Diagnosis and Classification of Diabetes Mellitus, 2005; WHO, 1994). Hypertension was defined as systolic pressure $\geq$ 140 mm/Hg and/or diastolic pressure $\geq$ 90 mm/Hg for people under 60 years of age. For those aged 60 years and over, hypertension was defined as systolic pressure $\geq$ 160 mm/Hg and/or diastolic pressure $\geq$ 90 mm/Hg. Hypercholesterolaemia was defined as fasting blood cholesterol concentrations of $\geq$ 200 mg/dl, and hypertriglyceridaemia as fasting triglyceride concentrations of $\geq$ 150 mg/dl (Expert Panel on Detection, Evaluation and Treatment of High Blood Cholesterol in Adults, 2001).

Trends in communicable and non-communicable disease mortality

The mortality indicators for the years 1950 to 2000 were obtained from estimations made by the Ministry of Health for the national health programme (Ministry of Health, 2001). Mortality rates for intestinal infectious diseases, acute respiratory diseases and undernutrition in children aged one to nine years, and ischaemic heart disease (IHD) and diabetes mellitus in adults aged 20 to 74 years were obtained from the National Institute of Informatics, Statistics and Geography (INEGI) using the International Classification of Diseases version 9 (ICD-9) for the years 1979 to 1995 (WHO/PAHO, 1978) and version 10 (ICD-10) for 2000 and 2002 (WHO, 1992).

TABLE 2
Women's energy and nutrient intakes and percentage adequacies by region and location, 1988 and 1999

| | Region | | | | | | | | | | Location | | | |
| | National | | North[a] | | Central[b] | | Mexico City[c] | | South[d] | | Urban[o] | | Rural | |
Intake	Median	Adequacy (%)	Median	Adequacy (%)	Median	Adequacy (%)	Median	Adequacy (%)	Median	Adequacy (%)	Median	Adequacy (%)	Median	Adequacy (%)
1988														
n	9 449		2 655		2 102		2 279		2 409		8 007		1 442	
Energy (kcal)	1 624	80.9	1 624	79.3	1 620	81.1	1 590	79.3	1 670	84.1	1 624	80.6	1 625	81.7
12 to 19 years	1 595	82.7	1 618	81.0	1 568	82.0	1 584	84.0	1 633	85.9	1 603	83.1	1 544	81.7
20 to 29 years	1 646	79.3	1 604	75.9	1 678	81.4	1 598	77.6	1 671	80.9	1 646	79.3	1 654	79.0
30 to 39 years	1 657	81.5	1 681	80.0	1 635	82.0	1 575	77.7	1 709	84.7	1 638	80.4	1 710	84.8
40 to 49 years	1 576	81.4	1 606	81.3	1 467	77.0	1 602	81.2	1 620	84.6	1 580	81.5	1 525	81.2
Fat (g)	44.8	66.6	45.3	66.5	44.5	66.2	46.2	68.4	43.5	65.9	45.6	67.8	40.6	61.3
Protein (g)	58.5	138.5	57.9	126.1	57.0	136.6	62.3	142.9	57.7	144.3	59.8	139.9	54.3	131.5
Vitamin A (mcg ER)	123.3	23.8	151.8	29.8	114.1	22.5	163.3	31.8	91.8	17.5	134.5	25.8	81.7	15.9
Vitamin B12 (mcg)	1.6	79.5	1.8	86.5	1.6	80.0	1.9	96.5	1.3	60.0	1.7	83.0	1.3	63.0
Vitamin D (mcg)	-	-	-	-	-	-	-	-	-	-	-	-	-	-
1999														
n	2 596		776		738		283		799		1 687		909	
Energy (kcal)	1 471	70.7	1 402[bcd]	64.2[bcd]	1 500[acd]	72.0[acd]	1 362[abd]	65.7[abd]	1 560[abc]	77.3[abc]	1 465[o]	69.8[o]	1 492	74.7
12 to 19 years	1 591	82.9	1 499	69.8	1 591	83.6	1 777	89.6	1 616	86.4	1 614	85.0	1 563	81.3
20 to 29 years	1 488	70.6	1 467	64.2	1 520	71.6	1 279	60.5	1 696	81.9	1 475	69.7	1 560	75.4
30 to 39 years	1 436	68.8	1 347	60.0	1 492	70.1	1 377	69.8	1 455	73.6	1 436	68.0	1 421	72.5
40 to 49 years	1 338	65.0	1 225	55.7	1 337	61.4	1 191	57.8	1 442	73.6	1 338	61.6	1 324	70.7
Fat (g)	48.6	69.9	50.9[bcd]	69.4[bcd]	51.9[acd]	72.9[acd]	49.8[abd]	72.4[abd]	45.3[abc]	66.4[abc]	52.0[o]	73.2[o]	37.4	56.3
Protein (g)	47.2	111.6	46.0[bcd]	99.4[bcd]	48.1[acd]	113.3[acd]	46.3[abd]	110.0[abd]	48.8[abc]	121.3[abc]	48.4[o]	111.3[o]	45.4	113.2
Vitamin A (mcg ER)	360.3	68.7	326.6[cd]	61.4[bcd]	343.0[cd]	64.9[acd]	468.8[abd]	92.7[abd]	341.8[abc]	62.9[abc]	403.0[o]	76.7[o]	244.3	47.2
Vitamin B12 (mcg)	1.6	84.6	1.7[bcd]	86.8[bcd]	1.7[acd]	86.7[acd]	2.0[abd]	100.2[abd]	1.3[abc]	66.4[abc]	1.9[o]	95.5[o]	0.8	38.4
Vitamin D (mcg)	3.6	71.2	7.2[bcd]	143.4[bcd]	1.3[acd]	25.0[acd]	5.6[abd]	112.5[abd]	3.5[abc]	70.0[abc]	4.3[o]	85.8[o]	<1.0	<1.0

a, b, c, d Different superindices represent statistically significant differences among regions. o Statistically different from rural locations.
Sources: MNS–1, 1988; MNS–2, 1999.

TABLE 3

Women's energy and nutrient intakes and percentage adequacy, by socio-economic status and education, 1988 and 1999

Intake	Socio-economic status						Education			
	Low[a]		Medium[b]		High[c]		Primary school and less[▲]		Middle and higher	
	Median	Adequacy (%)	Median	Adequacy (%)	Median	Adequacy (%)	Median	Adequacy (%)	Median	Adequacy (%)
1988										
N	3 254		2 638		3 153		5 179		4 230	
Energy (kcal)	1 654	82.3	1 623	81.1	1 592	79.3	1 655	82.4	1 591	79.1
12–19 years	1 585	83.4	1 600	82.6	1 595	82.5	1 623	85.5	1 568	80.6
20–29 years	1 670	78.6	1 669	81.6	1 583	77.9	1 665	79.8	1 624	78.4
30–39 years	1 734	86.2	1 596	78.6	1 605	78.9	1 699	83.3	1 598	78.7
40–49 years	1 563	83.2	1 550	81.2	1 575	79.7	1 584	82.6	1 539	79.1
Fat (g)	39.4	59.6	45.8	67.0	50.3	74.9	41.9	63.1	48.4	72.2
Protein (g)	55.3	138.5	58.9	135.6	62.0	140.1	57.6	136.1	60.0	141.3
Vitamin A (mcg ER)	82.4	15.6	129.1	24.9	169.2	33.6	93.8	18.5	158.3	31.2
Vitamin B12 (mcg)	1.2	58.0	1.6	81.5	1.9	96.5	1.4	70.0	1.8	90.0
Vitamin D (mcg)	-	-	-	-	-	-	-	-	-	-
1999										
N	877		905		814		1 341		1 249	
Energy total (kcal)	1 455.7[bc]	74.4[bc]	1 432.6[ac]	68.4[ac]	1 510.7[ab]	70.9[ab]	1 435.9[▲]	70.1[▲]	1 505.3	71.1
12–19 years	1 528.3	77.7	1 634.7	83.6	1 776.8	88.5	1 547.8	81.8	1 683.0	85.0
20–29 years	1 528.7	76.9	1 425.7	65.5	1 556.7	71.1	1 448.1	71.2	1 517.0	70.3
30–39 years	1 401.0	72.9	1 374.9	63.5	1 494.1	70.1	1 435.9	68.8	1 433.7	68.0
40–49 years	1 288.6	65.7	1 382.7	66.0	1 365.2	61.6	1 288.6	62.9	1 437.8	69.0
Fat (g)	37.0[bc]	56.9[bc]	49.1[ac]	70.2[ac]	56.4[ab]	78.4[ab]	41.3[▲]	61.7[▲]	54.6	78.0
Protein (g)	45.0[bc]	114.5[bc]	46.5[ac]	107.3[ac]	50.3[ab]	114.1[ab]	45.5[▲]	107.2[▲]	50.2	118.4
Vitamin A (mcg ER)	237.3[bc]	45.8[bc]	315.4[ac]	60.1[ac]	493.7[ab]	95.5[ab]	254.3[▲]	48.6[▲]	468.8	87.8
Vitamin B12 (mcg)	0.7[bc]	36.4[bc]	1.6[ac]	84.6[ac]	2.2[ab]	113.2[ab]	1.2[▲]	60.8[▲]	2.0	101.9
Vitamin D (mcg)	<1.0[bc]	<1.0[bc]	4.0[ac]	80.0[ac]	5.0[ab]	99.1[ab]	0.8[▲]	15.3[▲]	5.6	112.5

Sample sizes: children < 11 years of age, 1 249; females 12 to 49 years of age – 1988, 9 449; 1999, 2 596.
[a,b,c] Different superindices represent statistically significant differences among socio-economic quintiles.
[▲] Statistically different from middle and higher education.
Sources: MNS–1; MNS–2.

Macronutrient intake

The case study results show that there was an apparent decrease of 12.6 percent in total energy adequacy between 1988 and 1999. This reduction was observed across all regions and socio-economic status quintiles, and in both urban and rural locations (Table 2). Rural locations had higher adequacies than urban ones, and the South had higher adequacies than the other three regions. However, differences across regions and locations were higher in 1988 than in 1999. It should be noted that the dietary intake data of the 1988 and 1999 surveys are not directly comparable. Different food composition databases were used in the analysis of each survey. Also, the availability of food outside the home increased dramatically between 1988 and 1999, and the data indicate that in 1999 people ate away from home more often. As food consumption outside the home is often underreported, underreporting in 1999 can be expected. In addition, the case study team had clear indications of large rates of underreporting among overweight and obese women, probably resulting from a slim ideal body shape in Mexican society. According to case study estimates, obese women were 1.51 times more likely to underreport than women within the normal range of reference body weight (95 percent confidence interval = 1.35, 1.69) (Campirano *et al.*, 2001). The prevalence of high BMI (> 25) in women increased from 35 percent in 1988 to 59 percent in 1999; therefore, greater underreporting is expected in 1999. Thus it is clear that these surveys are not directly comparable and that the 1999 survey has greater underreporting.

Despite the evidence for underreporting of energy intakes, both fat intake and fat adequacy showed increases between 1988 and 1999 in all but rural locations and populations in the lowest socio-economic status quintile (Tables 2 and 3). A similar trend was seen for the percentage of energy derived from fat, where the increase between surveys was far smaller in rural and poor populations. This increase apparently occurred at the expense of both protein and carbohydrate intakes (Table 4). Protein adequacy at the national level was above the adequacy rate, and decreased from 1988 to 1999 across all groups.

TABLE 4
Nutrient intake by age group, 1988 and 1999

Gender	Age (years)	Total dietary energy intake (kcals)		% dietary energy from fat		% dietary energy from protein		% dietary energy from carbohydrates	
		1988	1999	1988	1999	1988	1999	1988	1999
Male	0–4	-	995	-	33.4	-	13.9	-	53.2
	5–11	-	1 439	-	31.8	-	12.8	-	56.7
Female	0–4	-	912	-	33.3	-	13.7	-	52.5
	5–11	-	1 319	-	32.2	-	12.6	-	56.2
	12–19	1 595	1 591	25.1	31.4	13.9	12.5	62.5	57.4
	20–29	1 646	1 488	26.1	31.7	14.3	12.9	60.7	55.8
	30–39	1 657	1 436	26.3	31.6	14.4	13.5	60.6	55.8
	40–49	1 576	1 338	26.1	27.4	14.2	12.7	61.6	60.8
Overall	**12–49**	**1 624**	**1 471**	**25.8**	**31.3**	**14.2**	**13.0**	**61.3**	**56.9**

Sources: MNS–1, 1988; MNS–2, 1999.

Micronutrient intake

At the national level, the adequacy of intakes of vitamins A and B12 and folate increased between the 1988 and 1999 surveys (Tables 2, 3 and 5). The magnitude of the increase was substantial for both vitamin A (from 23.8 to 68.7 percent) and folate (from 18.0 to 67.0 percent). While the intake adequacy of these vitamins increased similarly across all stratification levels, the absolute adequacy of intake of vitamin A (but not folate) remained much lower in the lowest socio-economic quintile (45.5 percent) than in the highest (95.5 percent); regional differences for vitamin A adequacy were minor. The adequacy of iron intake, on the other hand, decreased by about 30 percent at the national level, and reductions were observed in all the stratification levels. Intake data for neither vitamin D nor zinc were available in MNS–1 (1988) (Tables 5 and 6). Vitamin D adequacy at the national level in MNS–2 was 71.2 percent, but there was a large discrepancy between the lowest and the highest socio-economic status tertiles. The median adequacy for zinc intake in MNS–2 was 82.8 percent, and varied little among regions and socio-economic status quintiles.

TABLE 5
Women's mineral intakes and percentage adequacy, by region and location, 1988 and 1999

Intake	National		North[a]		Central[b]		Mexico City[c]		South[d]		Urban[o]		Rural	
	Median	Adequacy (%)	Median	Adequacy (%)	Median	Adequacy (%)	Median	Adequacy (%)	Median	Adequacy (%)	Median	Adequacy (%)	Median	Adequacy (%)
1988														
n	9 449		2 655		2 102		2 279		2 409		8 007		1 442	
Iron (mg)	11.8	144.3	10.9	131.4	12.1	148.8	11.5	141.3	12.2	151.0	11.6	141.5	12.8	157.8
Calcium (mg)	643.2	60.6	619.5	58.8	697.7	64.7	687.9	65.3	580.4	55.5	648.6	61.2	622.0	57.8
Zinc (mg)	-	-	-	-	-	-	-	-	-	-	-	-	-	-
Folate (mcg)	60.9	18.0	67.7	20.3	54.6	15.8	87.2	26.1	48.6	14.6	65.4	19.4	42.6	12.7
1999														
n	2 596		776		738		283		799		1 687		909	
Iron (mg)	8.3	101.2	8.5[bcd]	99.2[bcd]	8.4[acd]	103.2[acd]	6.8[abd]	82.3[abd]	9.2[abc]	112.5[abc]	7.9[o]	96.8[o]	9.4	116.1
Calcium (mg)	673.2	64.5	513.0[bcd]	50.0[bcd]	714.1[acd]	68.8[acd]	665.9[abd]	64.9[abd]	733.0[abc]	69.1[abc]	652.9[o]	63.3[o]	729.6	68.3
Zinc (mg)	6.0	82.8	5.7[bcd]	77.6[bcd]	6.0[acd]	83.4[acd]	5.6[abd]	77.5[abd]	6.3[abc]	87.2[abc]	6.0[o]	83.1[o]	6.0	82.6
Folate (mcg)	220.9	67.0	215.1[bcd]	64.5[bcd]	229.9[acd]	70.4[acd]	187.7[abd]	58.0[abd]	238.2[abc]	71.4[abc]	213.4[o]	64.5[o]	250.3	73.8

[a,b,c,d] Different superindices represent statistically significant differences among regions.
[o] Statistically different from rural locations.
Sources: MNS–1, 1988; MNS–2, 1999.

TABLE 6
Women's mineral intakes and percentage adequacy, by socio-economic status and education, 1988 and 1999

Intake	Socio-economic status						Education			
	Low[a]		Medium[b]		High[c]		Primary school and less[▲]		Middle and higher	
	Median	Adequacy (%)	Median	Adequacy (%)	Median	Adequacy (%)	Median	Adequacy (%)	Median	Adequacy (%)
1988										
N	3 254		2 638		3 153		5 179		4 230	
Iron (mg)	12.8	155.4	11.8	147.3	10.8	131.1	12.6	154.7	10.9	133.2
Calcium (mg)	611.5	57.2	639.6	60.6	687.7	64.7	630.0	59.9	665.0	61.5
Zinc (mg)	-	-	-	-	-	-	-	-	-	-
Folate (mcg)	42.9	12.6	64.3	19.0	80.1	24.5	49.9	14.7	75.8	22.8
1999										
n	877		905		814		1 341		1 249	
Iron (mg)	9.2[bc]	109.2[bc]	7.8[ac]	98.7[ac]	8.1[ab]	96.1[ab]	8.3[▲]	101.6[▲]	8.2	100.1
Calcium (mg)	726.2[bc]	67.3[bc]	622.0[ac]	59.1[ac]	679.6[ab]	66.3[ab]	690.5[▲]	65.6[▲]	659.9	63.2
Zinc (mg)	5.9[bc]	79.2[c]	5.7[ac]	78.8[c]	6.4[ab]	87.9[ab]	5.8[▲]	79.4[▲]	6.2	86.7
Folate (mcg)	229.9[bc]	68.6[bc]	225.0[ac]	67.8[ac]	206.4[ab]	63.0[ab]	226.3[▲]	68.6[▲]	215.9	64.9

[a,b,c] Different superindices represent statistically significant differences among socio-economic index tertiles.
[▲] Statistically different from middle and higher education.
Sources: MNS–1, 1988; MNS–2, 1999.

TABLE 7
Mean food intake in Mexico

	National Mean	National SD	Location Urban[*] Mean	Location Urban[*] SD	Location Rural Mean	Location Rural SD	Socio-economic index Low[a] Mean	Socio-economic index Low[a] SD	Socio-economic index Medium[b] Mean	Socio-economic index Medium[b] SD	Socio-economic index High[c] Mean	Socio-economic index High[c] SD	Region North[d] Mean	Region North[d] SD	Region Central[e] Mean	Region Central[e] SD	Region Mexico City[f] Mean	Region Mexico City[f] SD	Region South[g] Mean	Region South[g] SD
Cereals	263.9	(169.6)	236.9[*]	(151.3)	348.8	(194.3)	347.1[ab]	(195.4)	249.8[ac]	(156.9)	212.5[ab]	(130.5)	203.7[efg]	(138.1)	279.2[dfg]	(159.7)	195.7[deg]	(109.4)	324.9[def]	(197.3)
Rice	13.9	(38.6)	13.9[*]	(38.1)	13.7	(40.2)	11.1[bc]	(32.8)	13.2[ac]	(42.9)	16.6[ab]	(38.7)	13.8[efg]	(34.8)	8.2[dfg]	(24.2)	12.8[deg]	(32.5)	20.2[def]	(52.5)
Wheat	63.3	(75.9)	68.1[*]	(74.6)	48.0	(77.7)	45.8[bc]	(66.5)	65.5[ac]	(78.1)	74.6[ab]	(78.2)	67.3[efg]	(90.1)	68.4[dfg]	(76.0)	66.4[deg]	(67.8)	53.8[def]	(69.8)
Maize	186.8	(169.3)	154.9[*]	(143.2)	287.1	(202.4)	290.1[bc]	(200.8)	171.1[ac]	(145.4)	121.3[ab]	(116.5)	122.6[efg]	(129.1)	202.6[dfg]	(158.5)	116.5[deg]	(92.3)	250.0[ef]	(203.8)
Breakfast cereals	3.8	(26.5)	4.8[*]	(29.9)	0.8	(8.4)	0.2[bc]	(3.1)	3.7[ac]	(22.3)	6.8[ab]	(37.2)	7.4[efg]	(45.4)	4.5[dfg]	(23.6)	2.7[de]	(17.2)	1.7[de]	(16.1)
Starchy roots and tubers	12.0	(41.3)	11.6[*]	(40.8)	13.3	(42.8)	9.7[bc]	(34.1)	13.0[a]	(44.7)	13.0[a]	(43.1)	12.4[efg]	(38.8)	15.9[dfg]	(47.9)	12.1[deg]	(44.9)	7.9[def]	(31.8)
Potato	10.9	(35.0)	10.4[*]	(33.5)	12.3	(39.2)	8.7[bc]	(29.9)	11.9[ac]	(38.4)	11.7[ab]	(35.3)	11.3[efg]	(31.7)	14.5[dfg]	(41.0)	10.1[deg]	(32.5)	7.5[def]	(30.9)
Meat	81.3	(96.3)	88.0[*]	(100.8)	60.2	(76.7)	63.2[bc]	(78.0)	75.4[ac]	(84.8)	100.3[ab]	(113.4)	89.1[efg]	(111.4)	70.1[dfg]	(89.2)	83.1[deg]	(86.3)	86.9[def]	(97.9)
Beef	24.4	(63.8)	28.0[*]	(68.6)	13.3	(44.0)	13.7[bc]	(43.9)	22.5[ac]	(57.2)	34.3[ab]	(78.9)	35.6[efg]	(86.0)	23.8[dfg]	(61.5)	20.9[deg]	(47.3)	20.5[def]	(57.9)
Pork	10.4	(40.7)	11.7[*]	(43.9)	6.5	(28.1)	8.1[bc]	(30.3)	9.8[ac]	(39.8)	12.8[ab]	(47.7)	5.0[efg]	(22.7)	14.0[dfg]	(51.2)	9.5[deg]	(31.9)	10.7[def]	(41.3)
Poultry	23.4	(58.4)	25.2[*]	(60.8)	17.9	(49.4)	15.6[bc]	(42.6)	20.0[ac]	(53.9)	32.4[ab]	(70.2)	24.7[efg]	(70.9)	16.1[dfg]	(42.7)	25.3[deg]	(52.5)	29.0[def]	(65.9)
Eggs	23.0	(46.4)	23.2[*]	(48.6)	22.5	(38.9)	25.8[bc]	(48.4)	23.1[ac]	(41.3)	20.8[ab]	(48.9)	23.8[efg]	(37.6)	16.3[dfg]	(36.4)	27.4[deg]	(62.6)	26.7[def]	(48.3)
Processed meat	9.7	(30.1)	11.0[*]	(31.1)	5.6	(26.2)	6.0[bc]	(23.7)	8.6[ac]	(26.5)	13.4[ab]	(36.3)	14.8[efg]	(39.7)	9.3[dfg]	(27.9)	10.3[deg]	(32.5)	6.7[def]	(22.9)
Fresh fish	5.0	(34.5)	5.3[*]	(36.5)	3.9	(27.2)	3.3[bc]	(25.8)	5.7[ac]	(38.7)	5.6[ab]	(36.4)	3.4[efg]	(31.8)	4.8[dfg]	(38.7)	5.2[deg]	(31.8)	5.9[def]	(33.1)
Processed fish	0.9	(11.2)	0.9[*]	(10.3)	1.2	(13.8)	1.0[bc]	(12.6)	1.1[ac]	(12.9)	0.8[ab]	(8.2)	1.5[efg]	(11.9)	0.5[dg]	(6.4)	0.5[dg]	(6.4)	1.3[def]	(15.9)
Dairy products	137.6	(204.0)	159.1[*]	(214.3)	70.2	(148.7)	54.5[bc]	(131.9)	137.1[ac]	(194.7)	201.8[ab]	(232.4)	112.3[efg]	(166.8)	168.5[dfg]	(214.9)	180.3[deg]	(223.3)	96.5[def]	(190.5)
Fresh milk	118.6	(190.4)	136.0[*]	(199.8)	63.9	(144.0)	47.2[bc]	(122.1)	122.0[ac]	(186.2)	170.4[ab]	(217.7)	97.8[efg]	(156.1)	144.3[dfg]	(197.9)	159.4[deg]	(216.0)	81.1[def]	(176.2)
Cheese	10.4	(40.0)	12.0[*]	(43.2)	5.4	(27.1)	4.4[bc]	(18.2)	9.8[ac]	(32.5)	15.6[ab]	(54.7)	9.6[efg]	(31.0)	12.7[dg]	(48.2)	11.5[dg]	(43.4)	8.0[def]	(32.8)
Yoghurt	8.6	(47.4)	11.0[*]	(53.6)	0.9	(13.4)	2.9[bc]	(24.5)	5.3[ac]	(42.9)	15.8[ab]	(61.4)	4.9[ef]	(35.9)	11.5[dfg]	(61.2)	9.5[deg]	(41.6)	7.4[ef]	(39.6)
Nuts	1.3	(15.6)	1.4[*]	(15.5)	1.2	(15.9)	0.7[bc]	(6.5)	1.6[ac]	(16.5)	1.6[ab]	(19.3)	1.2[efg]	(10.2)	1.6[dfg]	(16.3)	2.4[deg]	(26.6)	0.5[def]	(9.0)
Legumes	35.3	(64.6)	28.3[*]	(55.0)	57.2	(84.4)	52.5[bc]	(82.2)	36.9[ac]	(63.7)	20.6[ab]	(42.7)	40.9[efg]	(70.0)	36.8[dfg]	(58.8)	14.5[deg]	(43.3)	42.5[def]	(73.9)
Processed/canned fruits, vegetables	2.4	(21.9)	2.9[*]	(24.1)	1.0	(12.2)	0.5[bc]	(6.1)	1.6[ac]	(12.3)	4.6[ab]	(33.1)	4.1[efg]	(20.1)	2.0[dfg]	(17.1)	2.9[deg]	(31.3)	1.6[def]	(20.4)
Fresh vegetables	68.4	(94.0)	71.2	(93.9)	59.8	(93.6)	55.9[bc]	(84.5)	73.2[ac]	(103.6)	73.9[ab]	(91.1)	53.8[efg]	(88.7)	77.7[dfg]	(94.0)	65.3[deg]	(78.2)	69.5[def]	(103.7)
Green leafy vegetables	1.2	(12.4)	1.1[*]	(11.1)	1.5	(15.9)	1.3[b]	(12.5)	1.1[ac]	(13.7)	1.3[b]	(11.1)	1.0[fg]	(9.3)	0.7[fg]	(8.0)	1.1[deg]	(12.8)	2.0[def]	(16.7)
Fresh fruit	84.7	(163.6)	90.3[*]	(169.5)	67.2	(142.4)	52.9[bc]	(118.8)	72.0[ac]	(145.3)	120.3[ab]	(198.1)	68.3[efg]	(150.9)	82.6[dfg]	(172.0)	102.5[deg]	(170.8)	86.4[def]	(156.8)
Citrus	47.1	(125.8)	49.4[*]	(129.3)	39.8	(113.5)	33.0[bc]	(100.5)	37.4[ac]	(112.2)	66.4[ab]	(149.6)	41.2[efg]	(118.9)	45.4[dfg]	(133.5)	49.5[deg]	(110.8)	50.9[def]	(129.6)
Fats and oils	10.0	(17.8)	9.7[*]	(17.3)	10.8	(19.1)	10.2[bc]	(19.4)	9.7[ac]	(15.5)	10.0[ab]	(18.4)	7.8[efg]	(11.5)	12.5[dfg]	(20.6)	9.5[deg]	(18.5)	9.0[def]	(17.1)
Animal fat (butter, lard)	2.0	(9.3)	1.6[*]	(8.3)	3.1	(11.9)	2.8[bc]	(11.7)	1.3[ac]	(5.1)	2.0[ab]	(10.0)	1.6[efg]	(6.2)	3.6[dfg]	(13.7)	0.4[deg]	(2.9)	1.5[def]	(7.3)
Vegetable oil	8.0	(15.3)	8.1[*]	(15.4)	7.7	(15.0)	7.4[bc]	(15.2)	8.5[ac]	(15.2)	8.0[ab]	(15.5)	6.2[efg]	(10.2)	8.9[dfg]	(16.3)	9.2[deg]	(17.9)	7.5[def]	(15.0)
Sweet drinks and sugar	204.7	(274.1)	230.8[*]	(285.5)	122.6	(215.1)	139.8[bc]	(235.9)	190.4[ac]	(240.1)	266.8[ab]	(313.2)	253.1[efg]	(272.0)	184.7[dfg]	(243.5)	245.8[deg]	(325.0)	172.1[def]	(265.1)
Soft drinks	184.8	(275.8)	210.7[*]	(288.1)	103.4	(213.4)	120.8[bc]	(234.6)	167.8[ac]	(241.4)	248.7[ab]	(316.6)	238.0[efg]	(271.3)	165.1[dfg]	(244.9)	223.3[deg]	(329.3)	150.7[def]	(266.3)
Sugar	13.7	(30.0)	13.3[*]	(30.9)	14.7	(26.8)	15.8[bc]	(34.4)	14.2[ac]	(27.8)	11.6[ab]	(28.0)	9.0[efg]	(19.6)	14.2[dfg]	(32.7)	12.2[deg]	(24.3)	16.8[def]	(34.5)
Confectionery	6.2	(27.7)	6.7[*]	(29.2)	4.5	(22.0)	3.3[bc]	(15.8)	8.3[ac]	(33.5)	6.6[ab]	(29.0)	6.1[efg]	(30.1)	5.4[dfg]	(22.1)	10.4[deg]	(36.0)	4.6[def]	(25.4)

Mean g or ml of purchased food

[a,b,c] Different superindices represent statistically significant differences among socio-economic index tertiles.

[*] Statistically different from rural.

[d,e,f,g] Different superindices represent statistically significant differences among regions.

Sources: MNS–1, 1988; MNS–2, 1999.

Food intake

Food intake information was not available from MNS–1. However, some trends in food intake among stratification groups were observed with data from MNS–2 (Table 7). Consumption rates of both maize products and legumes were substantially greater in the lowest socio-economic quintile (290.1 and 52.5 g, respectively) than in the highest (121.3 and 20.6 g, respectively). Similar differences in maize and legume consumption were also apparent among regions, with the highest intakes occurring in the South and the lowest in Mexico City. In contrast, women of higher socio-economic status consumed more meat than those of lower socio-economic status (100.3 versus 63.3 g). Of the regions, Mexico City had the highest meat consumption (89.1 g) and the Central region the lowest (70.1 g). Milk intake showed a similar pattern to meat, although with more dramatic differences: the highest socio-economic quintile consumed about four times more milk products than the lowest (201.8 versus 54.5 g). Fresh vegetable and fruit intakes, as well as soft drink consumption were also greater among the highest socio-economic quintile than the lowest. At the national level, a total of 204.7 g of sweet drinks and sugar were consumed daily, with a higher intake in the North (253.1 g) than the South region (172.1 g). Urban locations consumed almost twice the amount consumed in rural locations. The average daily fats and oils consumption was 10.0 g, and did not differ substantially among stratification groups.

Trends in national food expenditure 1989 to 2002

The most notable trends in terms of grams of food or food group purchased per capita at the national level were a decrease in purchases of cereals and legumes, and an increase in purchases of meats, milk and dairy products, and vegetables. Some of these trends were not universal, however. The decline in cereal purchase was apparent in the lowest income quintile, but not in the highest, with the result that cereal purchase per AE in the lowest quintile (301 to 326 g/d/per AE) was more similar to that in the higher quintile in 2002 (337 g/d/per AE) than it had been in previous years (316 and 412 g/d/per AE, respectively). Per capita legume purchase showed a decreasing trend from 1989 to 2002 across all income quintiles. For meat and vegetable purchases, the increases observed at the national level were observed in the lowest but not the highest income quintile. In this period, fruit consumption increased by 29.0 g in the highest quintile, but by only 2.0 g in the lowest (Table 8). Although there was no clear trend in egg purchase at the national level, there was an apparent increase among the lowest quintile group.

Looking at regional trends, cereal purchase was higher in the South region and rural locations, showing a decreasing trend in the North region, Mexico City and urban locations. The decrease in legume purchase, on the other hand, was similar across the regions. Per capita meat purchases increased, particularly in Mexico City. The South region consumed less fruit, milk and dairy products and more sugar and cereals than the other three regions. Mexico City consumed more meat, fruit and vegetables than the other regions, and urban locations showed higher expenditures on fruit, vegetables, milk and dairy products and meat, and lower expenditures on sugar, fats and oils, legumes and cereal than rural ones (Annex 2).

TABLE 8
Mean daily consumption per AE and percentages of total expenditure on food, by food group, national total and extreme income quintiles, 1989 to 2002

Food group	Year*	National (total)					Income quintile per AE									
							I					V				
		$\%^1$	$\%^2$	g/d^3	$(RC)_4$	Per capita $(g/d)^5$	$\%^1$	$\%^2$	g/d^3	$(RC)_4$	Per capita $(g/d)^5$	$\%^1$	$\%^2$	g/d^3	$(RC)^4$	Per capita $(g/d)^5$
Cereals (g)	1989	94.1	16	438	(1.00)	412	90	27	459	(1.00)	412	91	9	352	(1.00)	320
	1992	94.3	17	399	(0.91)	377	90	27	402	(0.88)	360	92	11	327	(0.93)	301
	1994	94.3	18	365	(0.83)	344	92	27	344	(0.75)	316	89	12	337	(0.96)	301
	1996	95.7	20	390	(0.89)	373	93	30	370	(0.81)	346	93	13	352	(1.00)	326
	1998	94.6	20	368	(0.84)	348	90	29	363	(0.79)	326	92	13	330	(0.94)	304
	2000	95.3	19	380	(0.87)	362	94	28	418	(0.91)	393	91	12	327	(0.93)	299
	2002	96.0	19	362	(0.83)	347	93	27	361	(0.79)	337	94	12	347	(0.99)	324
Meats (g)	1989	78.5	33	119	(1.00)	93	53	26	48	(1.00)	26	84	35	176	(1.00)	147
	1992	80.1	29	122	(1.02)	97	52	25	60	(1.25)	31	85	31	178	(1.01)	151
	1994	82.8	30	125	(1.05)	104	60	25	58	(1.20)	34	86	31	192	(1.09)	165
	1996	82.9	26	112	(0.94)	93	60	20	47	(0.98)	28	85	28	171	(0.97)	146
	1998	80.6	26	119	(1.00)	96	56	21	53	(1.11)	30	83	26	173	(0.98)	144
	2000	84.5	25	130	(1.09)	110	70	23	70	(1.45)	49	83	24	190	(1.08)	157
	2002	85.1	25	129	(1.08)	110	74	23	69	(1.43)	51	82	22	179	(1.02)	147
Eggs (g)	1989	61.9	5	55	(1.00)	34	53	8	36	(1.00)	19	55	3	73	(1.00)	40
	1992	62.3	5	57	(1.02)	35	53	8	38	(1.06)	20	59	3	75	(1.02)	44
	1994	60.2	5	58	(1.04)	35	54	8	39	(1.10)	21	55	3	75	(1.03)	41
	1996	65.8	6	54	(0.98)	36	59	9	33	(0.94)	20	58	4	72	(0.99)	42
	1998	60.9	5	56	(1.01)	34	55	8	39	(1.08)	21	50	4	74	(1.02)	37
	2000	63.8	4	60	(1.07)	38	67	6	44	(1.24)	30	52	3	77	(1.06)	40
	2002	59.9	4	60	(1.08)	36	62	7	47	(1.30)	29	47	2	77	(1.07)	36
Milk and dairy products (g)	1989	72.8	13	266	(1.00)	194	45	12	123	(1.00)	55	83	13	366	(1.00)	304
	1992	72.2	12	271	(1.02)	195	40	13	118	(0.96)	47	83	13	374	(1.02)	311
	1994	73.5	13	267	(1.00)	196	40	12	110	(0.90)	44	84	13	379	(1.04)	319
	1996	75.1	13	250	(0.94)	188	44	11	107	(0.87)	47	87	14	356	(0.97)	311
	1998	73.9	14	261	(0.98)	193	38	12	107	(0.87)	40	85	15	373	(1.02)	318
	2000	77.3	14	259	(0.97)	200	52	12	115	(0.94)	60	84	15	383	(1.05)	323
	2002	78.1	13	273	(1.02)	213	52	10	149	(1.22)	77	85	13	384	(1.05)	328
Legumes (g)	1989	55.1	5	72	(1.00)	40	65	12	76	(1.00)	50	35	3	84	(1.00)	29
	1992	56.0	6	69	(0.95)	39	63	12	67	(0.87)	42	37	3	69	(0.82)	25
	1994	53.3	5	68	(0.94)	36	62	12	68	(0.89)	42	36	3	75	(0.89)	27
	1996	59.0	7	66	(0.91)	39	67	13	61	(0.80)	41	39	4	71	(0.84)	28
	1998	54.0	6	66	(0.91)	35	62	13	63	(0.82)	39	37	3	73	(0.87)	27
	2000	52.5	4	66	(0.92)	35	67	8	68	(0.89)	46	32	2	71	(0.84)	23
	2002	47.9	5	64	(0.88)	31	65	9	65	(0.85)	42	26	3	69	(0.82)	18
Fats and oils (g)	1989	45.6	5	49	(1.00)	23	53	9	36	(1.00)	19	31	3	74	(1.00)	23
	1992	43.1	4	52	(1.05)	22	50	8	35	(0.98)	18	31	3	71	(0.96)	22
	1994	44.5	5	55	(1.11)	25	51	8	38	(1.07)	19	33	3	82	(1.11)	27
	1996	47.1	6	50	(1.02)	24	50	8	32	(0.88)	16	35	4	72	(0.98)	25
	1998	40.6	5	54	(1.09)	22	48	7	37	(1.04)	18	30	3	78	(1.06)	23
	2000	43.3	4	59	(1.19)	26	53	6	42	(1.17)	22	33	3	86	(1.16)	28
	2002	36.9	4	59	(1.18)	22	51	5	44	(1.22)	22	24	3	84	(1.14)	20
Vegetables (g)	1989	85.1	9	144	(1.00)	122	79	11	79	(1.00)	62	79	7	216	(1.00)	170
	1992	83.9	10	145	(1.01)	122	77	13	75	(0.96)	58	79	8	206	(0.95)	164
	1994	83.4	10	147	(1.02)	122	79	14	80	(1.02)	63	76	8	208	(0.96)	158
	1996	85.8	8	159	(1.11)	136	80	10	81	(1.03)	64	81	7	228	(1.05)	184
	1998	82.8	10	151	(1.05)	125	78	12	79	(1.01)	62	76	8	220	(1.02)	166
	2000	83.5	9	163	(1.14)	136	84	11	96	(1.22)	80	76	7	228	(1.05)	172
	2002	83.2	9	173	(1.20)	144	84	12	103	(1.31)	87	74	7	235	(1.09)	173

Fruits (g)	1989	53.7	6	151	(1.00)	81	29	5	71	(1.00)	21	65	6	246	(1.00)	160
	1992	53.4	5	178	(1.18)	95	26	5	78	(1.10)	20	66	6	272	(1.10)	179
	1994	55.3	6	179	(1.18)	99	27	5	91	(1.28)	25	66	6	271	(1.10)	179
	1996	54.6	5	162	(1.07)	88	28	4	69	(0.97)	19	68	6	260	(1.06)	178
	1998	50.8	5	154	(1.02)	78	25	5	95	(1.35)	24	63	6	240	(0.98)	152
	2000	57.5	6	193	(1.28)	111	38	5	88	(1.25)	33	67	6	312	(1.27)	210
	2002	52.6	5	178	(1.18)	94	34	5	81	(1.14)	28	60	7	300	(1.22)	181
Sugar (g)	1989	39.8	3	76	(1.00)	30	57	6	67	(1.00)	38	24	2	118	(1.00)	28
	1992	38.4	3	76	(1.01)	29	52	7	68	(1.02)	36	24	2	97	(0.83)	23
	1994	39.0	4	76	(1.01)	30	54	7	66	(0.98)	35	25	2	100	(0.85)	25
	1996	41.5	4	68	(0.90)	28	53	7	55	(0.82)	29	27	3	95	(0.80)	26
	1998	37.3	3	72	(0.95)	27	48	7	59	(0.88)	28	27	2	113	(0.95)	30
	2000	39.2	3	72	(0.95)	28	54	5	61	(0.92)	33	29	2	102	(0.86)	30
	2002	36.1	3	79	(1.05)	29	55	6	71	(1.06)	39	23	2	112	(0.95)	26

Data weighted by the expansion factors.

Sample sizes: 1989, 11 531 (expanded cases, 15 947 773); 1992, 10 508 (expanded cases, 17 798 635); 1994, 12 815, (expanded cases, 19 440 278); 1996, 14 042 (expanded cases, 20 467 038); 1998, 10 952 (expanded cases, 22 163 568); 2000, 10 089 (expanded cases, 23 452 319); 2002, 17167 (expanded cases, 24 650 169).

[1] Percentage of families reporting expenditure during the seven-day survey period.
[2] Percentage of total food expenditure.
[3] Mean grams per AE among families reporting expenditure.
[4] Relative change.
[5] Mean grams per capita.
Source: MHIES, 1989 to 2002.

While there was no apparent time trend in the per capita purchase of free sugar, there was a large per capita increase in the purchase of soda, particularly among the highest income group (Tables 8 and 9). Soda expenditure per AE in Mexico increased by 19 percent over the 13-year period. By income, it increased by 20 percent in the lowest quintile and by 21 percent in the highest. By region, soda expenditure showed the highest increasing trend in the Central region (27 percent). In 2002, however, the North was the region with the highest soda consumption (315 ml/AE), which was 57.5 percent higher than that of the South. Tobacco expenditure showed an increasing trend, particularly in the North region, rural locations and the highest income quintile (Annex 3). The trends observed for the extreme upper and lower income quintiles were somewhat similar when the data were disaggregated by urban and rural residence.

In summary, trends in per capita food expenditure have led to cereal and egg intakes in the lowest and highest income groups becoming more similar; food expenditures in the lowest income quintile are moving closer to those in higher income groups, but there are still large gaps in meats, milk and dairy products, vegetables and fruits. There are no apparent trends in the per capita purchases of fats and oils, or sugar, although the purchase of sugar is consistently greater among the lowest income group. Overall, the purchasing habits of the highest income quintile changed little between 1989 and 2002.

Food expenditure outside the home

In 2002, food expenditure outside the home accounted for 25.4 percent of total food expenditure by AE. Relative to 1989, this expenditure had increased across all regions, locations and income quintiles. However, it was more than twice as large in the highest income quintile than in the lowest (Table 10).

TABLE 9

Mean daily consumption per AE and percentages of total expenditure on soda, alcohol and tobacco, by national total and extreme income quintiles, 1989 to 2002

Food groups	Year*	National (total)					Income quintile per AE									
							I					V				
		%[1]	%[2]	ml/d[3]	(RC)[4]	Per capita (ml/d)[5]	%[1]	%[2]	ml/d[3]	(RC)[4]	Per capita (ml/d)[5]	%[1]	%[2]	ml/d[3]	(RC)[4]	Per capita (ml/d)[5]
Soda (ml)	1989	49.5	5	203	(1.00)	100	29	7	102	(1.00)	30	58	4	276	(1.00)	159
	1992	51.8	6	211	(1.04)	109	27	8	104	(1.03)	28	60	6	296	(1.07)	179
	1994	53.3	5	228	(1.12)	121	33	4	104	(1.02)	35	60	4	319	(1.15)	193
	1996	51.4	7	200	(0.98)	103	31	7	91	(0.89)	28	61	6	283	(1.02)	171
	1998	58.2	8	232	(1.14)	135	33	10	128	(1.26)	43	66	8	317	(1.15)	210
	2000	60.7	8	256	(1.26)	155	40	8	129	(1.26)	51	67	7	354	(1.28)	238
	2002	61.5	8	242	(1.19)	149	39	9	122	(1.20)	48	69	8	335	(1.21)	232
Alcohol (ml)	1989	5.8	10	168	(1.00)	10	5	7	89	(1.00)	4	9	9	207	(1.00)	19
	1992	5.2	9	201	(1.20)	10	4	9	167	(1.87)	7	9	11	249	(1.21)	22
	1994	6.9	10	189	(1.13)	13	6	12	86	(0.96)	5	10	10	282	(1.37)	28
	1996	5.4	9	187	(1.12)	10	5	11	196	(2.20)	9	9	9	230	(1.11)	21
	1998	6.6	9	187	(1.12)	12	5	11	271	(3.04)	14	10	10	208	(1.00)	20
	2000	6.9	11	172	(1.02)	12	4	13	153	(1.72)	6	11	13	213	(1.03)	24
	2002	4.3	12	252	(1.51)	11	2	11	196	(2.20)	5	7	12	350	(1.70)	25
Tobacco (g)	1989	15.7	5	3.4	(1.00)	0.54	11	5	1.6	(1.00)	0.18	19	5	4.3	(1.00)	0.83
	1992	21.1	6	2.8	(0.82)	0.60	14	6	1.6	(1.01)	0.23	26	6	4.1	(0.94)	1.06
	1994	11.3	7	3.4	(1.00)	0.39	7	9	2.1	(1.30)	0.14	15	7	5.2	(1.19)	0.76
	1996	9.2	5	3.3	(0.95)	0.30	6	6	1.6	(1.00)	0.10	12	5	4.8	(1.11)	0.58
	1998	8.7	5	3.8	(1.10)	0.33	5	6	1.5	(0.97)	0.08	11	5	5.9	(1.37)	0.63
	2000	9.1	6	3.7	(1.06)	0.33	5	6	1.7	(1.04)	0.08	11	5	5.5	(1.26)	0.62
	2002	7.1	6	4.9	(1.44)	0.35	2	6	3.0	(1.87)	0.07	11	6	6.8	(1.58)	0.77

TABLE 10

Median daily food expenditure outside the home as percentage of total food expenditure, 1989 to 2002.

Year*	National (total)		Income quintile per AE			
			I		V	
	%[1]	(RC)[2]	%[1]	(RC)[2]	%[1]	(RC)[2]
1989	23	(1.00)	13	(1.00)	34	(1.00)
1992	24	(1.04)	19	(1.46)	29	(0.85)
1994	26	(1.13)	15	(1.15)	39	(1.15)
1996	22	(0.96)	16	(1.23)	31	(0.91)
1998	22	(0.96)	15	(1.15)	32	(0.94)
2000	24	(1.04)	13	(1.00)	35	(1.03)
2002	25	(1.09)	15	(1.15)	37	(1.09)

Data weighted by the expansion factors.
Sample sizes: 1989, 11 531 (expanded cases, 15 947 773); 1992, 10 508 (expanded cases, 17 798 635); 1994, 12 815, (expanded cases, 19 440 278); 1996, 14 042 (expanded cases, 20 467 038); 1998, 10 952 (expanded cases, 22 163 568); 2000, 10 089 (expanded cases, 23 452 319); 2002, 17167 (expanded cases, 24 650 169).
[1] Percentage of total food expenditure.
[2] Relative change.
Source: MHIES, 1989 to 2002.

Breastfeeding patterns in Mexico

In Mexico, the average duration of breastfeeding is nine months, but only 25.7 percent of mothers reported exclusive breastfeeding for four months, and 20.3 percent for six months. Among the socio-demographic factors associated with shorter periods of exclusive breastfeeding are living in urban locations, being a non-indigenous family, and having a BMI above the mean (Table 11).

TABLE 11
Breastfeeding by socio-economic, demographic and anthropometric characteristics, 1999

	Duration of breastfeeding (months, median)	Ever breastfed (%)	Exclusive breastfeeding[1] (%)	
			4 months (< 123 days)	6 months (< 183 days)
N			502	750
National	9	92.3	25.7	20.3
Region				
North	6	91.8	16.5	10.5
Central	8	91.6	25.0	19.1
Mexico City	7	92.0	11.6	12.3
South	15	93.5	36.5[4]	30.5[4]
Location				
Urban	7	92.3	20.9	15.0
Rural	14	92.2	36.1[4]	33.2[4]
Ethnicity[2]				
Indigenous	>24	93.5	48.2	48.4
Non-indigenous	8	92.3	23.2[4]	17.8[4]
Socio-economic status[3]				
Low	15	92.3	39.8	33.8
Middle	8	91.6	17.3	14.2
High	6	93.1	20.7[4]	14.3[4]
Number of children				
1	7	94.1	22.8	16.6
2	8	91.6	26.1	19.9
≥ 3	12	91.5	27.8	23.6
Maternal age				
> 19 years	12	92.2	27.6	23.1
19 to < 25 years	10	93.5	24.5	21.6
25 to < 35 years	8	92.2	25.9	18.3
≥ 35 years	9	89.9	26.5	20.8
BMI (kg/m^2)				
< mean (25.7)	10	93.6	33.2	25.7

[1] Exclusive breastfeeding = receiving *only* breastmilk (consumption of pharmaceutical products – medicines or vitamin/mineral preparations – was not explored).
[2] Indigenous = mother speaks a native language.
[3] Calculated through principal components analysis.
[4] $p < 0.05$.
Source: Gonzalez-Cossio *et al.*, 2003.

Nutritional status of children under five years of age

Table 12 presents the prevalence of low HAZ, WAZ and WHZ in 1988 and 1999. In 1988, almost one-quarter of children under five years of age in Mexico were stunted (HAZ < -2.0 SD of the NCHS reference population) and 6.3 percent were wasted (WHZ < -2.0 SD of the NCHS reference population). Eleven years later, in 1999, wasting was no longer a public health concern in Mexico, with only 2.1 percent of children being wasted, but a substantial percentage remained stunted – almost 18 percent. The low prevalence of wasting in Mexico runs parallel to an equally low prevalence of this condition in almost all Latin American countries, which have an average prevalence of less than 3 percent (de Onis and Blössner, 2003). In contrast, stunting continues to be a public health problem in several Latin American countries (ACC/SCN, 2000). Relative to countries with similar per capita GNP (Chile, Brazil and Argentina), Mexico had a higher prevalence of stunting in 1999. Moreover, the reduction of 5.1 percentage points in the 11 years between surveys (from 22.9 percent in 1988 to 17.8 percent in 1999) is below the reduction rate experienced by several other Latin American countries during the same period (Hernandez *et al.,* 2003). Wasting declined to less than 2.5 percent in all regions, in urban and rural areas and in all socio-economic quintiles. The largest drop was observed in the North[1] and Central regions. As mentioned earlier, this condition is no longer a public health problem in Mexico.

On the other hand, stunting rates in 1999 were not only high at the national level but also heterogeneous in the different regions, in urban and rural locations and across socio-economic categories. Stunting rates in the lowest socio-economic quintile were six times those of the highest; rates were almost three times as high in rural as in urban areas and in the South (the poorest region) than in Mexico City and the North (the wealthiest regions). The decline in stunting rates between 1988 and 1999 was almost totally accounted for by the changes observed in the lowest socio-economic group, and was more pronounced in the Central region and in urban areas (Table 12). It should be noted that localities that were classified as rural in 1988 might have become urban by 1999 owing to population growth; changes in stunting rates between the two data points may therefore be partially explained by the urbanization process. Similarly, geographic regions that were regarded as being within the metropolitan area of Mexico City in 1999 were considered part of the Central region in 1988. This may partially explain the increase in stunting rates in Mexico City – which has incorporated more poor populations into its surrounding metropolitan area – and the sharp decline in stunting in the Central region. Parallel to the sharp drop in wasting and the slow decline in stunting, overweight (WAZ > +2 SD of the NCHS reference population) in children under five years of age has increased slightly at the national level and in all regions, with the highest increases in the South and Mexico City, a smaller increase in the North and a decline in the Central region. Despite the lower increase in overweight rates, the North has the highest prevalence (Figure 2).

---

[1] The apparent prevalence of wasting in the North region in 1988 has been questioned because it was too high for the level of development of the northern states of Mexico at that time.

TABLE 12

Prevalence of low HAZ, WAZ and WHZ in children (0 to four years) by region, urban or rural location and socio-economic quintile, 1988 and 1999

	HAZ				WAZ				WHZ			
	< -2 SD		< -3 SD		< -2 SD		< -3 SD		< -2 SD		< -3 SD	
	1988	1999	1988	1999	1988	1999	1988	1999	1988	1999	1988	1999
National	22.9	17.8	9.3	5.7	13.9	7.6	2.9	1.2	6.3	2.1	1.6	0.6
Region												
North[1]	11.0	7.1	3.9	1.7	10.5	3.3	1.4	0.8	10.1	2.2	2.9	0.6
Central[2]	25.1	14.5	9.6	4.4	13.8	6.1	3.0	1.3	7.1	2.3	1.5	1.0
Mexico city[3]	9.8	13.1	2.6	3.7	6.1	6.8	0.6	0.3	3.6	2.3	1.0	0.2
South[4]	34.1	29.2	15.6	10.2	20.5	12.0	4.7	1.8	5.3	1.7	1.4	0.4
Location												
Rural[5]	34.7	32.2	17.1	10.9	19.6	12.3	4.5	2.2	5.9	2.1	1.7	0.6
Urban[6]	18.8	11.7	14.2	3.5	12.3	5.7	2.4	0.8	6.4	2.0	1.6	0.6
Socio-economic status												
Low[7]	42.0	35.3	20.4	13.3	24.0	15.6	6.0	2.5	5.7	2.6	1.4	0.8
Medium[8]	16.9	15.0	5.0	3.8	11.1	6.5	1.5	1.0	6.8	2.4	1.5	0.8
High[9]	6.2	6.0	2.8	1.2	5.7	2.8	1.4	0.4	6.1	1.4	2.0	0.4

Sample sizes: 1988, 5904 (weight, 7 101 607); 1999, 8 011 (weight, 10 612 397).
[1] Sample sizes: 1988, 1 430 (weight, 1 097 654); 1999, 2 317 (weight, 1 984 629).
[2] Sample sizes: 1988, 1 411 (weight: 2 235 041); 1999, 2 533 (weight, 3 648 563).
[3] Sample sizes: 1988, 1 478 (weight, 1 422 801); 1999, 571 (weight, 1 492 824).
[4] Sample sizes: 1988, 1 585 (weight, 2 346 111); 1999, 2 590 (weight, 3 486 381).
[5] Sample sizes: 1988, 1 022 (weight, 5 526 366); 1999, 3 312 (weight, 3 161 671).
[6] Sample sizes: 1988, 4 882 (weight, 1 575 241); 1999, 4 699 (weight, 7 450 726).
[7] Sample sizes: 1988, 1 531 (weight, 2 229 853); 1999, 2 414 (weight, 2 882 015.
[8] Sample sizes: 1988, 2 862 (weight, 3 267 560); 1999, 2 804 (weight, 3 454 492).
[9] Sample sizes: 1988, 1 511 (weight, 1 604 194); 1999, 2 572 (weight, 4 025 820).
Sources: MNS–1, 1988; MNS–2, 1999.

FIGURE 2

Prevalence of overweight in children aged 0 to 4.9 years, national total, by region and by residence, 1988 and 1999

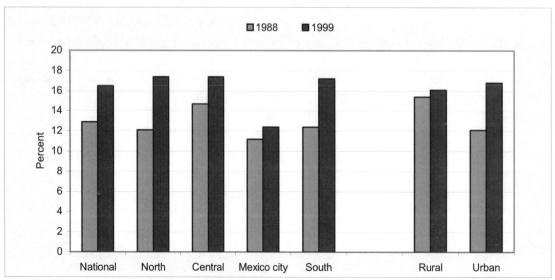

Sources: MNS, 1988; 1999.

Prevalence of overweight in school-age children

The prevalence of overweight in children aged five to 11 years was analysed from MNS–2 in 1999. No data were available on the anthropometry of school-age children from MNS–1 in 1988. Approximately one-quarter of children were overweight according to the reference proposed by Must, Dallal and Dietz (1991), while according to the Cole *et al.* (2000) classification, the prevalence was almost 20 percent. Prevalence was substantially higher in the wealthier North and Mexico City relative to the South and Central regions; it was twice as high in urban as in rural areas, higher in females and in the children of more educated women, and lower in indigenous populations (Table 13).

TABLE 13
Prevalence of overweight in school-age children (five to 11 years) by region, residence, gender, maternal education level and ethnicity

Variable		n	Cole %	Must %
National		**10 901**	**19.5**	**27.3**
Region	North	3 188	25.6	34.9
	Central	3 292	18.0	25.6
	Mexico City	855	26.6	33.4
	South	3 566	14.3	22.2
Location	Urban	6 142	22.9	30.6
	Rural	4 759	11.7	19.9
Sex	Female	5 505	21.2	28.7
	Male	5 396	17.7	25.9
Maternal education	No education	2 415	12.0	19.8
	Elementary school	5 087	17.6	25.1
	Middle school	1 839	25.6	34.1
	High school or more	1 560	25.6	33.3
Indigenous ethnicity	No	9 750	20.4	19.8
	Yes	1 151	12.1	11.5

Sources: Cole *et al.,* 2000; Must, Dallal and Dietz, 1999; MNS–1, 1988; MNS–2, 1999.

Prevalence of adult overweight, obesity and non-communicable chronic diseases

The changes in prevalence of overweight and obesity in Mexican adults were studied by comparing the results of MNS–1 (1988) and MNS–2 (1999), which included only women, and the results of MCDS (1994) and MHS (2000), which included both men and women.

Between 1988 and 1999, the prevalence of overweight and obesity increased in women by almost 70 percent (from 35 to 59 percent) (Table 14): overweight (BMI of 25 to 29.9) by almost 50 percent (from 24 to 35 percent), and obesity (BMI $\geq$ 30) by 150 percent (from 9 to 24 percent). These dramatic increases were observed in all regions, in both urban and rural areas and in all socio-economic groups. The prevalence of BMI < 18.5, indicating low weight in adults, was less than 2 percent in women in 1999, indicating that undernutrition in women is no longer a public health concern in Mexico.

Adult underweight is not a public health problem among males either, as observed in MHS, which recorded prevalence of about 2 percent in both men and women. The prevalence of adequate weight in men and women decreased from 21.9 percent in 1994 to

21.2 percent in 2000. Stratifying by age, only 22 percent of adults aged 40 to 59 years had adequate weight in 2000. This age group also had the highest prevalence of obesity (35.4 percent) in 2000, representing a relative increase of 2.6 percentage points (about 8 percent) since 1994. However, the highest relative increases in obesity were observed in the youngest age group (20 to 39 years), where it increased by 6.9 percentage points (47 percent) over the study period, followed by the oldest group (60 to 75 years), which showed a 7.6 percentage point increase (36 percent). As expected, urban locations and the North region had the highest prevalence of overweight and obesity. Obesity increased more in the North and Central regions (by about 8 percentage points during the six-year period), followed by the South (about 6 percentage points) and Mexico City (3 percentage points) (Table 15).

Diabetes mellitus and hypertension have increased dramatically in Mexico. According to the case study analysis, between 1994 and 2000, diabetes mellitus increased by 3.3 percentage points in males and by 4.6 in females. Hypertension did not show relevant increases by sex, but substantial increases were observed in the 40 to 59 years age group, in urban locations and in the North region. High cholesterol and triglyceride concentrations were more prevalent in men than in women. The prevalence of these increased between 1994 and 2000 in males and females, all age groups, urban and rural locations, and all regions (Table 16). Awareness of these conditions is an issue. Prior to the survey, only 41 percent of the people with hypertension and 77 percent of those with diabetes were aware of their condition (NHS, 2000; Olaiz, Rojas and Barquera, 2003).

TABLE 14
BMI trends in women aged 20 to 49 years, by residence and socio-economic status, 1988 and 2000

		BMI							
		Underweight (< 18.5 kg/m²)		Normal (18.5–24.9 kg/m²)		Overweight (> 25 kg/m²)		Obese (> 30 kg/m²)	
		1988	2000	1988	2000	1988	2000	1988	2000
National		7.7	1.8	55.7	33.4	36.6	64.7	9.4	29.0
	Urban	7.5	1.8	55.7	32.0	36.7	66.2	9.6	30.7
Location[1]	Rural	8.7	1.8	55.4	34.9	35.9	63.2	9.1	27.2
Socio-economic status	Low	9.3	2.4	55.8	37.7	34.9	59.9	9.7	25.1
	Medium	7.0	1.5	51.7	30.2	41.3	68.3	10.6	32.8
	High	6.8	1.6	59.2	32.1	34.0	66.4	8.4	29.3

Sample sizes: 1988, 10 746; 2000, 21 481.
[1] Location: rural = < 15 000 inhabitants; urban = > 15 000 inhabitants.
Sources: MNS–1, 1988; MHS, 2000.

TABLE 15
BMI trends in adults aged 20 years and over, by gender, age, residence and region, 1994 and 2000

		BMI							
		Underweight (< 18.5 kg/m^2)		Normal (18.5–24.9 kg/m^2)		Overweight (25–29.9 kg/m^2)		Obese (> 30 kg/m^2)	
		1994	2000	1994	2000	1994	2000	1994	2000
National		**1.7**	**1.8**	**42.2**	**32.5**	**35.9**	**37.5**	**20.2**	**28.3**
Sex	Male	1.9	1.8	46.0	36.1	36.1	40.5	15.9	21.6
	Female	1.5	1.7	39.4	30.8	35.8	36.1	23.4	31.3
Age (years)	20–39	2.2	2.1	49.4	38.5	33.6	37.7	14.8	21.7
	40–59	0.4	1.0	24.4	22.1	42.4	41.5	32.8	35.4
	60–75	1.8	1.9	33.0	28.3	43.8	40.8	21.4	29.0
Location[1]	Urban	1.6	1.6	40.9	29.4	37.7	40.3	19.8	28.7
	Rural	-	1.9	-	35.5	-	38.4	-	24.2
Region	North	0.9	1.7	38.8	28.0	36.7	39.1	23.6	31.2
	Central	2.4	1.8	45.6	31.6	33.8	40.1	18.2	26.5
	Mexico City	1.5	1.3	44.1	32.3	33.9	42.9	20.5	23.5
	South	1.9	1.7	38.2	36.2	42.6	38.5	17.3	23.6

Sample sizes: 1994, 2 125; 2000, 45 294.
[1] Location: rural = < 15 000 inhabitants; urban = > 15 000 inhabitants. The 1994 survey did not include rural areas.
Sources: MCDS, 1994; MHS, 2000.

TABLE 16
Prevalence of diabetes mellitus, hypertension, high blood cholesterol and high triglycerides in adults, by gender, age group, residence and region, 1994 and 2000

		Diabetes mellitus[1]		Hypertension[2]		High cholesterol (> 200 mg/dl)		High triglycerides (> 150 mg/dl)	
		1994	2000	1994	2000	1994	2000	1994	2000
Sex	Male	4.3	7.6	39.3	39.2	29.1	48.2	47.4	53.5
	Female	3.7	8.3	27.8	30.9	23.5	42.2	34.1	45.0
Age (years)	20–39	1.9	2.0	18.6	20.9	19.8	33.3	33.5	42.5
	40–59	7.2	12.5	38.3	45.2	38.4	69.2	53.6	63.5
	60–75	14.0	21.1	53.1	53.5	43.8	65.0	50.9	67.0
Location[3]	Urban	4.0	8.8	26.1	34.2	26.0	42.2	39.7	45.6
	Rural	-	7.2	-	33.0	-	43.0	-	53.1
Region	North	3.4	9.8	25.4	38.4	21.7	39.5	36.3	39.9
	Central	5.0	7.6	30.0	33.7	28.2	48.2	32.2	53.5
	Mexico City	1.7	8.9	23.7	27.9	29.8	53.5	46.7	30.0
	South	5.2	7.3	23.6	30.4	23.7	33.4	47.7	45.2

Sample sizes: 1994, 2 125; 2000, 2 422.
[1] Diabetes mellitus = fasting glucose > 126 mg/dl, or post-prandial glucose > 200 mg/dl (WHO), or previous medical diagnosis of diabetes mellitus.
[2] Hypertension = systolic blood pressure ≥ 140 mm/Hg, and/or diastolic blood pressure ≥ 90 mm/Hg in adults < 60 years, and systolic blood pressure ≥160 mm/Hg, and/or diastolic blood pressure ≥ 90 mm/Hg in adults ≥ 60 years.
[3] Location: rural = < 15 000 inhabitants; urban = > 15 000 inhabitants.
Sources: MCDS, 1994; MHS, 2000.

Biochemical indicators of anaemia status

Results from MNS–1 (1988) and MNS–2 (1999) show increases in the prevalence of anaemia over the 11-year period in pregnant women (from 18.2 to 27.8 percent) and non-pregnant women (from 15.4 to 20.8 percent) (Table 17) (Martinez *et al.,* 1995; Shamah-Levy *et al.,* 2003). Child anaemia was not evaluated until MNS–2, which recorded a prevalence of 27.2 percent at the national level (Table 17). A number of factors could explain the increase in anaemia; for example, haemoglobin was measured *in situ* with a portable photometer in 1999, but not in 1988, when venous blood was used. Changes in feeding patterns among the population also partially explain the increase. The total protein intake decreased over this period, from 58.5 to 47.2 g (Table 2), while data on expenditure show almost no change in meat purchases at the national level between 1989 and 2002 (Table 8). Another important factor could be that comprehensive national interventions oriented to reduce micronutrient deficiencies in poor locations, such as the Progresa/Oportunidades programmes, did not start until 1999, when their design and targeting were improved by the results MNS–2.

The highest prevalence of anaemia in women was observed in rural locations, particularly in those with indigenous populations. The main socio-economic factors associated with high prevalence of anaemia were number of children, lower socio-economic status, indigenous background and residence in rural locations. As reported in other studies, these factors are closely associated with poverty (ACC/SNC, no date; Becerra *et al.,* 1998; Diallo *et al.,* 1995; Frith-Terhune, Cogswell and Kettel Khan, 2000; Zavaleta, Caulfield and Garcia, 2000).

TABLE 17
Prevalence of anaemia in women aged 12 to 49 years and children aged 0 to five years, by region and residence, 1988 and 1999

	Non-pregnant (%)		Pregnant (%)		Children (%)
	1988	**1999**	**1988**	**1999**	**1999**
n	*15 146*	*16 496*	*7 420*	*6 970*	*5 526*
National	**15.4**	**20.8**	**18.2**	**27.8**	**27.2**
Region					
North	19.7	20.9	21.6	21.1	26
Central	12.4	20.6	13.9	27.7	27.5
Mexico City	13.4	14.9	15.1	12.3	27.2
South	17.5	23.2	22.8	29.9	27.6
Location					
Urban	15.6	20.2	18.5	27.7	26.1
Rural	14	22.6	16.8	28	29.5

Anaemia = < 12 g/dl haemoglobin in non-pregnant and < 11 g/dl in pregnant women.
Sources: MNS–1, 1988; MNS–2, 1999.

Mortality trends

The case study's analysis of the mortality register found decreasing trends in child mortality and in mortality among the 15 to 59 years age group. All-cause mortality per thousand inhabitants decreased from 16 in 1950 to 4.5 in 2000. Mortality due to communicable diseases, undernutrition and reproduction represented 49.8 percent of all-cause mortality in 1950, decreasing to 14 percent in 2000. In contrast, mortality due to non-communicable chronic diseases has been increasing in the last five decades, contributing 43.7 percent of all-cause mortality in 1950 and 73 percent in 2000 (Figure 3). Thus, a decreasing trend in mortality due to infectious gastrointestinal diseases, acute respiratory infections and undernutrition was observed, while non-communicable chronic diseases such as diabetes mellitus, hypertension and IHD show a steady increase over time, which is consistent with the epidemiologic transition theory (Ministry of Health, 2001).

FIGURE 3

Mortality trends: percentage contributions to all-cause mortality of non-communicable chronic diseases and acute infectious diseases, 1950 to 2000

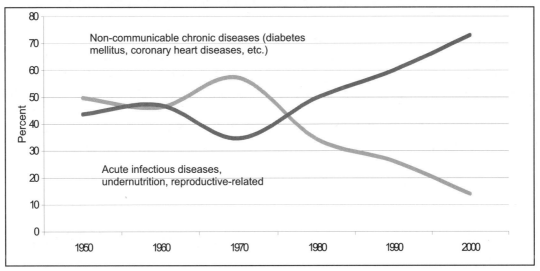

Physical activity in Mexico

There is only limited information on the physical activity of the Mexican population. Using data from MNS–2 (1999), Hernández *et al.* (2003) concluded that females aged from 12 to 49 years have very limited physical activity. Only 16 percent reported the regular practice of sports. Several socio-demographic factors are associated with this, and women were more likely to practise sports if they were less than 20 years of age, had no children and were of high socio-economic status.

FOOD AND NUTRITION PROGRAMMES IN MEXICO

Social policy in Mexico has included diverse food aid programmes designed to improve nutritional status in the country. Since the 1990s, the government has changed its food policy substantially, moving from generalized to selective targeting programmes, which have been demonstrated to be a more effective strategy for transferring resources and inputs to the poor. Among current programmes are ones for food distribution, micronutrient supplementation and fortification. Most of these include health and nutrition education components. The two most important national poverty alleviation integrated nutrition programmes are Oportunidades and Liconsa. In addition, the government has national food fortification and food coupon programmes directed to vulnerable populations. Several other initiatives are being implemented to address the double burden of disease: the Mexican Institute of Social Security's Preven-IMSS is an integrated health programme with an important nutrition and physical activity component; and the Ministry of Health has a programme for adults and elderly people that emphasizes prevention of non-communicable chronic diseases as one of its objectives.

The Oportunidades programme

The current comprehensive national programme for human development – Oportunidades – has three main components: nutrition, education and health. Among its diverse inputs are cash transfers, food coupons, food supplements for preschool children and pregnant women, and medical services (Barquera, Rivera-Dommarco and Gasca-Garcia, 2001). This programme has the general objective of supporting families that are suffering from extreme poverty by increasing the capacities of their members and increasing their education, health care and food options (Ministry of Social Development, 2000). In addition, it acts as a link to new services and development programmes to improve socio-economic conditions and quality of life.

The education component supports the registration and regular assistance of participating children through scholarships and school materials support. The health component has four specific strategies: delivering free health care services; preventing child undernutrition at the pre-gestational age through the delivery of food supplements; promoting and improving self-sufficiency through education; and improving families' health care and nutrition status. The food component provides direct cash transfer supports to beneficiary families in order to improve dietary quantity, quality and diversity with the aim of improving nutritional status. Supplement delivery and nutrition education are designed to reinforce adequate nutrition among infants and women.

In 2004, the programme had an annual budget of about US$2 273 million, and covered 5 million families in rural and urban areas in more than 70 000 locations of Mexico's 31 states. In order to measure the programme's impact on beneficiary families, external academic institutions designed evaluations (Bautista *et al.,* 2003; Behrman and Hoddinott, 2000; Parker, 2004; Rivera *et al.,* 2004b). Among the impacts observed during these evaluations are: a 12 percent reduction in the prevalence of disease in children under five years of age; an 8 percent increase in pregnant women's attendance at health care centres; a 59 percent increase in attendance at health care centres among the programme's beneficiaries; a 19 percent reduction in the number of days of morbidity among adults; a height increase in children under three years of age; and a 23.9 percent decrease in anaemia prevalence in children under two years of age.

The Liconsa programme

Iron deficiency anaemia (IDA) is a public health problem in Mexican children. Among children aged 12 to 23 months, MNS–2 (1999) found prevalence of anaemia of 49 percent, with iron deficiency (percentage transferrin saturation < 16) at 66 percent. Thus, approximately two-thirds of anaemic children were iron-deficient (Shamah-Levy *et al.,* 2003). Although total dietary iron intake in Mexican children is high relative to recommendations, the intake of haem iron is low, while the consumption of foods that inhibit iron absorption – such as phytates – is high.

Since 1944, a Federal Government programme – Liconsa – has been distributing low-cost milk to low-income families with children aged one to 11 years (Barquera, Rivera Dommarco and Gasca-Garcia, 2001). Since 1970, the milk distributed by this programme has been fortified with vitamins A and D according to sanitary norms. No further nutritional improvements were introduced until 2002, when in response to the high prevalence of IDA and its detrimental effects the government decided to fortify further the milk that Liconsa was distributing to about 5 million children. Every 400 ml daily ration of milk now contains 6.6 mg of iron (as gluconate), 6.6 mg of zinc (as oxide), 60 mg of vitamin C, 40.2 mcg of folic acid, and 0.55 mcg of vitamin B12.

The effectiveness and efficacy of the new fortified milk was assessed in 2003 among children aged 12 to 30 months at baseline by the National Institute of Public Health (Rivera *et al.,* 2005; Villalpando *et al.,* 2005). A double blind effectiveness trial was carried out at 17 milk distribution centres located in four states in Central Mexico. Baseline prevalence of anaemia fell in both the non-fortified (from 43.9 to 23.9 percent) and fortified (from 47.6 to 17.8 percent) groups by 20.0 and 29.8 percentage points, respectively. Thus, 33 percent of the reduction in the group receiving the fortified milk was attributable to the programme. The programme was effective in reducing the prevalence of anaemia in 12 to 30-month-old children over a six-month period. Extrapolating these results to all the children who were exposed to the programme during the course of the study, it is estimated that more than 50 000 cases of anaemia were prevented during the six-month period. A far larger number of older children (ages not evaluated) probably also benefited as a result of the programme. Based on these results, the National Institute of Public Health recommended that distribution of fortified milk be continued and incorporated into other food assistance programmes that distribute milk.

The Preven-IMSS programme

The Mexican Institute for Social Security (MISS) provides health services to approximately 50 percent of the population. As part of recent efforts to improve these services, MISS designed and implemented an integrated strategy for health programmes called Preven-IMSS, which focuses on a portfolio of preventive actions aimed at improving the health status of target populations. This is the first massive prevention programme to be launched by MISS. Starting in 2002, actions were organized for different age groups and vulnerable populations: children up to ten years of age; adolescents aged ten to 19 years; women aged 20 to 59 years; men aged 20 to 59 years; and elderly adults over 60 years of age. Activities include major food and nutrition, physical activity and health education components (MISS, 2005).

The main preventive actions among *children* focus on health promotion; nutrition education; disease control and prevention; early identification of diseases; oral health; vaccination; and miscellaneous issues such as personal hygiene, breastfeeding issues and fever control. For *adolescents* activities include physical activity; prevention of accidents, violence and addiction; oral health; sexual health and education; nutrition education; overweight and obesity detection and control; parasite treatment; vaccination; condom use; prevention of human immunodeficiency virus (HIV) and sexually transmitted diseases (STD); visual, auditory and postural defects; and reproductive health.

Activities directed to *women,* include health care education; physical activity; oral health; sexual education; prevention of addiction, accidents and family violence; nutrition education; detection and control of overweight and obesity; detection of anaemia; prevention of HIV and STD; prevention of tuberculosis; mammary cancer; cervical and uterine cancer; diabetes mellitus; high blood pressure; reproductive health; post-pregnancy care; climaterium attention and prevention of menopause complications; and vaccination. Activities for *men* focus on health care education; nutrition education; physical activity; diabetes mellitus; high blood pressure; obesity; prevention of accidents and violence; prevention of HIV and STD; prevention of tuberculosis; oral health; sexual education; and vaccination.

Among *older adults* the main preventive actions focus on health care education; physical activity; oral health; prevention of accidents and family violence; sexual education; prostate disease; detection and control of undernutrition, overweight and obesity; vaccination; prevention of tuberculosis; post-menopause care; mammary, cervical and uterine cancer; diabetes mellitus; and high blood pressure.

For each preventive action there is a set of activities and objectives designed for each age group. As part of the promotion strategy, this programme produces a magazine with health care information related to its activities, which is sold at newspaper shops nationwide. In addition, television advertisements are broadcast every day, focusing on lifestyles, nutrition and obesity, and promoting the magazine to the general public.

Ministry of Health programmes for non-communicable chronic diseases

The Ministry of Health has a number of programmes that include prevention as a component. Rather than being integrated health or nutrition programmes, these focus on the most relevant public health problems such as obesity, diabetes mellitus, high blood pressure and cancer. For each of these diseases there is a programme providing general management and prevention guidelines for government health service providers to follow.

DISCUSSION

At present, as in the past, there are many clear differences in dietary patterns and disease risk among different subpopulations of Mexico, including among different socio-economic groups, between rural and urban locations and among regions. As this case study makes clear, trends or rates of change in dietary patterns and disease risk over the last decade and a half also differ along the same lines. Many trends in dietary intake, food expenditure and health status are very clearly differentiated according to socio-economic status or income level, suggesting that poverty continues to play an important role in dietary patterns – perhaps more so than cultural differences by region or locality.

The case study found that total energy consumption dropped by about 9 percent between 1988 and 1999, but there is clear indication that underreporting was greater in 1999 than in 1988. Given the increases in per capita GNP, food availability and the prevalence of obesity observed in the country, the case study team consider that total energy intake is not decreasing in Mexico. Furthermore, the increase in total fat intake observed over the period is very likely to be underestimated, given the issues described earlier. Despite the marked underreporting of intakes in MNS–2, both fat intake and percentage of energy derived from fat had increased since MNS–1, 11 years earlier. This implies that the overall energy density of the diet also increased, which is consistent with the important shift in BMI distribution towards overweight and obesity. There is also consistency in the time-based trends observed: among women, the increase in percentage of energy intake from fat that occurred between MNS–1 and MNS–2 was greater among women of higher socio-economic status, as was the increase in prevalence of overweight and obesity that was determined from the same surveys. Nonetheless, in the absence of comparative data on physical activity, the relative contribution to weight gain of increased energy intake and decreased energy expenditure in the population cannot be assessed adequately. In order more fully to understand the contribution of dietary changes in this phenomenon, it is necessary to collect reliable information on physical activity and related lifestyle factors.

Vegetable fat was the greatest source of dietary fat in both rural and urban populations, with the second most important sources being milk in urban and maize products in rural areas. As the purchase of milk products continues to rise, a good public health measure to help reduce fat intake may be to promote greater availability of reduced-fat milk and milk products. Although maize is not likely to be an important source of fat *per se*, maize products are often prepared with fat (e.g., tortillas are fried in vegetable oil and tamales are prepared with lard). Education campaigns are the only way of achieving changes in such food preparation or selection practices.

While there is much concern about sugar intake and its likely contributions to obesity and chronic diseases, there is no satisfactory way of quantifying total sugar intake in Mexico. Dietary intake data derived from national surveys and food expenditure data are largely confined to capturing the intake of sugar added at the table or to dishes prepared at home, thereby omitting sugar derived from industrialized foods (e.g., sweet drinks, cookies, cakes), which may often be consumed outside the home. Soda may well be a sentinel food for total sugar intake, but other sources may be important contributors. In order adequately to quantify and monitor the intakes and specific food sources of sugar, it is necessary to include sugar in the food composition database used for dietary intake assessment in the future.

The gap that remains between lower- and upper-income quintiles in the purchase of micronutrient-rich foods (meats, milk and dairy products, vegetables and fruit) suggests that there will also remain inequalities in the micronutrient adequacy of the diet among socio-economic status groups. When expressed as percentage adequacy of intakes there was a clear trend of greater adequacies at higher socio-economic levels for vitamins A, D and B12, while the adequacies of iron, zinc, folate and calcium showed no apparent trend with socio-economic level. This can be explained by the fact that the foods that contribute most to intakes of vitamins A, D and B12 are also those for which the greatest intake and purchase discrepancies occur (i.e., meat, dairy products and vegetables). On the other hand, the foods that contribute most to intakes of calcium, iron, zinc and folate come from food groups with similar intakes or purchase distributions among different socio-economic or income groups (i.e., maize products, legumes). Biochemical indicators for micronutrient status determined in MNS–2 conform with the dietary data. Most notable is the apparent increase in the prevalence of anaemia with an apparent decrease in the adequacy of iron intakes among women.

While the adequacy of intakes of vitamins A and B12 and folate has improved substantially, iron adequacy decreased by about 30 percent. (Although the iron adequacy estimate according to United States dietary recommendations was > 100 percent, the case study team considers this to be an overestimate of the true adequacy because the bioavailability of iron from the Mexican diet – about 7.5 percent [Rivera *et al.,* 2005] – is far lower than the 18 percent assumed for the United States population [Institute of Medicine, 2001].) Tortillas and beans have high contents of phytic acid and other food components that inhibit iron absorption, so percentage iron adequacies are not useful predictors of iron intakes without accounting for bioavailability.

Owing to the underreporting of intakes in MNS–2, it is likely that the changes in nutrient intakes and adequacy were underestimated. The case study team therefore thought that expressing nutrient intakes as density (nutrient/100 kcal) may be more indicative of the quality of the diet. It was found that the density of iron was also lower in MNS–2 than in MNS–1, which could be attributable either to differences in the iron content of some key foods in the food composition tables used in each of the surveys, or to the increased energy density of the diet, as suggested by the greater percentage of energy derived from fats in MNS–2. Vitamin A and folate showed large increases in total intake, and higher densities of these nutrients were also found in MNS–2, despite the underreporting and the increased energy density of the diet. Interestingly, the trend was reversed for the folate densities recorded in MNS–1 and MNS–2; while folate densities were higher in higher socio-economic levels and urban areas in MNS–1, the opposite was true in MNS–2. This is difficult to interpret, as biochemical data for overt folate deficiency do not suggest that such a trend exists (Shamah-Levy *et al.,* 2003).

Although large quantities of resources are being directed to programmes to prevent micronutrient deficiencies among the poorest populations (e.g., Oportunidades and Liconsa), certain micronutrient deficiencies – such as those of iron, zinc and folate – still persist in populations of moderate to high socio-economic status levels. The fortification of maize flour with iron and folate is mandatory in Mexico, but only about half the population consumes maize products made from flour. The other half derives maize products from a nixtamalized maize dough, which is currently not fortified because of technological and logistic difficulties. One possible public health measure would be to encourage industry to fortify additional basic foods with micronutrients in order to reach the entire population.

Prevalence of child stunting, which is a result of chronic undernutrition early in life, showed a substantial decrease (23 percent) between the two surveys. This change was not homogeneous, however, and prevalence was as high as 38 percent in the South region, 40.1 percent in rural locations and 40.8 percent in the lowest socio-economic quintile. Stunting therefore continues to be a main public health and nutrition challenge. Mexico has a higher prevalence of stunting than the average for Latin American countries (Rivera *et al.,* 2004a). This problem coexists with another common form of malnutrition – overweight and obesity, which is present in high prevalence in not only developed regions but also in rural locations and the South. Overall, 62.3 percent of men and 67.6 percent of women over 20 years of age are overweight or obese. This represents relative increases of 19.8 and 13.6 percent, respectively, in only seven years. Diabetes mellitus, which is commonly associated with overweight and obesity, has also doubled in recent years (Barquera, Rivera Dommarco and Gasca-Garcia, 2001).

Although the collection and interpretation of data on nutritional and health status may have become more standardized, there is a great need to adapt and improve methods of data collection on dietary habits. The important impact of underreporting on the interpretation of dietary intake data is of concern, and efforts should be made to develop innovative methods of quantifying food consumption, both inside and outside the home. This is of great concern because underreporting appears to be intimately linked with degree of overweight. Trends in the quality of food consumed outside the home may be of special concern, but these cannot be assessed with the data that are available at present; food consumption outside the home may be underestimated in the food intake surveys, and the types of foods consumed outside the home are not captured by food expenditure studies. Although food expenditure data may reflect consumption in urban areas fairly accurately, they are less reliable among rural populations, where domestic agricultural production contributes more to total intakes. Surveys combining food intake data for both inside and outside the home, expenditure data and food production data would be useful for monitoring dietary trends and informing the design of dietary and food policy interventions.

CONCLUSIONS

Although this analysis used cross-sectional surveys that lack the conditions necessary to establish causal relationships, the information obtained can be used to identify opportunities for action and research aimed at reducing and controlling nutrition-related diseases. The double burden of disease related to under- and overnutrition represents one of Mexico's most challenging public health problems (Ministry of Health, 2001). Anaemia and other micronutrient deficiencies coexist with rising levels of obesity, type-2 diabetes, high blood pressure and dislipidaemias. Clearly, nutritional recommendations must be developed to avoid collateral negative effects, but this is not a simple task. For example, there is a need for interventions that promote higher energy intakes, particularly among schoolchildren from marginal communities and among vulnerable groups. This situation needs to be addressed through targeted interventions with educational messages promoting adequate calorie intakes that include the consumption of a variety of fruits and vegetables, and not only energy-dense foods as these can be a factor in the development of future nutrition-related chronic diseases. Funds for the prevention and control of obesity in children and adults should become a health expenditure priority in order to avoid the higher costs generated by cardiovascular risk factors associated with excess body fat and adiposity.

In Mexico, the diet is changing rapidly and becoming more homogeneous across regions, locations and socio-economic groups. The same is happening with morbidity and mortality patterns. Increasing urbanization and modernization could reduce, for better or worse, the polarization currently observed in the country. The national food fortification policy (i.e., folate, zinc, iron) and the distribution of micronutrient supplements to vulnerable groups are playing a key role in reducing the prevalence of stunting and micronutrient deficiencies. The importance of MNS–2's recommendation to improve the targeting of nutrition inputs to the most vulnerable populations has been recognized, as has the importance of evaluating the impact of food and nutrition programmes in order to distribute scarce resources more efficiently.

Overweight, obesity and other diet-related non-communicable diseases are currently the main nutrition and public health problem. The success of focusing health policy on preventing infectious diseases, improving reproductive health and preventing some micronutrient deficiencies has modified the shape of Mexico's population pyramid. It is now necessary to adapt the health systems to face a relatively new type of disease, which can only be prevented and controlled by organized responses involving not only policy planners, but also communities, families and people interacting with the health and education sectors to regulate, promote and inform about diseases. The coexistence of obesity and undernutrition has been documented in diverse Latin American countries (Garret and Ruel, 2003; Popkin, Richards and Montiero, 1996; Sawaya *et al.,* 2003).

In Mexico, an estimated 6.1 percent of overweight mothers have a stunted child under five years of age (Barquera, 2005). This fact, together with the high prevalence of obesity in adults, suggests that programmes aimed at improving nutrition should always consider the high risk of obesity. Thus, nutrition programmes must address the double burden of disease, and focus on comprehensive integrated approaches – including the promotion of adequate nutrition through education and environmental changes – rather than trying to solve the problem though one-dimensional interventions such as the use of supplements or food coupons. The health sector, which for a long time was concerned exclusively with infections and other acute health problems, must now pay attention to nutrition-related chronic diseases, which are a very different type of health problem. Thus, health professionals require training so that they can encourage appropriate behavioural change in the population (WHO, 2002).

Among the topics that should be addressed through integrated nutrition programmes are general education on health and nutrition in order to foster a culture where healthy eating practices are promoted, increasing the consumption of fruits and vegetables, and implementing regulatory measures focused on food and nutrition in public schools (Kennedy, Nantel and Shetty, 2004). Studies need to be carried out in order to identify cost-effective policies aimed at preventing, reducing and controlling nutrition-related diseases, including behavioural change and environmental modifications. Such interventions could use the experiences and data from previous studies (mostly conducted in developed countries) as a reference. However, given the unique characteristics of Mexico – in terms of heterogeneous socio-economic development, infrastructure and cultural background – it will be necessary to evaluate the feasibility and impact of these. Improved methods of data collection for evaluation and monitoring purposes should also be emphasized.

Various institutions, universities and government bodies are implementing a wide range of research projects in Mexico to improve the understanding of and to prevent nutrition-related and other emerging diseases. The results of these studies will contribute to ameliorating and controlling these health challenges (Fernald, Gertler and Olaiz, 2005; Fernald *et al.*, 2004; Rivera *et al.*, 2005; 2004b).

REFERENCES

ACC/SCN. 2000. *Fourth Report of the World Nutrition Situation.* Geneva, Administrative Committee on Coordination/Subcommittee on Nutrition (ACC/SCN) in collaboration with the International Food Policy Research Institute (IFPRI).

ACC/SNC. No date. *The world nutrition situation. Nutrition life cycle.* Geneva, in collaboration with IFPRI.

Barquera, S. 2005. *The nutrition and epidemiologic transition in Mexico: analysis of three national surveys. Article 3: Coexistence of maternal central adiposity and child stunting in Mexico.* Boston, Massachusetts, USA, Tufts University, Friedman School of Nutrition Science and Policy. (Ph.D. thesis)

Barquera, S., Rivera-Dommarco, J. & Gasca-Garcia, A. 2001. Policies and programs of food and nutrition in Mexico. *Salud Publica Mex.,* 43(5): 464–77.

Bautista, S., Martínez, S., Bertozzi, S. & Gertler, P. 2003. *Evaluación del efecto de Oportunidades sobre la utilización de servicios de salud en el medio rural. Evaluación de resultados de impacto del Programa Oportunidades de Desarrollo Humano Oportunidades.* Mexico City, Ministry of Social Development.

Becerra, C., Gonzalez, G.F., Villena, A. & de la Cruz, D. 1998. Prevalencia de anemia en gestantes. Hospital Regio. *Rev. Panam. Salud Publica,* 3(5): 285–291.

Behrman, J. & Hoddinott, J. 2000. *An evaluation of the impact of Progresa on pre-school child height.* Washington, DC, International Food Policy Research Institute (IFPRI).

Bobadilla, J., Frenk, J., Lozano, R., Frejka, T. & Stern, C. 1993. The epidemiologic transition and health priorities. *In* D. Jamison, ed. *Disease control priorities in developing countries.* New York, Oxford University Press.

Campirano, F., Barquera, S., Rivera, J., Hernández-Prado, B., Flores, M. & Monterrubio, E. 2001. Estimation of energy under-reporting in obese and non-obese Mexican women using different equations: Analysis of the Mexican Nutrition Survey. *Ann. Nutr. Metabol.,* 45(s1): 146.

Cole, T., Bellizzi, M., Flegal, K. & Dietz, W. 2000. Establishing a standard definition for child overweight and obesity worldwide: international survey. *BMJ,* 320: 1240–1243.

de Onis, M. & Blössner, M. 2003. The World Health Organization Global Database on Child Growth and Malnutrition: methodology and applications. *Int. J. Epidemiol.,* 32: 518–526.

Diallo, M.S., Diallo, T.S., Diallo, F.B., Diallo, Y., Camara, A.Y., Onivogui, G., Keita, N. & Diawo, S.A. 1995. Anemia and pregnancy. Epidemiologic, clinical and prognostic study at the university clinic of the Ignace Deen Hospital, Conakry (Guinea). *Rev. Fr. Gynecol. Obstet.,* 90(3): 138–141.

Expert Committee on the Diagnosis and Classification of Diabetes Mellitus. 2005. Report on the diagnosis and classification of diabetes mellitus. *Diabetes Care,* 26 (suppl. 1 January).

Expert Panel on Detection, Evaluation and Treatment of High Blood Cholesterol in Adults. 2001. Excecutive summary of the third report of the national cholesterol education program (NCEP) expert panel on detection, evaluation and treatment of high blood cholesterol in adults (adult treatment panel III). *JAMA,* 287: 356–359.

Fernald, L., Gertler, P. & Olaiz, G. 2005. Impacto de mediano plazo del Programa Oportunidades sobre la obesidad y las enfermedades crónicas en áreas rurales. *In* B. Hernandez, ed. *Evaluación externa de impacto del programa oportunidades 2004,* Vol. 2. Cuernavaca, Mexico, National Insitute of Public Health.

Fernald, L., Gutierrez, J., Neufeld, L., Olaiz, G., Bertozzi, S., Mietus-Snyder, M. & Gertler, P. 2004. High prevalence of obesity among the poor in Mexico. *JAMA,* 291(21): 2544–2545.

Flores, M., Melgar, H., Cortés, C., Rivera, M., Rivera-Dommarco, J. & Sepulveda, J. 1998. Consumo de energía y nutrimentos en mujeres mexicanas en edad reproductiva. *Salud Publica Mex.,* 40: 161–171.

Frenk, J., Bobadilla, J.L., Stern, C., Frejka, T. & Lozano, R. 1991. Elements for a theory of transition in health. *Salud Publica Mex.,* 33(5): 448–462. (in Spanish)

Frith-Terhune, A., Cogswell, M. & Kettel Khan, L. 2000. Iron deficiency anemia: higher prevalence in Mexican American than in non-Hispanic white females in the third National Health and Nutrition Examination Survey, 1988–1994. *Am. J. Clin. Nutr.,* 72: 963–968.

Garret, J. & Ruel, M. 2003. *Stunted children–overweight mother pairs: an emerging policy concern?* Washington DC, International Food Policy Research Institute (IFPRI).

González-Cossío, T., Moreno-Macías, H., Rivera, J., Villalpando, S., Shamah-Levy, T., Monterrubio, E. & Hernández-Garduño, A. 2003. Breast-feeding practices in Mexico: Results from the Second National Nutrition Survey, 1999. *Salud Publica Mex.,* 45(suppl. 4): S477–S489.

Hernandez-Diaz, S., Peterson, K., Dixit, S., Hernandez, B., Parra, S., Barquera, S., Sepulveda, J. & Rivera, J.A. 1999. Association of maternal short stature with stunting in Mexican children: common genes vs common environment. *Euro. J. Clin. Nutr.,* 53: 938–945.

Hernandez, B., de Haene, J., Barquera, S., Monterrubio, E., Rivera, J., Shamah, T., Sepulveda, J., Haas, J. & Campirano, F. 2003. Factors associated with physical activity among Mexican women of childbearing age. *Rev. Panam. Salud Publica,* 14(4): 235–245.

INEGI. 2002. *La salud y la atención de la salud en el campo mexicano. Programa Emergente de Salud para el Campo 2003–2006.* Mexico City. National Institute of Informatics, Statistics and Geography (INEGI).

Institute of Medicine. 2000a *Dietary reference intakes for calcium, phosphorus, magnesium, vitamin D and fluoride.* Washington, DC, Institute of Medicine/National Academy Press.

Institute of Medicine. 2000b. *Dietary reference intakes for thiamin, riboflavin, niacin, vitamin B6, folate, vitamin B12, panthothenic acid, biotin and choline.* Washington, DC, Institute of Medicine/National Academy Press.

Institute of Medicine. 2001. *Dietary reference intakes for vitamin A, vitamin K, arsenic, boron, chromium, copper, iodine, iron, manganese, molybdenum, nickel, silicon, vanadium, and zinc.* Washington, DC, Institute of Medicine/National Academy Press.

Institute of Medicine. 2002. *Dietary reference intakes for energy, carbohydrate, fiber, fat, fatty acids, cholesterol, protein, and amino acids (macronutrients).* Washington, DC, Institute of Medicine/National Academy Press.

Kennedy, G., Nantel, G. & Shetty, P. 2004. Globalization of food systems in developing countries: a synthesis of country case studies. *In* FAO. *Globalization of food systems in developing countries: impact on food security and nutrition,* FAO Food and Nutrition Paper No. 83. Rome, FAO.

Long-Dunlap, K., Rivera-Dommarco, J., Rivera-Pasquel, M., Hernández-Avila, M. & Lezana, M. 1995. Feeding patterns of Mexican infants recorded in the 1988 National Nutrition Survey. *Salud Publica Mex.,* 37: 120–129.

Martinez, H., Gonzalez-Cossío, T., Flores, M., Rivera, J., Lezana, M. & Sepulveda, J. 1995. Anemia en edad reproductiva. Resultados de una encuesta probabilistica nacional. *Salud Publica Mex.,* 37: 108–119.

Ministry of Health. 2001. *Programa Nacional de Salud 2001–2006. La democratización de la salud en México; hacia un sistema universal de salud.* Mexico City.

Ministry of Social Development. 2000. *Programa Institucional Oportunidades, Plan Nacional de Desarrollo.* Mexico City.

MISS. 2005. *Preven-IMSS.* Available at www.imss.gob.mx/imss/imss_sitios/dpm/servicios/prevenimss. Mexican Institute of Social Security (MISS).

Muñoz, M., Chávez, A., Pérez-Gil, F., Roldán, J., Ledesma, J. & Hernández-Cordero, S. 1996. *Tablas de valor nutritivo de los alimentos de mayor consumo en México.* Mexico City, Federal Government of Mexico.

Must, A., Dallal, G. & Dietz, W. 1991. Reference data for obesity: 85th and 95th percentiles of body mass index (wt/ht^2) and triceps skinfold thickness. *Am. J. Clin. Nutr.,* 53: 839–846.

National Research Council. 1989. *Recommended dietary allowances.* Washington, DC, National Academy Press.

Olaiz, G., Rojas, R. & Barquera, S. 2003. *Encuesta Nacional de Salud 2000. Tomo 2. La salud de los adultos.* Cuernavaca, Mexico, National Institute of Public Health.

Parker, S. 2004. *Evaluación de impacto de Oportunidades sobre la inscripción, reprobación y abandono escolar. Resultados de la Evaluación Externa del Programa de Desarrollo Humano Oportunidades 2003.* Mexico City, Ministry of Social Development.

Popkin, B., Richards, M. & Montiero, C. 1996. Stunting is associated with overweight in children of four nations that are undergoing the nutrition transition. *J. Nutrition,* 126(12): 3009–3016.

Resano-Perez, E., Mendez-Ramirez, I., Shamah-Levy, T., Rivera, J. & Sepulveda-Amor, J. 2003. Methods of the National Nutrition Survey 1999. *Salud Publica Mex.,* 45(suppl. 4): S558–S564.

Rivera, J., Barquera, S., Campirano, F., Campos, I., Safdie, M. & Tovar, V. 2002. Epidemiological and nutritional transition in Mexico: rapid increase of non-communicable chronic diseases and obesity. *Public Health Nutrition,* 14(44): 113–122.

Rivera, J., Barquera, S., Gonzalez-Cossio, T., Olaiz, G. & Sepulveda, J. 2004a. Nutrition transition in Mexico and other Latin American countries. *Nutrition Reviews,* 62(7): s1–s9.

Rivera, J.A., Sotres-Alvarez, D., Habicht, J.P., Shamah, T. & Villalpando, S. 2004b. Impact of the Mexican program for education, health, and nutrition (Progresa) on rates of growth and anemia in infants and young children: a randomized effectiveness study. *JAMA,* 291(21): 2563–2570.

Rivera, J., Shamah, T., Villalpando, S., Cuevas, L. & Mundo, V. 2005. Effectiveness of an iron-fortified milk distribution program in reducing the rates of anemia of infants and young children in Mexico. *FASEB Journal,* Abstract No. 848.3.

Rivera-Dommarco, J., Shamah, T., Villalpando-Hernández, S., González de Cossío, T., Hernandez, B. & Sepulveda, J. 2001. *Encuesta Nacional de Nutrición 1999.* Cuernavaca, Mexico, National Institute of Public Health, Ministry of Health, INEGI.

Sawaya, A., Martins, P., Hoffman, D. & Roberts, S. 2003. The link between childhood undernutrition and risk of chronic diseases in adulthood: a case study of Brazil. *Nutr. Rev.,* 61(5 Pt 1): 168–175.

Sepulveda-Amor, J., Angel Lezana, M., Tapia-Conyer, R., Luis Valdespino, J., Madrigal, H. & Kumate, J. 1990. Nutritional status of pre-school children and women in Mexico: results of a probabilistic national survey. *Gaceta Medica de Mexico,* 126(3): 207–224.

Shamah-Levy, T., Villalpando, S., Rivera, J.A., Mejia-Rodriguez, F., Camacho-Cisneros, M. & Monterrubio, E.A. 2003. Anemia in Mexican women: a public health problem. *Salud Publica Mex.,* 45(suppl. 4): S499–S507.

Souci, S., Fachmann, W. & Kraut, H. 2000. *Food composition and nutrition tables.* sixth edition. Stuttgart, Germany, Medpharm Scientific Publishers, CRC Press.

University of California. 1998. *Food composition database.* Davis, California, USA.

USDA-ARS. 1999. USDA National Nutrient Database for Standard Reference, Release 13. Nutrient Data Laboratory Home. United States Department of Agriculture, Agricultural Research Service (USDA-ARS)

Villalpando, S., Shamah, T., Robledo, R., Rivera, J., Merlos, C. and Lara, Y. 2005. Efficacy of iron fortified milk in the rates of anemia and iron status of infants and young children in Mexico. *FASEB Journal,* Abstract No. 848.5.

WHO. 1983. *Measuring change in nutrition status: Guidelines for assessing the nutritional impact of supplementary feeding programmes.* Geneva, World Health Organization (WHO).

WHO. 1992. *International statistical classification of diseases and related health problems (ICD-10).* Geneva.

WHO. 1994. *Study Group. Prevention of diabetes mellitus.* WHO Technical Report Series No. 844. Geneva.

WHO. 1995. *Physical status: The use and interpretation of anthropometry.* Report of a WHO Expert Consultation, WHO Technical Report Series No. 854. Geneva.

WHO. 2002. *Non-communicable diseases and mental health. Innovative care for chronic conditions: building blocks for action.* Geneva.

WHO/PAHO. 1978. *International classification of diseases.* Revision 9 (ICD-9). Washington, DC, WHO/Pan-American Health Organization (PAHO).

World Bank. 2005. *World Development Indicators.* New York.

Wuleung, W. & Flores, M. 1962. *Tabla de Composición de Alimentos para uso en América Latina.* Guatemala, Institute of Nutrition of Central America and Panama, Inter-Departmental Committee on Nutrition for National Protection (INCAP-ICNND).

Zavaleta, N., Caulfield, L. & Garcia, T. 2000. Changes in iron status during pregnancy in Peruvian women receiving prenatal iron and folic acid supplements with or without zinc. *Clinical Nutr.,* 71(4): 956–961.

ANNEX 1 :ACHIEVEMENT OF POPULATION NUTRIENT INTAKE GOALS, 1988 AND 1999

Gender	Age group (years)	% of population with 15–30% energy intake from fat		% of population with < 10% energy intake from free sugars[1]	% of population with 55–75% energy intake from carbohydrate		% of population consuming ≥ 400 g/day fresh fruits and vegetables
		1988	1999	1999	1988	1999	1999
Male	10–11	-	36.7	99.4	-	45.1	-
Female	10–11	-	30.5	99.4	-	41.7	-
	12–19	41.2	36.9	95.0	43	47.2	9.3
	20–29	41.8	37.6	98.1	45.1	41.9	8.6
	30–39	39.4	40.3	97.3	44.9	43.2	10.7
	40–49	41.2	45.0	98.5	42.8	48.2	8.3
	12–49	40.9	39.6	97.4	44.2	44.3	9.3

[1] Determined from intakes of sugar added to foods or beverages in the household only. Will be recalculated in a future report to include sugar derived from composite dishes and industrialized foods.
Sources: MNS–1, 1988; MNS–2, 1999.

ANNEX 2: MEAN DAILY CONSUMPTION PER AE AND PERCENTAGE OF TOTAL EXPENDITURE ON FOOD, BY FOOD GROUP AND REGION, 1989 TO 2002

Food group	Year	North					Central					Mexico City					South				
		%¹	%²	g/d³	(RC)⁴	Per capita (g/d)⁵	%¹	%²	g/d³	(RC)⁴	Per capita (g/d)⁵	%¹	%²	g/d³	(RC)⁴	Per capita (g/d)⁵	%¹	%²	g/d³	(RC)⁴	Per capita (g/d)⁵
Cereals (g)	1989	94.3	15	346	(1.00)	326	94.7	17	428	(1.00)	406	94.7	12	361	(1.00)	341	93.0	20	545	(1.00)	507
	1992	92.5	16	332	(0.96)	307	95.7	17	403	(0.94)	385	95.2	13	342	(0.95)	325	93.5	20	458	(0.84)	428
	1994	94.4	19	333	(0.96)	314	94.7	18	362	(0.85)	343	95.2	12	312	(0.87)	297	93.3	21	409	(0.75)	381
	1996	95.1	18	346	(1.00)	329	96.6	22	395	(0.92)	382	96.6	16	363	(1.01)	351	94.4	23	434	(0.80)	410
	1998	94.4	19	317	(0.92)	299	94.5	21	372	(0.87)	351	96.7	15	334	(0.93)	323	93.5	22	418	(0.77)	391
	2000	95.4	18	328	(0.95)	313	96.2	20	366	(0.86)	352	95.1	15	321	(0.89)	306	94.4	22	463	(0.85)	437
	2002	95.6	19	312	(0.90)	298	96.2	21	380	(0.89)	365	97.7	16	324	(0.90)	317	94.9	21	401	(0.74)	381
Meats (g)	1989	80.1	29	116	(1.00)	93	78.4	32	102	(1.00)	80	90.3	38	147	(1.00)	133	72.2	34	127	(1.00)	92
	1992	76.0	26	127	(1.10)	97	82.6	28	112	(1.10)	93	92.7	33	160	(1.08)	148	75.0	29	114	(0.90)	86
	1994	80.8	29	134	(1.16)	109	83.9	29	114	(1.12)	96	92.1	34	163	(1.11)	151	79.3	31	119	0.94	95
	1996	82.3	24	117	(1.01)	96	80.9	23	92	(0.90)	75	93.0	31	139	(0.95)	129	78.5	27	107	(0.84)	84
	1998	78.8	24	118	(1.02)	93	79.7	24	102	(0.99)	81	93.3	30	148	(1.00)	138	75.4	28	117	(0.92)	88
	2000	82.6	23	140	(1.21)	116	84.5	23	112	(1.09)	94	90.5	27	148	(1.00)	134	82.0	29	129	(1.01)	106
	2002	81.7	24	134	(1.16)	110	83.1	22	109	(1.06)	90	93.7	30	157	(1.07)	147	84.1	28	126	(0.99)	106
Eggs (g)	1989	61.7	6	72	(1.00)	44	60.5	5	53	(1.00)	32	66.3	4	63	(1.00)	42	61.6	5	44	(1.00)	27
	1992	56.8	5	68	(0.94)	38	60.1	4	56	(1.06)	34	69.8	4	66	(1.04)	46	66.0	6	48	(1.09)	32
	1994	57.2	6	72	(1.00)	41	59.7	4	56	(1.06)	33	67.6	4	68	(1.07)	46	60.4	5	47	(1.06)	29
	1996	62.1	7	67	(0.92)	41	64.0	6	48	(0.91)	31	74.6	6	63	(1.00)	47	64.1	7	45	(1.01)	29
	1998	56.8	6	65	(0.91)	37	60.7	5	53	(0.99)	32	70.9	4	62	(0.98)	44	57.9	5	50	(1.12)	29
	2000	58.5	5	69	(0.96)	41	62.6	4	55	(1.05)	35	69.5	4	68	(1.08)	47	64.9	4	52	(1.17)	34
	2002	54.5	5	72	(0.99)	39	57.2	4	56	(1.06)	32	66.5	3	62	(0.99)	41	62.1	5	55	(1.24)	34
Milk and dairy products (g)	1989	82.4	14	264	(1.00)	218	75.1	15	301	(1.00)	226	85.4	10	304	(1.00)	260	57.7	13	183	(1.00)	106
	1992	77.7	14	283	(1.07)	220	76.8	13	306	(1.02)	235	87.3	11	319	(1.05)	279	57.6	11	176	(0.96)	101
	1994	83.8	16	277	(1.05)	232	75.9	13	294	(0.98)	223	88.3	11	328	(1.08)	289	58.5	11	178	(0.97)	104
	1996	83.2	15	243	(0.92)	202	76.5	15	279	(0.93)	213	88.6	12	295	(0.97)	262	58.5	11	170	(0.93)	99
	1998	83.3	16	242	(0.92)	202	76.1	15	301	(1.00)	229	90.3	12	305	(1.00)	275	55.7	12	186	(1.01)	103
	2000	85.7	16	258	(0.98)	221	81.6	15	297	(0.99)	243	87.5	13	309	(1.02)	271	61.6	11	167	(0.91)	103
	2002	85.1	16	263	(1.00)	224	82.3	14	297	(0.99)	244	89.0	12	369	(1.22)	329	62.4	10	163	(0.89)	102
Legumes (g)	1989	41.4	5	87	(1.00)	36	57.1	5	71	(1.00)	40	46.1	3	51	(1.00)	24	65.3	7	75	(1.00)	49
	1992	38.0	5	78	(0.90)	30	58.2	6	70	(1.00)	41	48.0	3	53	(1.02)	25	67.3	7	68	(0.90)	46
	1994	39.7	5	76	(0.87)	30	57.0	5	67	(0.95)	38	45.1	3	55	(1.07)	25	60.0	7	68	(0.90)	41
	1996	51.4	7	74	(0.85)	38	64.5	8	71	(1.00)	46	52.7	4	52	(1.02)	27	63.0	7	64	(0.85)	40
	1998	42.8	5	77	(0.88)	33	57.4	6	68	(0.96)	39	51.7	4	53	(1.03)	27	59.3	9	65	(0.86)	38
	2000	39.4	4	73	(0.84)	29	55.8	4	65	(0.92)	36	45.8	3	57	(1.10)	26	61.9	5	69	(0.92)	43
	2002	29.3	5	73	(0.84)	21	49.5	5	65	(0.91)	32	42.9	3	50	(0.98)	21	61.7	7	66	(0.88)	41
Fats and oils (g)	1989	41.5	5	62	(1.00)	26	44.9	5	48	(1.00)	22	34.8	3	49	(1.00)	17	54.2	6	45	(1.00)	24
	1992	37.7	5	73	(1.18)	28	42.8	4	50	(1.03)	21	36.4	3	56	(1.15)	20	49.4	5	43	(0.96)	21

Year																			
1996	49.6	6	62	(1.01)	31	48.9	6	48	(1.00)	24	40.0	4	53	(1.09)	21	48.2	6	43	(0.95)	21
1998	38.5	5	63	(1.02)	24	41.1	4	51	(1.05)	21	35.0	4	56	(1.15)	20	44.9	5	50	(1.11)	22
2000	43.0	4	73	(1.18)	31	43.0	4	53	(1.10)	23	43.3	3	66	(1.36)	29	43.9	4	52	(1.15)	23
2002	31.6	4	66	(1.06)	21	34.2	4	59	(1.22)	20	32.2	3	57	(1.16)	18	46.0	4	56	(1.24)	26

Data weighted by the expansion factors.

Sample sizes: 1989, 11 531 (expanded cases, 15 947 773); 1992, 10 508 (expanded cases, 17 798 635); 1994, 12 815, (expanded cases, 19 440 278); 1996, 14 042 (expanded cases, 20 467 038); 1998, 10 952 (expanded cases, 22 163 568); 2000, 10 089 (expanded cases, 23 452 319); 2002, 17167 (expanded cases, 24 650 169).

[1] Percentage of families reporting expenditure during the seven-day survey period.

[2] Percentage of total food expenditure.

[3] Mean grams per AE among families reporting expenditure.

[4] Relative change.

[5] Mean grams per capita.

Source: MHIES, 1989 to 2002.

ANNEX 3: MEAN DAILY CONSUMPTION PER AE AND PERCENTAGE OF TOTAL EXPENDITURE ON FOOD, BY FOOD GROUP AND REGION, 1989 TO 2002

Food group	Year	Region North					Central					Mexico City					South				
		%1	%2	g/d3	(RC)4	Per capita (g/d)5	%1	%2	g/d3	(RC)4	Per capita (g/d)5	%1	%2	g/d3	(RC)4	Per capita (g/d)5	%1	%2	g/d3	(RC)4	Per capita (g/d)4
Vegetables (g)	1989	80.0	8	126	(1.00)	101	87.3	9	145	(1.00)	127	87.2	9	213	(1.00)	185	84.5	9	118	(1.00)	100
	1992	72.2	8	130	(1.03)	94	86.1	9	147	(1.01)	126	90.1	11	236	(1.11)	212	86.4	11	119	(1.00)	103
	1994	74.0	9	133	(1.06)	99	86.2	11	153	(1.05)	132	87.5	11	217	(1.02)	190	84.4	11	120	(1.02)	102
	1996	78.6	7	139	(1.10)	109	87.6	8	150	(1.03)	131	90.8	10	229	(1.08)	208	85.4	9	130	(1.10)	111
	1998	71.1	8	122	(0.97)	87	86.4	9	148	(1.02)	128	89.6	10	216	(1.01)	193	83.1	11	128	(1.08)	106
	2000	73.8	8	140	(1.11)	104	86.7	9	165	(1.14)	143	86.8	9	212	(1.00)	184	84.5	10	143	(1.21)	121
	2002	68.7	7	141	(1.12)	97	84.2	8	167	(1.15)	140	90.4	10	231	(1.08)	209	87.3	10	158	(1.34)	138
Fruits (g)	1989	44.9	5	125	(1.00)	56	57.4	6	147	(1.00)	84	73.4	7	211	(1.00)	155	44.9	5	129	(1.00)	58
	1992	44.3	4	147	(1.18)	65	60.4	6	171	(1.17)	103	79.4	7	243	(1.16)	193	41.3	5	169	(1.32)	70
	1994	46.2	5	148	(1.19)	69	62.4	5	169	(1.15)	105	76.2	7	253	(1.20)	193	44.4	6	174	(1.35)	77
	1996	49.6	4	132	(1.06)	66	55.2	5	150	(1.03)	83	74.9	5	207	(0.98)	155	43.4	4	147	(1.14)	64
	1998	42.9	4	119	(0.96)	51	54.6	5	149	(1.01)	81	73.0	6	197	(0.93)	144	39.3	5	138	(1.08)	54
	2000	47.8	5	160	(1.29)	77	61.3	6	200	(1.37)	123	79.3	7	233	(1.11)	185	46.4	5	163	(1.27)	76
	2002	38.3	5	166	(1.33)	63	56.5	5	177	(1.21)	100	73.8	6	221	(1.05)	163	44.8	5	143	(1.11)	64
Sugar (g)	1989	26.4	3	78	(1.00)	21	41.8	3	67	(1.00)	28	26.5	3	94	(1.00)	25	51.7	4	80	(1.00)	41
	1992	27.2	3	80	(1.02)	22	37.4	3	68	(1.01)	25	30.1	2	84	(0.88)	25	49.6	5	82	(1.03)	41
	1994	27.4	3	76	(0.98)	21	38.7	3	71	(1.06)	28	28.8	3	89	(0.94)	25	50.5	5	79	(0.99)	40
	1996	34.1	4	74	(0.95)	25	43.4	4	59	(0.88)	26	33.5	3	69	(0.73)	23	50.1	5	74	(0.92)	37
	1998	27.6	3	69	(0.89)	19	40.6	3	62	(0.93)	25	31.3	3	79	(0.84)	25	44.1	4	79	(0.99)	35
	2000	28.5	3	79	(1.01)	22	42.0	3	64	(0.96)	27	33.3	2	74	(0.78)	25	46.7	4	75	(0.94)	35
	2002	23.2	3	86	(1.10)	20	37.2	3	71	(1.06)	26	29.6	2	72	(0.76)	21	47.4	5	86	(1.08)	41
Soda (ml)	1989	72.6	8	259	(1.00)	188	51.6	5	174	(1.00)	90	46.7	4	226	(1.00)	106	33.8	4	169	(1.00)	57
	1992	71.5	10	274	(1.06)	196	56.5	5	182	(1.05)	103	46.6	4	234	(1.04)	109	35.4	6	177	(1.05)	63
	1994	71.1	5	299	(1.15)	213	55.4	4	197	(1.13)	109	52.0	4	237	(1.05)	123	39.3	4	198	(1.17)	78
	1996	69.2	9	248	(0.96)	172	54.9	6	177	(1.02)	97	42.9	5	201	(0.89)	86	41.3	7	174	(1.02)	72
	1998	73.4	11	281	(1.09)	207	62.4	9	221	(1.27)	138	53.4	6	217	(0.96)	116	47.0	8	206	(1.22)	97
	2000	80.4	12	335	(1.29)	269	64.8	8	231	(1.33)	150	57.0	6	236	(1.04)	134	46.7	8	217	(1.28)	101
	2002	78.4	12	315	(1.22)	247	66.0	8	221	(1.27)	146	58.7	6	231	(1.02)	136	47.7	8	200	(1.18)	96
Alcohol (ml)	1989	7.0	10	262	(1.00)	18	4.8	7	148	(1.00)	7	4.9	10	82	(1.00)	4	6.6	12	154	(1.00)	10
	1992	7.1	11	239	(0.91)	17	4.2	9	169	(1.14)	7	4.9	8	165	(2.01)	8	5.4	8	211	(1.37)	11
	1994	8.1	12	255	(0.98)	21	7.2	8	201	(1.36)	15	4.7	6	98	(1.19)	5	6.5	10	141	(0.91)	9
	1996	7.1	9	209	(0.80)	15	5.8	8	209	(1.41)	12	3.5	5	103	(1.25)	4	5.2	10	180	(1.17)	9
	1998	10.7	10	181	(0.69)	19	6.2	7	134	(0.91)	8	4.7	8	113	(1.38)	5	5.5	12	290	(1.88)	16
	2000	8.9	12	208	(0.79)	18	7.3	10	174	(1.17)	13	7.3	11	93	(1.13)	7	5.0	12	199	(1.29)	10

Tobacco (g)																				
1989	18.8	7	6.0	(1.00)	1.12	16.9	5	2.9	(1.00)	0.50	24.2	4	2.9	(1.00)	0.71	8.2	4	1.8	(1.00)	0.15
1992	29.2	9	3.8	(0.64)	1.11	23.7	6	2.6	(0.87)	0.61	25.5	5	3.2	(1.08)	0.81	11.3	4	1.7	(0.91)	0.19
1994	15.7	9	3.1	(0.53)	0.49	13.1	7	3.4	(1.17)	0.45	11.2	6	5.1	(1.73)	0.57	6.1	6	2.9	(1.58)	0.17
1996	10.7	6	3.5	(0.59)	0.37	12.4	5	3.4	(1.14)	0.42	7.6	5	3.9	(1.31)	0.29	5.9	4	2.3	(1.27)	0.14
1998	11.3	7	3.5	(0.58)	0.39	10.9	6	3.5	(1.17)	0.38	9.0	4	5.7	(1.92)	0.51	4.6	4	2.8	(1.56)	0.13
2000	11.2	7	4.0	(0.68)	0.45	11.4	7	3.6	(1.22)	0.41	9.6	4	4.0	(1.36)	0.39	5.3	6	2.8	(1.56)	0.15
2002	9.0	10	15.9	(2.66)	1.42	9.0	6	6.4	(2.17)	0.58	9.8	4	5.2	(1.75)	0.51	2.2	5	7.4	(4.10)	0.17

Data weighted by the expansion factors.

Sample sizes: 1989, 11 531 (expanded cases, 15 947 773); 1992, 10 508 (expanded cases, 17 798 635); 1994, 12 815, (expanded cases, 19 440 278); 1996, 14 042 (expanded cases), 20 467 038; 1998, 10 952 (expanded cases, 22 163 568); 2000, 10 089 (expanded cases, 23 452 319); 2002, 17167 (expanded cases, 24 650 169).

[1] Percentage of families reporting expenditure during the seven-day survey period.

[2] Percentage of total food expenditure.

[3] Mean grams or millilitres per AE among families reporting expenditure.

[4] Relative change.

[5] Mean grams or millilitres per capita.

Source: MHIES, 1989 to 2002.

ANNEX 4: MEDIAN DAILY FOOD EXPENDITURE OUTSIDE THE HOME AS PERCENTAGE OF TOTAL FOOD EXPENDITURE, 1989 TO 2002

Year*	Region								Location[1]			
	North		Central		Mexico City		South		Urban		Rural	
1989	2	(1.00)	21	(1.00	28	(1.00	19	(1.00)	24	(1.00)	16	(1.00)
1992	2	(1.00)	25	(1.19	28	(1.00	19	(1.00)	25	(1.04)	20	(1.25)
1994	2	(0.96)	26	(1.24	34	(1.21	24	(1.26)	28	(1.17)	20	(1.25)
1996	2	(1.09)	18	(0.86	28	(1.00	21	(1.11)	24	(1.00)	18	(1.13)
1998	2	(1.00)	20	(0.95	27	(0.96	20	(1.05)	24	(1.00)	17	(1.06)
2000	2	(1.00)	22	(1.05	25	(0.89	24	(1.26)	25	(1.04)	19	(1.19)
2002	2	(1.22)	23	(1.10	31	(1.11	23	(1.21)	28	(1.17)	20	(1.25)

Data weighted by the expansion factors.

Sample sizes: 1989, 11 531 (expanded cases, 15 947 773); 1992, 10 508 (expanded cases, 17 798 635); 1994, 12 815, (expanded cases, 19 440 278); 1996, 14 042 (expanded cases, 20 467 038); 1998, 10 952 (expanded cases, 22 163 568); 2000, 10 089 (expanded cases, 23 452 319); 2002, 17167 (expanded cases) 24 650 169).

[1] Location: urban > 15 000 inhabitants; rural ≤ 15 000 inhabitants.

Source: MHIES, 1989 to 2002.

ANNEX 5: MEAN DAILY CONSUMPTION PER AE AND PERCENTAGE OF TOTAL EXPENDITURE ON FOOD, BY FOOD GROUP AND LOCATION, 1989 TO 2002

| Food groups | Year | Location[1] | | | | | | | | | |
| | | Urban | | | | | Rural | | | | |
		%[2]	%[3]	g/d[4]	(RC)[5]	Per capita (g/d)[6]	%[2]	%[3]	g/d[4]	(RC)[5]	Per capita (g/d)[6]
Cereals (g)	1989	95.8	14	387	(1.00)	371	91.1	22	534	(1.00)	486
	1992	95.3	15	358	(0.92)	341	92.7	22	470	(0.88)	436
	1994	94.9	16	335	(0.87)	318	93.4	24	412	(0.77)	385
	1996	96.1	18	354	(0.91)	340	95.0	25	452	(0.85)	429
	1998	95.8	17	333	(0.86)	319	92.5	24	427	(0.80)	395
	2000	96.0	17	335	(0.86)	321	94.1	23	461	(0.86)	434
	2002	97.0	18	325	(0.84)	315	94.3	24	428	(0.80)	403
Meats (g)	1989	87.9	35	132	(1.00)	116	61.5	29	86	(1.00)	53
	1992	88.2	30	136	(1.04)	120	66.5	25	89	(1.04)	59
	1994	90.0	32	141	(1.07)	127	71.5	26	94	(1.09)	67
	1996	88.8	27	124	(0.94)	110	73.1	23	87	(1.01)	64
	1998	88.1	27	132	(1.01)	117	68.4	24	92	(1.06)	63
	2000	88.6	26	141	(1.07)	125	77.4	24	108	(1.25)	83
	2002	89.1	26	142	(1.08)	127	78.2	23	102	(1.19)	80
Eggs (g)	1989	66.1	5	60	(1.00)	40	54.1	6	45	(1.00)	24
	1992	67.4	4	60	(0.99)	40	54.0	6	51	(1.14)	28
	1994	63.8	4	61	(1.01)	39	54.7	6	52	(1.15)	28
	1996	69.2	6	59	(0.98)	41	60.1	7	45	(1.01)	27
	1998	64.1	5	60	(0.99)	38	55.6	6	49	(1.11)	28
	2000	64.3	4	63	(1.04)	40	63.0	5	54	(1.21)	34
	2002	61.3	4	62	(1.02)	38	57.6	5	57	(1.28)	33
Milk and dairy products (g)	1989	83.9	13	296	(1.00)	249	52.5	13	179	(1.00)	94
	1992	84.2	12	302	(1.02)	254	52.2	13	187	(1.05)	98
	1994	85.8	13	302	(1.02)	259	54.2	13	178	(1.00)	97
	1996	85.6	14	277	(0.94)	237	57.5	11	181	(1.01)	104
	1998	85.8	14	283	(0.95)	242	54.4	13	206	(1.15)	112
	2000	86.6	14	282	(0.95)	244	61.0	13	203	(1.14)	124
	2002	86.6	13	303	(1.02)	262	63.2	12	200	(1.12)	127
Legumes (g)	1989	52.1	4	63	(1.00)	33	60.6	9	87	(1.00)	53
	1992	53.3	4	63	(1.00)	33	60.5	9	78	(0.89)	47
	1994	49.3	4	60	(0.96)	30	59.5	9	77	(0.89)	46
	1996	55.9	6	59	(0.94)	33	64.3	10	76	(0.87)	49
	1998	51.2	5	59	(0.95)	30	58.4	10	75	(0.85)	44
	2000	48.4	3	60	(0.95)	29	59.9	7	76	(0.87)	45
	2002	42.2	4	57	(0.90)	24	57.8	7	73	(0.83)	42
Fats and oils (g)	1989	41.4	4	51	(1.00)	21	53.3	8	47	(1.00)	25
	1992	38.4	3	54	(1.05)	21	51.0	6	50	(1.05)	25
	1994	39.8	3	57	(1.11)	23	51.8	6	53	(1.12)	28
	1996	42.7	5	52	(1.02)	22	54.4	7	48	(1.02)	26
	1998	36.8	4	54	(1.06)	20	47.0	6	53	(1.13)	25
	2000	40.3	3	64	(1.25)	26	48.5	5	53	(1.11)	25
	2002	31.4	3	57	(1.11)	18	46.4	5	61	(1.29)	28

Vegetables (g)	1989	86.7	8	166	(1.00)	144	82.3	9	101	(1.00)	83
	1992	85.2	9	168	(1.01)	144	81.8	11	105	(1.04)	86
	1994	83.8	10	166	(1.00)	139	82.8	12	115	(1.14)	96
	1996	86.6	8	181	(1.09)	157	84.4	9	122	(1.20)	103
	1998	83.5	9	170	(1.03)	142	81.8	11	118	(1.17)	97
	2000	83.0	8	178	(1.07)	148	84.4	11	138	(1.36)	116
	2002	82.7	8	184	(1.11)	153	84.1	10	154	(1.52)	129
Fruits (g)	1989	62.6	6	166	(1.00)	104	37.4	6	107	(1.00)	40
	1992	63.2	5	195	(1.18)	123	37.1	5	132	(1.23)	49
	1994	64.7	6	194	(1.17)	126	40.7	5	141	(1.32)	57
	1996	64.0	5	180	(1.08)	115	38.9	4	114	(1.06)	44
	1998	59.3	5	166	(1.01)	99	37.0	5	120	(1.12)	45
	2000	63.8	6	208	(1.26)	133	46.5	6	157	(1.47)	73
	2002	57.6	5	195	(1.18)	112	43.9	5	140	(1.31)	61
Sugar (g)	1989	32.2	2	74	(1.00)	24	53.4	4	78	(1.00)	42
	1992	31.5	3	74	(1.01)	23	49.9	5	79	(1.01)	39
	1994	31.1	3	71	(0.97)	22	51.3	6	81	(1.04)	42
	1996	35.0	3	65	(0.88)	23	52.3	5	72	(0.93)	38
	1998	33.2	3	72	(0.98)	24	44.0	5	72	(0.92)	32
	2000	33.7	2	72	(0.97)	24	48.7	4	73	(0.93)	35
	2002	29.3	3	70	(0.95)	20	47.9	5	89	(1.15)	43

Data weighted by the expansion factors.

Sample sizes: 1989, 11 531 (expanded cases, 15 947 773); 1992, 10 508 (expanded cases, 17 798 635); 1994, 12 815, (expanded cases, 19 440 278); 1996, 14 042 (expanded cases, 20 467 038); 1998, 10 952 (expanded cases, 22 163 568); 2000, 10 089 (expanded cases, 23 452 319); 2002, 17167 (expanded cases, 24 650 169).

[1] Location: urban > 15 000 inhabitants; rural ≤ 15 000 inhabitants.

[2] Percentage of families reporting expenditure during the seven-day survey period.

[3] Percentage of total food expenditure.

[4] Mean grams per AE among families reporting expenditure.

[5] Relative change.

[6] Mean grams per capita.

Source: MHIES, 1989 to 2002.

ANNEX 6: MEAN DAILY CONSUMPTION PER AE AND PERCENTAGE OF TOTAL EXPENDITURE ON FOOD, BY FOOD GROUP AND LOCATION, 1989 TO 2002

Food group *	Year	Location[1]									
		Urban					Rural				
		%[2]	%[3]	ml/d[4]	(RC)[¥]	Per capita (ml/d)[6]	%[2]	%[3]	ml/d[4]	(RC)[5]	Per capita (ml/d)[6]
Soda (ml)	1989	70.8	5	224	(1.00)	122	29.2	6	150	(1.00)	61
	1992	70.9	6	226	(1.01)	133	29.1	8	173	(1.15)	70
	1994	67.6	5	251	(1.12)	148	32.4	4	178	(1.19)	79
	1996	69.2	6	217	(0.97)	123	30.8	7	161	(1.07)	68
	1998	70.0	8	245	(1.09)	161	30.0	9	202	(1.35)	93
	2000	70.9	8	273	(1.22)	185	29.1	9	212	(1.41)	103
	2002	70.9	8	259	(1.16)	178	29.1	9	201	(1.34)	99
Alcohol (ml)	1989	62.1	8	169	(1.00)	9	37.9	12	165	(1.00)	10
	1992	69.7	9	195	(1.15)	11	30.3	10	215	(1.30)	9
	1994	59.9	9	177	(1.05)	12	40.1	13	206	(1.25)	15
	1996	63.9	8	162	(0.95)	9	36.1	11	233	(1.41)	12
	1998	65.9	8	151	(0.89)	11	34.1	13	258	(1.56)	15
	2000	67.8	11	161	(0.95)	12	32.2	12	193	(1.17)	12
	2002	68.5	12	269	(1.59)	12	31.5	11	215	(1.31)	8
Tobacco (g)	1989	71.7	5	3.7	(1.00)	0.65	28.3	6	2.8	(1.00)	0.34
	1992	73.0	6	2.9	(0.78)	0.72	27.0	8	2.6	(0.96)	0.40
	1994	64.6	6	3.3	(0.90)	0.40	35.4	9	3.6	(1.32)	0.37
	1996	66.4	5	3.6	(0.98)	0.35	33.6	6	2.6	(0.95)	0.22
	1998	69.0	5	4.1	(1.11)	0.40	31.0	6	3.0	(1.10)	0.21
	2000	68.7	5	3.9	(1.04)	0.38	31.3	6	3.2	(1.17)	0.25
	2002	75.0	6	9.5	(2.57)	0.80	25.0	9	5.7	(2.09)	0.28

Data weighted by the expansion factors.
Sample sizes: 1989, 11 531 (expanded cases, 15 947 773); 1992, 10 508 (expanded cases, 17 798 635); 1994, 12 815, (expanded cases, 19 440 278); 1996, 14 042 (expanded cases, 20 467 038); 1998, 10 952 (expanded cases, 22 163 568); 2000, 10 089 (expanded cases, 23 452 319); 2002, 17167 (expanded cases, 24 650 169).
[1] Location: urban > 15 000 inhabitants; rural ≤ 15 000 inhabitants.
[2] Percentage of families reporting expenditure during the seven-day survey period.
[3] Percentage of total food expenditure.
[4] Mean grams or millilitres per AE among families reporting expenditure.
[5] Relative change.
[6] Mean grams or millilitres per capita.
Source: MHIES, 1989 to 2002.

ANNEX 7: MAIN CAUSES OF DEATH BY LOCATION, 1990 AND 2001

Cause	Rural[1]					Urban[1]					National				
	1990		2001			1990		2001			1990		2001		
	n	%	n	%	Change	n	%	n	%	Change	n	Rate[2]	n	Rate[2]	Change
Diabetes mellitus	7 936	4	14 976	9	88.7	17 711	8	34 829	13	96.7	25 647	29.9	49 805	49.1	64.2
Coronary heart disease	10 011	5	14 581	3	45.6	19 392	9	30 626	11	57.9	29 403	34.3	45 207	44.5	30.0
Cirrhosis and others hepatic chronic diseases	7 994	4	11 004	5	37.7	9 591	4	14 335	5	49.5	17 585	20.5	25 339	24.9	21.8
Cerebrovascular disease	8 591	4	9 859	4	14.8	11 076	5	15 729	6	42.0	19 667	22.9	25 588	25.2	10.0
Chronic obstructive pulmonary diseases	5 423	3	6 196	4	14.3	6 960	3	9 694	4	39.3	12 383	14.4	15 890	15.6	8.5
Acute respiratory infections low	13 636	7	5 672	3	-58.4	10 108	5	7 272	3	-28.1	23 744	27.7	12 944	12.7	-53.9
Malnutrition caloric protean	7 331	4	4 682	3	-36.1	4 309	2	3 873	1	-10.1	11 640	13.6	8 555	8.4	-37.9
Asphyxia and injury in during birth	5 984	3	4 225	3	-29.4	8 587	4	6 781	3	-21.0	14 571	17.0	11 006	10.8	-36.1
Aggression (homicide)	7 403	4	4 091	2	-44.7	6 382	3	5 695	2	-10.8	13 785	16.1	9 786	9.6	-40.0
Nephritis and nephrosis	3 477	2	3 992	2	14.8	4 752	2	6 457	2	35.9	8 229	9.6	10 449	10.3	7.4
Hypertensive diseases	2 858	1	3 847	2	34.6	-	-	-	-	-	-	-	-	-	-
Motor vehicle accidents	3 660	2	3 293	2	-10.0	4 585	2	4 888	2	6.6	8 245	9.6	8 181	8.1	-16.1
Intestinal infectious diseases	15 403	8	2 862	2	-81.4	6 674	3	-	-	-	22 077	25.7	-	-	-
Alcohol consumption	2 473	1	2 537	2	2.6	-	-	-	-	-	-	-	-	-	-
Malign bronchial or tracheal tumours	1 761	1	2 087	1	18.5	3 245	1	4 308	2	32.8	5 006	5.8	6 395	6.3	8.0

[1] Location: rural < 15 000 inhabitants; urban ≥ 15 000 inhabitants.
[2] Rate per 100 000 inhabitants.
Total population: 1990 = 85 784 220; 2001 = 101 453 433.
Source: INEGI. 2002.

Dietary changes and their health implications in the Philippines

M.R.A. Pedro and R.C. Benavides, Food and Nutrition Research Institute, and C.V.C. Barba, Institute of Human Nutrition and Food, University of the Philippines Los Baños

INTRODUCTION

In recent years, social, economic and demographic developments within the Southeast Asian region have accelerated to varying degrees. Nutritional status has improved widely in many countries, with some experiencing a transition in nutrition or the double burden of undernutrition and overnutrition. This report examines evidence of the dietary changes and whether or not the Philippines, in common with some of its neighbours in the region, is facing the double burden of under- and overnutrition.

The population of the Philippines was estimated at 85.5 million people in 2005, compared with 76.5 million in 2000. Growing at an annual 2.11 percent, the population is expected to reach 102.8 million in 2015. The Philippine economy has grown in recent years, with gross national product (GNP) expanding at an average of 5.05 percent and gross domestic product (GDP) at an average of 4.52 percent from 2001 to 2004 (NEDA, 2005). However, there has been a boom–bust pattern of growth over the 30 years from 1970 to 2000 (Figure 1). The sharp fall in growth of the economy from 1982 to 1984 coincided with political and economic crises. The dip from 1988 to 1990 reflected the impact of successive political shocks (i.e., coup attempts) and several natural disasters, as well as an economic slowdown that affected not only the Philippines but also the rest of the world; the Philippines was not spared the effects of the Asian crisis in 1997 (Templo, 2003).

FIGURE 1
Real GNP/GDP growth, 1970 to 2000

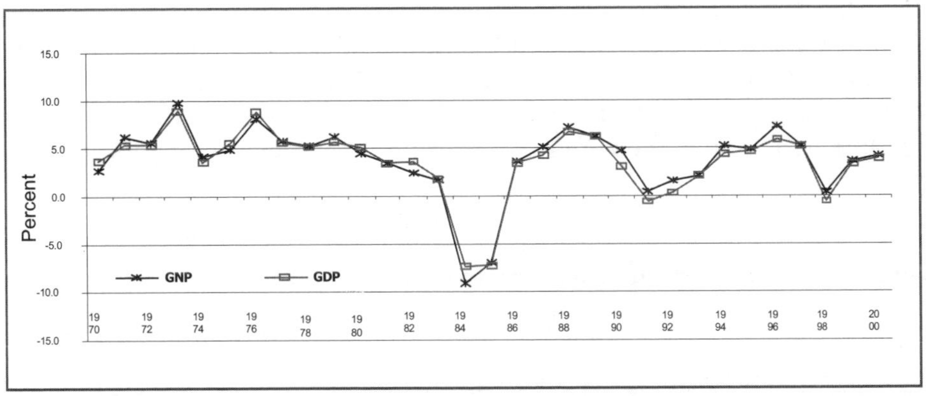

Source: Templo, 2003.

The Philippines has made remarkable progress in improving life expectancy and reducing infant mortality. Life expectancy has increased from 58 to about 70 years over the past 30 years, and infant mortality has decreased from 60 to 29 deaths per 1 000 live births

(UNDP, 2004). In addition to improvements in health care services, high levels of literacy (94 percent simple literacy rate), high primary school enrolment rates (90 percent elementary participation rate) and access to safe water (80 percent) have contributed to these remarkable reductions in infant mortality and increased life expectancy.

TABLE 1
Key development indicators

Indicator	Value	Year
Estimated total population	85.5 million	2005
Population growth rate	2.11%	2000–2005
Human development index (HDI), HDI rank	0.753, 83rd	2002
Gender development index (GDI), GDI rank	0.751, 66th	2002
GDP per capita (US$)	1 026	2004
Social sector expenditure (as % of total expenditure)	42.81%	2003
Share of poorest quintile in income or consumption	4.7%	2003
Share of richest quintile in income or consumption	53.3%	2003
Male life expectancy: (at birth in years)	67.2	2003
Female life expectancy: (at birth in years)	72.5	2003
Unemployment rate	10.9%	2004
Underemployment rate	16.9%	2004
Poverty headcount ratio (% of families below national poverty line) (Preliminary)	24.7%	2003
Population with access to safe water supply	80%	2002
Simple literacy rate	94%	2003
Elementary school participation rate	90%	2002
Under-five mortality rate (per 1 000 children)	40	2003
Maternal mortality rate (per 100 000 live births)	172	1998

Sources: NEDA; UNDP, 2004; Family Income Expediture Survey (FIES), 2003

The age structure of the population is also shifting. The dependency ratio (defined as the ratio of people aged 0 to 14 years or over 64 years per 100 people aged 15 to 64 years) has decreased from 88 to 64 over the past 30 years. This decrease is due more to changes in the proportion of children, rather than elderly people. The child dependency ratio dropped from 88 to 64, while the elderly dependency ratio has remained constant at 6 (UN Population Division, 2004).

The last 30 years witnessed rapid urbanization in the Philippines, with the urban proportion of the population rising from 32 percent in 1970 to 54 percent in 1995. In 2001, 59 percent of the population lived in urban areas, and the urban growth rate was 5.14 percent (Table 2). The proportion of urban population is expected to increase to 68 percent in 2015.

TABLE 2
Trends in urban and rural growth rates, 1960 to 2001

Indicators	1960	1970	1975	1980	1990	1995	2001
Percentage urban	29.8	31.8	33.3	37.2	48.6	54.1	59.1
Urban growth (%)	2.7	4.0	3.0	4.9	5.0	5.0	5.14
Rural growth (%)	2.5	2.6	2.6	1.5	0.3	0.3	-

Source: Population Commission, 2002.

A new methodology for estimating poverty was adopted in 1997. Figure 2 illustrates the trends in prevalence of poverty among Philippine families over the last 17 years, and compares the estimates made with the earlier official methodology, which applied a constant Engel's coefficient (i.e., the proportion of food expenditure to total expenditure), with estimates from the new methodology, which employs a changing Engel's coefficient (i.e., depending on the year). Poverty decreased between 1991 and 1997, while GNP and GDP were increasing (Figure 1), and then increased slightly or remained unchanged (depending on the method used to estimate poverty) during a short period of growth slump brought on by the Asian economic crisis. The estimates indicate that in 2003, 24.7 percent of Philippine families were considered poor (measured as income below the poverty threshold of 12 267 Philippine pesos [p]), compared with 28.4 percent in 2000.

FIGURE 2
Trends in prevalence of poverty among Philippine families, 1988 to 2000

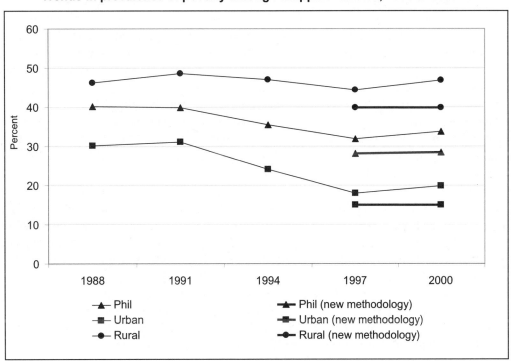

Source: Reyes, 2003.

While poverty has decreased in urban areas, it persists essentially as a rural phenomenon. Three out of four poor people reside in rural areas. In 2000, 13 percent of urban and 36 percent of rural families were considered poor, or had income below the poverty threshold of 12 267 p per year (Reyes, 2003). Disparities in poverty are also seen across different regions of the country, with the autonomous region of Muslim Mindanao, the Caraga region and the Zamboanga Peninsula – all in Mindanao or Southern Philippines – being the poorest (NEDA, 2005).

Income distribution in the Philippines has remained largely unequal as measured by the GINI ratio, which assigns values ranging from 0 to 1 – the closer to 1 the more unequal. Compared with its Asian neighbours, the Philippines has wider disparity in terms of income distribution. Between 1998 and 2000, the Philippine GINI ratio worsened from 0.4446 to 0.4822, but then improved slightly to reach 0.4660 in 2003.

DATA SOURCES USED IN THE CASE STUDY

The major sources of data used in this case study are the surveys of the Food and Nutrition Research Institute, Department of Science and Technology (FNRI-DOST). These are periodic National Nutrition Surveys (NNS), and regional updating of the nutritional status of Philippine children. The dietary data reported here were obtained from the 1978, 1982, 1987, 1993 and 2003 NNS, while the data on nutritional status of various population groups and nutrition-related risk factors for non-communicable diseases (NCDs) among adults come from Regional Updating of the Nutritional Status of Children and the 1993, 1998 and 2003 NNS. Data on mortality trends are from the Field Health Service Information System (FHSIS) of the Department of Health. These are components of the Philippine Statistical System, and provide vital inputs to the country's nutrition, health and development programmes.

National Nutrition Surveys

FNRI-DOST conducts NNS every five years to obtain information on the nutritional status of the Philippine population through recording food consumption in households and using 24-hour recall for children and pregnant and lactating women. Surveys were carried out in 1978, 1982, 1987, 1993, 1998 and 2003, each of which included anthropometric, biochemical and clinical assessment of nutritional status. A food consumption survey component was carried out in all the surveys except for that of 1998.

Nutritional status is assessed by anthropometric measurements of all age groups, biochemical indicators (serum retinol and haemoglobin) in children aged 0 to five years and pregnant and lactating women, and urinary iodine excretion of children aged six to 12 years and pregnant and lactating women. Anthropometric measurements include weight and height for children and adults, and recumbent length for children under two years of age. Nutritional status of children 0 to ten years of age is assessed using the World Health Organization/National Center for Health Statistics (WHO/NCHS) growth curves (WHO, 1995); for pre-adolescents and adolescents aged 11 to 19 years body mass index (BMI)-for-age is used (Must, Dallal and Dietz, 1991), and for adults aged 20 years and over WHO's recommendations for BMI are used (WHO, 1995). The nutritional status of pregnant women is based on a Philippine reference population (Magbitang *et al.,* 1988).

The fifth (1998) and sixth (2003) NNS also included measurements of blood pressure, fasting blood glucose and blood lipids (triglyceride, cholesterol, HDL and LDL) for individuals aged 20 years and over in order to assess hypertension, diabetes and dyslipidaemia as nutritional factors associated with chronic degenerative diseases among adults.

Household food consumption data are collected through one-day household food weighing, which involves weighing all foods in "as-purchased" (AP) form before they are cooked. Food is weighed before breakfast, lunch and dinner. Food waste (i.e., edible and inedible food parts that are thrown away, given to pets, etc.) and plate waste are weighed after meals. Beginning and end inventories of all non-perishable food items such as coffee, sugar, salt and other condiments are taken, and food recall by all household members for foods eaten outside the home is recorded. The information generated is the aggregated measure of the foods eaten and the energy and nutrient intakes of all household members, which are divided by the number of people in the household during the reference period in order to derive per capita intakes. Energy and nutrient intakes from the foods consumed are based on the Philippines Food Composition Table (FCT); nutrient values of fortified foods, particularly of vitamin A, iron and iodine, are from food labels. The nutrient values in the latest Philippine FCT (1997) were revised using results from interlaboratory food composition analyses. The revision included new iron values for about 30 food items, many of which were fresh and processed fish.

Per capita percentage adequacies of energy and nutrient intakes were estimated for each household, after computing for the mean recommended dietary allowances (RDAs) or recommended energy and nutrient intakes (RENI), by summing the RDAs of each household member and dividing by the number of household members. There have been two revisions to the original 1976 RDAs for the Philippines, one in 1989 and the other in 2002. The original 1976 RDAs were used in the 1978, 1982 and 1987 NNS, the 1989 revision was used to determine energy and nutrient adequacy in the 1993 survey, and the 2002 revision was used in 2003. (For more details see Annexes 1, 2 and 3.)

Assessment of the dietary intake of children aged 0 to five years and of pregnant and lactating women was included in the 1987, 1993 and 2003 NNS. Information on the food intake of these groups is obtained through 24-hour food recall. Mothers are asked to recall all the foods and beverages consumed by their children in the previous 24 hours. Aids to assist the estimation of portion sizes include using standard household measures, such as cups and spoons, and an album of standard food portion sizes, which the mother can look at to estimate the amount consumed by the child.

Sampling design of NNS
All the NNS employed a multi-stage stratified sampling design, and covered all regions of the country. In the 1978, 1982, 1987 and 1993 NNS, the number of sample provinces or cluster areas for each of the regions and Metro Manila was selected based on probability proportional to the number of households. From each sample province, an equal allocation of urban and rural barangays[1] (i.e., four urban and four rural barangays) were selected at random. In the case of Metro Manila, eight barangays – all urban – were selected per cluster. A systematic sample of ten households per barangay, with replacements, were then selected in the final stage of sampling. In the 1998 and 2003 surveys, all provinces were covered and the number of barangays or enumeration areas was based on probability proportional to the number of households. The 2003 NNS adopted the Master Sample developed by the Philippine Statistical System for the 2003 Family Income and Expenditure Survey (FIES) and other national surveys.

For the 1978, 1982, 1987, 1993 and 2003 NNS, the final sampling unit was the household, and all the members of each household were included. In the 1998 NNS (when there was no household food consumption survey), the final sampling unit was the individual – i.e., subjects or respondents aged 0 to five years, six to 12 years, 13 to 19 years and 20 years and over were sampled within sample barangays.

Regional Updating of the Nutritional Status of Children
The nutritional status of children aged 0 to ten years is updated two to three years after each NNS, using anthropometry. The first updating survey was carried out in 1989/1990. The sampling design of the regional updating surveys is similar to that of the 1998 NNS, in which the barangay was the primary sampling unit and children aged 0 to ten years were the secondary sampling units. The update surveys generate national- and regional-level estimates.

---

[1] A barangay is the smallest local government unit in the Philippines, and is similar to a village.

TABLE 3
Sampling design of NNS and the Regional Updating of the Nutritional Status of Children, 1978 to 2003

	1978[1]	1982[1]	1987[1]	1989/ 1990[2]	1993[1]	1996[2]	1998[1]	2001[2]	2003[1]
Sampling design	Stratified 3-stage	Stratified 3-stage	Stratified 3-stage	Stratified 2-stage	Stratified 3-stage	Stratified 2-stage	Stratified 2-stage	Stratified 2-stage	Stratified 2-stage
Stratification	Region Urban/rural	Region Urban/rural	Region Urban/rural	Region Province Urban/rural	Region Province Urban/rural	Region Province Urban/rural	Region Province Urban/rural	Region Province Urban/rural	Region Province
Sampling units	Province Barangay Household	Province Barangay Household	Province Barangay Household	Barangay Individual	Barangay Household	Barangay Individual	Barangay Individual	Barangay Individual	Barangay Household
Sample size									
Households	2 800	2 280	3 200		4 050		–		5 514
0–5 years				6 932	4 977	10 385	28 698	10 634	4 111
6–10 years				5 382	3 223	15 530	3 040	1 791	3 436
11–19 years					4 111		6 079		4 856
≥ 20 years					8 480		9 299		11 685
Pregnant women					850		2 880		593
Lactating mothers					1 105		2 990		1 201

[1] NNS: there was no food consumption survey component in NNS 1998.
[2] Regional Updating of the Nutritional Status of Children included anthropometry among Philippine children only.

The Field Health Service Information System and Philippine Health Statistics

FHSIS is a nationwide compilation of health indicators collected by city and provincial health offices from health facilities such as district hospitals, rural health units (RHUs) and barangay health stations (BHS). The indicators collected reflect the state of health programmes: Maternal and Child Health, Family Planning, the Expanded Programme on Immunization, Nutrition, Dental, Communicable and Non-Communicable Disease Prevention and Control, and Environmental Health. Philippine Health Statistics (PHS) provides summary statistical data of births and deaths registered and reported in a given year, as well as the notified diseases reported in FHSIS.

DIETARY CHANGES 1978 TO 2003
Trends in food consumption

Food consumption in Philippine households has been analysed in two forms: as per capita intake in grams, and converted into kilocalories (kcal) of dietary energy. Food consumption recorded as raw as-purchased (AP) weight in grams has not changed significantly over the last 25 years. However, when converted into dietary energy, the mean daily per capita energy intake increased from 1 804 kcal in 1978 to 1 905 kcal in 2003 (Figure 3). Thus, while food intake has not increased in terms of weight, the energy density of diets is increasing. Figure 3 also demonstrates fluctuations in intake as measured both in grams and in kcal. The decreasing food intakes from 1982 to 1987 and from 1987 to 1993 may be related to the negative growth of the Philippine economy up to 1986 and from 1988 to 1991, the modest progress in reducing poverty, and lingering income inequality. The positive growth from 1991 to 1996 and from 1998 to 2003, on the other hand, reflects the increasing food intake from 1993 to 2003.

FIGURE 3
Trends in mean per capita food intake (g/day and kcal/day) in Philippine households, 1978 to 2003

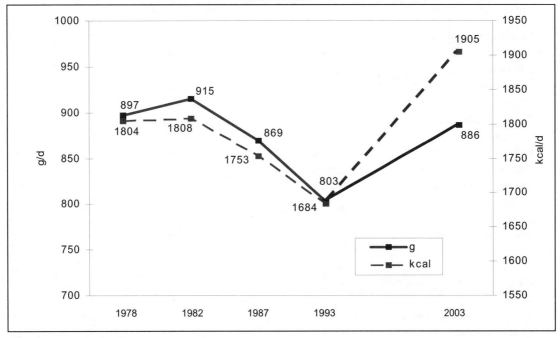

Sample sizes: 1978, 2 800; 1982, 2 280; 1987, 3 200; 1993, 4 050; 2003, 5 514.
Sources: NNS, 1978; 1982; 1987; 1993; 2003.

Trends in per capita food consumption (in grams) by food group

Generally, the overall dietary pattern in Philippine households remains that of rice, vegetables and fish (Table 4), which contributed 34, 13 and 12 percent, respectively, of food weight in 2003. The proportional contributions of rice and fish have remained similar over the past 25 years, while the proportion of vegetables has declined slightly.

TABLE 4
Trends in mean daily per capita food consumption, by food group, 1978 to 2003

Food group/sub-group	Consumption (g/day, raw, AP)				
	1978	**1982**	**1987**	**1993**	**2003**
Cereals and cereal products	367	356	345	340	364
Rice and products	308	304	303	282	303
Maize and products	38	34	24	36	31
Other cereals and products	21	18	18	22	30
Starchy roots and tubers	37	42	22	17	19
Sugars and syrups[1]	19	22	24	19	24
Fats and oils[2]	13	14	14	12	18
Fish, meat and poultry	133	154	157	147	185
Fish and products	102	113	111	99	104
Meat and products	23	32	37	34	61
Poultry	7	10	9	14	20
Eggs	8	9	10	12	13
Milk and milk products	42	44	43	44	49
Whole milk				35	35
Milk products				9	14
Dried beans, nuts and seeds[3]	8	10	10	10	10
Vegetables	145	130	111	106	111
Green leafy, yellow vegetables	34	37	29	30	31
Other vegetables	111	93	82	76	80
Fruits	104	102	107	77	54
Vitamin C-rich foods	30	18	24	21	12
Other fruits	74	84	83	56	42
Miscellaneous	21	32	26	19	39
Beverages[4]					26
Condiments					13
Total (g/day)	**897**	**915**	**869**	**803**	**886**

Sample sizes: 1978, 2 800; 1982, 2 280; 1987, 3 200; 1993, 4 050; 2003, 5 514.
[1] Includes soft drinks (sugar content), sherbet and similar preparations.
[2] Includes grated coconut and coconut milk (fat).
[3] Includes mung beans, soybeans, peanuts and other dried beans, nuts.
[4] Includes coffee, tuba (local wine), alcoholic beverages and others.
Numbers may not add up to totals owing to rounding off.
Sources: NNS, 1978; 1982; 1987; 1993; 2003.

Among the cereals, the intake of rice and its products has generally not changed; the mean per capita intake fluctuated from 282 g in 1993 – the lowest recorded intake in the 25-year period – to between 303 and 308 g during the other survey years, including 2003. The consumption of maize, which is more common as a staple in combination with rice in Central and Southern Philippines, particularly in rural areas, generally declined, except in 1993. The intake of starchy roots and tubers was half as much in 2003 (19 g/day) as in 1978 (37 g/day), reflecting the diminishing consumption of traditional and ethnic foods, such as snacks made from locally available yams and tubers.

FIGURE 4
Trends in per capita food intake (grams) by food group, 1978 to 2003

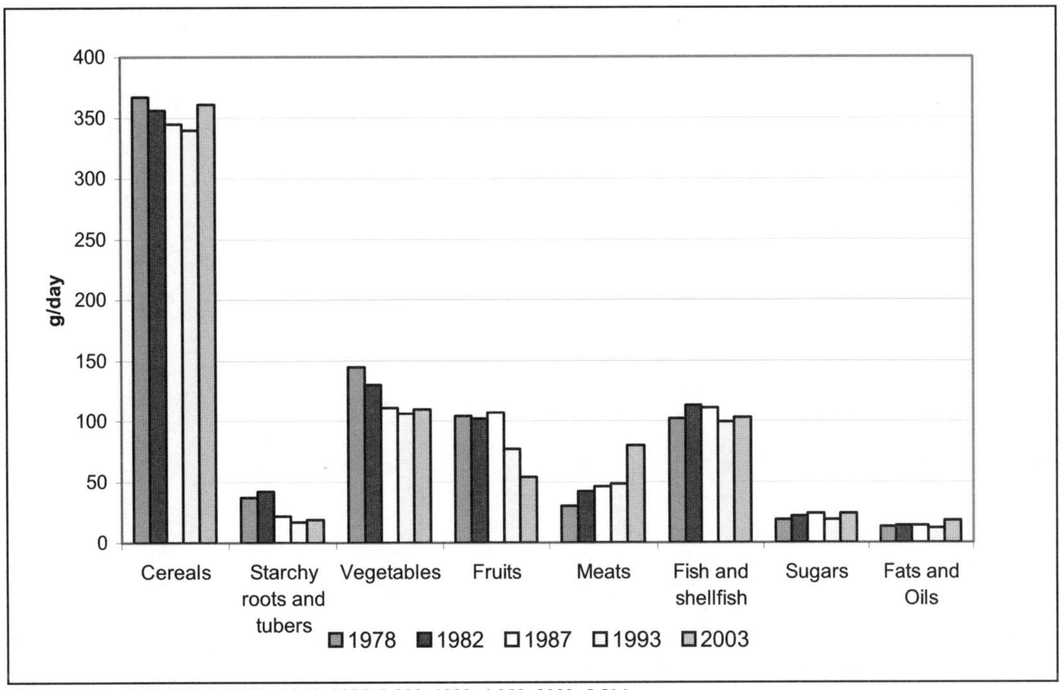

Sample sizes: 1978, 2 800; 1982, 2 280; 1987, 3 200; 1993, 4 050; 2003, 5 514.
Sources: NNS, 1978; 1982; 1987; 1993; 2003.

The consumption of other cereals and cereal products, which include breads and bakery products, noodles and snack foods made from wheat flour, peaked at 30 g in 2003 – an increase of 36 percent on the 22 g of 1993. The intake of sugars and syrups, including soft drinks, increased. The consumption of soft drinks increased by 150 percent, from 2 g in 1993 to 5 g in 2003.

Other food groups for which major increases in mean per capita intake between 1993 and 2003 were recorded include fats and oils (50 percent higher in 2003), meat and meat products (79 percent higher), poultry (43 percent higher), milk and milk products (11 percent higher) and miscellaneous food items (105 percent higher). With regard to meat and meat products, in 2003 the intake of pork (32 g) – whether fresh meat or popular processed meat products (e.g., hotdogs, meatloaf, sausages) and cooked foods – was greater than that of fresh beef (5 g) or organ meats (6 g). In 2003, processed meat products represented nearly 30 percent of meat intake. Among the miscellaneous food items, 33 percent (13 g) of the per capita daily intake in 2003 comprised alcoholic beverages. It will be important to track the trends in consumption of these foods and beverages over time, as excessive consumption of processed meat products (which contain more sodium and preservatives than fresh products) and alcoholic beverages may contribute to the incidence of hypertension and related NCDs.

TABLE 5
Comparison of fresh and processed meat intakes (g/day), 2003

Food group/sub-group	g/day
Fresh meat	38
Pork	32
Beef	5
Carabeef	N
Other fresh meat	1
Organ meat	6
Pig	2
Cow	1
Carabao	N
Chicken and other poultry	1
Other organ meats	N
Organ meat recipes	2
Liver spread	N
Processed meat	18
Popular processed meat	15
Canned	1
Cooked mixed recipes	2

Consumption of vegetables and fruits declined, as did their percentage contribution to total food intake. The intake of fruits, both vitamin C-rich and other, hit a low of 54 g in 2003, a decrease of 50 g since 1978 after a steady 30 percent reduction during the periods 1987 to 1993 and 1993 to 2003. Among vegetables, the intake of green leafy and yellow vegetables has remained the same since 1987, while that of other vegetables has increased – albeit by only 4 g – in the past decade.

Trends in per capita food consumption (in kilocalories) by food group
Rice and rice products continue to be the major source of dietary energy, but their contribution to total per capita dietary energy intake has declined, particularly in the last 13 years (Table 6). Between 1978 and 1987, this group provided 1 050 to 1 022 kcal per capita/day (58 to 56 percent of total per capita dietary energy intake), decreasing to 1 006 kcal (53 percent of total intake) in 2003. The contribution of other traditional staples such as maize and starchy roots and tubers also declined between 1978 and 2003: maize from 137 to 98 kcal per capita/day, and starchy roots and tubers from 40 to 23 kcal. These two food groups fell from providing 10 percent of total dietary energy in 1978 to providing 6 percent in 2003. Other cereals and cereal products, meat and meat products, poultry, fats and oils, sugars and syrups, and miscellaneous food items, including beverages, have been increasing. The contribution of other cereals and cereal products to dietary energy increased from 4 to 10 percent (or 3 to 6 kcal/g), while that of fish, meats and poultry rose from 8 to 12 percent (or 1.00 to 1.24 kcal/g).

In 1978, the energy intake from milk and milk products (94 kcal) was more than three times that of later surveys, even though the quantity of milk and milk products remained very similar (Table 4). Sweetened condensed milk was more frequently consumed in 1978 than in succeeding periods. The energy value of sweetened condensed milk is 321 kcal/100 g compared with 60 kcal/100 g for whole milk and 35 kcal/100 g for skim milk (USDA, no date).

TABLE 6
Trends in per capita dietary energy intake (kcal) by food group and sub-group, 1978 to 2003

Food group/sub-group	Consumption (kcal)				
	1978	**1982**	**1987**	**1993**	**2003**
Cereals and cereal products		1 262	1 213	1 196	1 286
Rice and products	1 050	1 032	1 022	950	1 006
Maize and products	137	130	82	114	99
Other cereals and products	70	99	109	131	181
Starchy roots and tubers	40	42	23	17	23
Sugars and syrups[1]	67	81	84	71	84
Fats and oils[2]	88	112	110	99	112
Fish, meat and poultry	135	155	166	160	229
Fish and products	68	65	70	62	65
Meat and products	58	78	86	82	141
Poultry	9	11	11	17	23
Eggs	11	13	14	17	19
Milk and milk products	94	27	23	24	27
Whole milk				22	23
Milk products				2	4
Dried beans, nuts and seeds[3]	20	24	23	22	21
Vegetables	34	29		25	32
Green leafy, yellow vegetables	9	9	7	7	10
Other vegetables	25	20	60[a]	18	23
Fruits	45	42		35	30
Vitamin C-rich foods	14	11	12	8	4
Other fruits	31	31		29	27
Miscellaneous	11	18	18	18	42
Beverages[4]					30
Condiments					8
Others					4
Total (kcal)	**1 804**	**1 808**	**1 753**	**1 684**	**1 905**

Sample sizes: 1978, 2 800; 1982, 2 280; 1987, 3 200; 1993, 4 050; 2003, 5 514.
[1] Includes soft drinks (sugar content), sherbet and similar preparations.
[2] Includes grated coconut and coconut milk (fat).
[3] Includes mung beans, soybeans, peanuts and other dried beans, nuts.
[4] Includes coffee, tuba (local wine), alcoholic beverages and others.
[a] Includes other fruits and other vegetables
Numbers may not add up to totals owing to rounding off.
Sources: NNS, 1978; 1982; 1987; 1993; 2003.

Trends in nutrient adequacy

Based on absolute intakes, the mean per capita intakes of energy, protein, vitamin A, calcium, thiamine, riboflavin and niacin increased in 2003 from the levels in 1993 and earlier years. Intakes for most other nutrients, however, remained inadequate, particularly those for iron, calcium, riboflavin and vitamin C, all of which were less than 80 percent of the recommended levels – an indication that these nutrients are probably inadequately provided for by the average food consumption pattern in Philippine households (see reference RENIs for 2002 in Annex 3).

TABLE 7
Trends in per capita energy and nutrient intakes and percentage adequacy based on Philippine RDAs and RENIs, 1978 to 2003

Nutrients	1978[1]	1982[1]	1987[1]	1993[2]	2003[3]
Energy					
Intake (kcal)	1 804	1 808	1 753	1 684	1 905
% adequacy	88.6	89.0	87.1	87.8	98.3
Protein					
Intake (g)	53.0	50.6	49.7	49.9	56.2
% adequacy	102.9	99.6	98.2	106.2	99.2
Iron					
Intake (mg)	11.0	10.8	10.7	10.1	10.1
% adequacy	91.7	91.5	91.5	64.7	60.1
Vitamin A					
Intake (ug RE)	-	-	389.7	391.9	455.2
% adequacy	-	-	75.9	88.1	91.4
Calcium					
Intake (g)	0.44	0.45	0.42	0.39	0.44
% adequacy		80.4	75.0	67.0	57.1
Thiamine					
Intake (mg)	0.73	0.74	0.68	0.67	0.88
% adequacy		71.8	66.7	68.4	86.3
Riboflavin					
Intake (mg)	0.53	0.58	0.56	0.56	0.73
% adequacy		56.3	54.4	57.1	68.0
Niacin					
Intake (mg)	15.3	16.4	16.3	16.1	20.6
% adequacy		119.7	119.9	68.0	156.4
Ascorbic acid					
Intake (mg)	66.8	61.6	53.6	46.7	46.5
% adequacy		91.1	80.0	73.2	75.0
Fats					
Intake (g)		30	30	29	38
Carbohydrates					
Intake (g)		327	313	310	333

Sample sizes: 1978, 2 800; 1982, 2 280; 1987, 3 200; 1993, 4 050; 2003, 5 514.
[1] 1976 RDA for Philippines (Annex 1).
[2] 1989 RDA for Philippines (Annex 2).
[3] 2002 RENI for Philippines (Annex 3).
Sources: NNS, 1978; 1982; 1987; 1993; 2003.

The contributions of animal and plant food sources to total energy, protein, vitamin A and iron intakes are shown in Figure 5. Plant foods, particularly cereals such as rice and rice products, continue to be the major contributors of energy, protein and iron in Philippine diets. Rice and rice products alone contributed 53, 37 and 29 percent, respectively, of total energy, protein and iron intakes in Philippine households.

FIGURE 5
Percentage contributions of animal and plant foods to total energy, protein, vitamin A and iron intakes, 2003

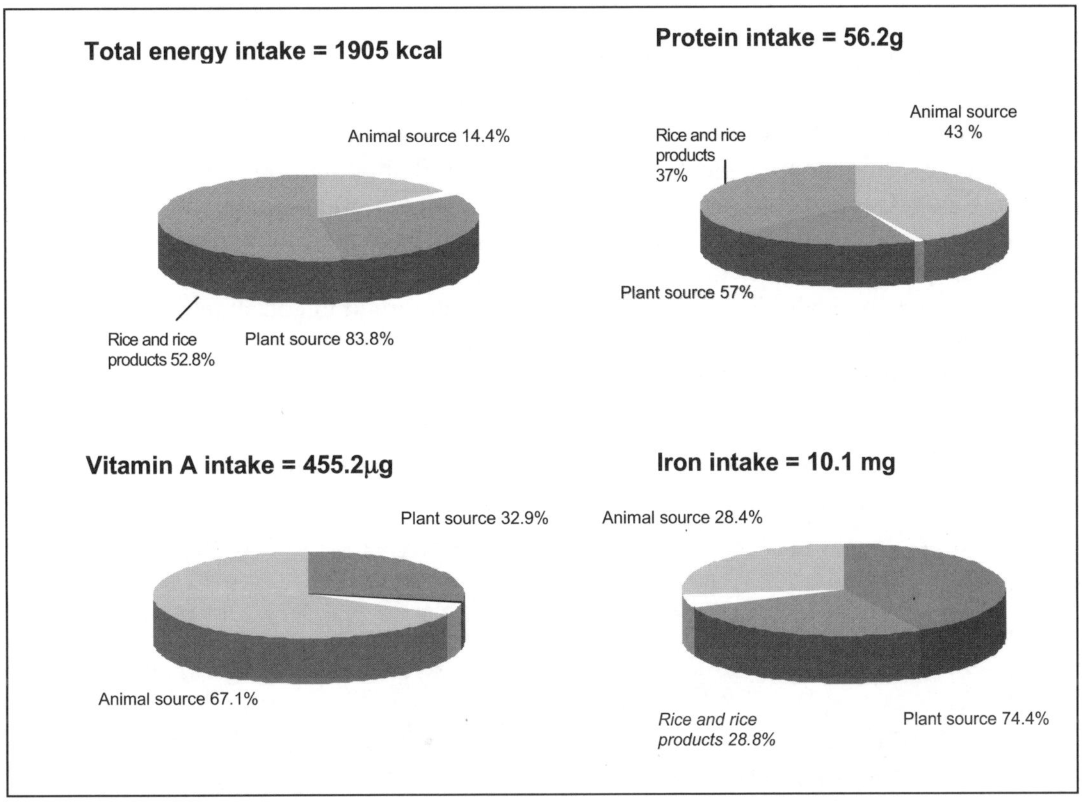

Total energy intake = 1905 kcal

Animal source 14.4%

Rice and rice products 52.8%   Plant source 83.8%

Protein intake = 56.2g

Animal source 43 %

Rice and rice products 37%

Plant source 57%

Vitamin A intake = 455.2μg

Plant source 32.9%

Animal source 67.1%

Iron intake = 10.1 mg

Animal source 28.4%

Rice and rice products 28.8%   Plant source 74.4%

Sample size: 5 514.
Source: NNS, 2003.

The declining intake of vitamin C over the years may be explained by the generally declining intake of vitamin C-rich fruits. There was also no increase in iron intake in 2003, in spite of the reported increased intake of meat, because most of this increase was in the form of pork, which in general has lower iron content (0.8 mg/100 g) than beef (2.8 mg/100 g). In addition, the revised iron values in the updated Philippine FCT – particularly those affecting about 30 food items, many of which were fresh and processed fish – were generally lower, as reflected in the lower iron contribution from fish in spite of an increased intake in 2003 (Annexes 6 and 7).

The remarkable drop in iron adequacy since 1987, from 91.5 to < 65 percent in 1993 and 2003 in spite of absolute intakes that remained nearly the same throughout the same period, is attributed to the revisions in recommended nutrient intakes already noted. Specifically for iron, differences in estimating the basal or obligatory losses and the requirements for growth among children resulted in higher requirements in the 1989 RDAs and 2002 RENIs compared with those of 1976. There were also notable changes in the niacin and calcium requirements. For niacin, the requirement in the 1976 RDAs and 2002 RENIs was based only on preformed niacin, and therefore lower than that in the 1989 RDA, which included the contribution of tryptophan. This explains the drop in mean per capita niacin adequacy in 1993, even though the absolute intake was virtually the same as in preceding years. With regard to calcium, the requirement was increased in the 2002 RENIs, primarily because of a shift in the paradigm for setting calcium requirements, i.e., a change in objective from that of attaining calcium balance to that of preventing osteoporosis. This also explains the drop in calcium adequacy in 2003, in spite of an increase in calcium intake.

Achievement of population nutrient intake goals

The increased intakes of fats and oils, fish, meats and poultry, and milk and milk products are consistent with the Nutritional Guidelines for the Philippines (Annex 4), which has called for specific improvements to the quality of Philippine diets by including more animal foods (Guideline no. 4), fats and oils (Guideline no. 6) and milk and milk products (Guideline no. 7). Overall, the proportion of animal foods in total food intake has increased – from 20 percent in 1978, to 25 percent in 1993 and to 28 percent in 2003 (Figure 6). These increases may also be attributed to the increasing trend in consumption of fast foods and could signal a detrimental increase in saturated fat and cholesterol, which will be discussed in the following sections.

FIGURE 6
Mean per capita food intake by source, 1993 and 2003.

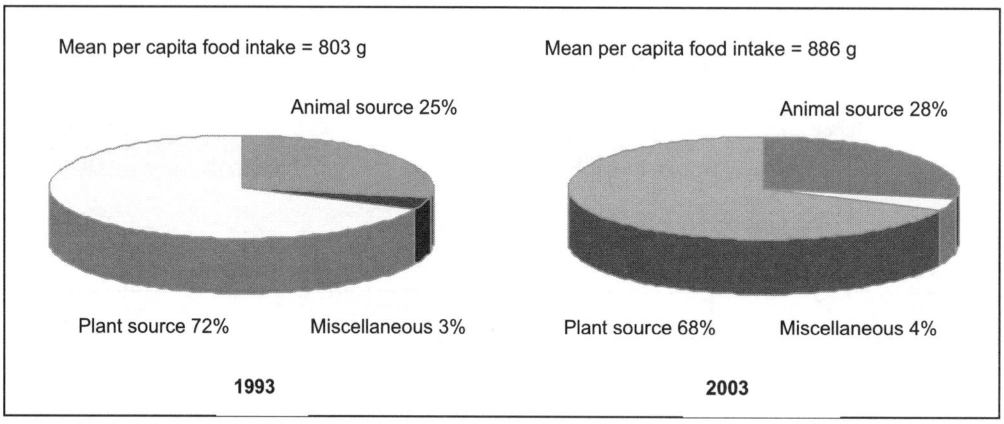

Mean per capita food intake = 803 g   Mean per capita food intake = 886 g

Animal source 25%   Animal source 28%

Plant source 72%   Miscellaneous 3%   Plant source 68%   Miscellaneous 4%

1993   **2003**

Sample sizes: 1993, 4 050; 2003, 5 514.
Sources: NNS, 1993; 2003.

The average contribution of fat to total dietary energy intake increased from 15 to 18 percent, and that of carbohydrate decreased from 74 to 70 percent. The proportion of households with per capita fat consumption or contribution within the WHO/FAO (2003) recommendations of 15 to 30 percent of energy intake increased from 38 percent in 1993 to 46 percent in 2003. The proportion of households with per capita carbohydrate consumption of between 55 and 75 percent of energy intake increased from 53 to 58 percent over the same period.

FIGURE 7
Percentage distribution of per capita dietary energy from fat, protein and carbohydrates, 1987, 1993 and 2003

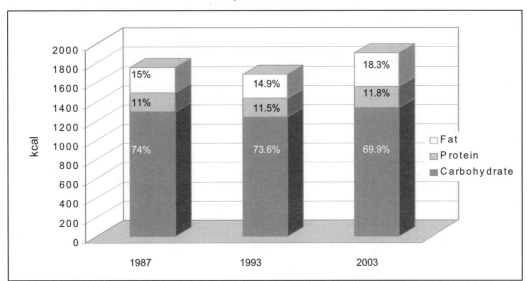

The continuing pattern of decreasing fruit and vegetable consumption is reflected in the declining proportion of households that consume ≥ 400 g fruits and vegetables per capita per day, particularly in the last ten years. In 1993, 11.5 percent of Philippine households had a per capita intake of ≥ 400 g fruits and vegetables a day; this figure had declined to 8.2 percent in 2003 – a drop of about one-third (Table 8).

TABLE 8
Trends in achievement of population nutrient intake goals, 1993 and 2003

Year	% of population with 15–30% energy intake from fat	% of population with < 10% energy intake from free sugars	% of population with 55–75% energy intake from carbohydrate	% of population consuming ≥ 400 g/day fruits and vegetables
1993	37.6	94.3	53.0	11.5
2003	46.2	92.1	57.9	8.2

Sample sizes: 1993, 4 050; 2003, 5 514.
Sources: NNS, 1993; 2003.

The proportion of households with less than 100 percent of mean per capita energy adequacy was 57 percent in 2003, an improvement from 1993's figure of 74 percent. The Millennium Development Goal (MDG) for hunger calls for halving the proportion of population below the minimum level of dietary energy consumption. Data collected by FAO to measure the proportion of undernourished people show a declining trend in the proportion of the population considered undernourished (FAO, 2003).

Trends in food and nutrient intakes in urban and rural areas

The 1987 and 1993 NNS show urban and rural differences in food (Table 9) and energy and nutrient intakes (Table 10). Generally, in both years, the intakes of cereals and cereal products, particularly rice and maize products, starchy roots and tubers, fish, and vegetables, including green leafy and yellow and other vegetables were higher in rural than in urban areas. Urban households, on the other hand, had higher per capita intakes of other cereals and cereal products (which include breads and bakery products, noodles and snack foods made from wheat flour), sugars and syrups, fats and oils, meat and poultry, eggs, milk and milk products, dried beans, nuts and seeds, and vitamin C-rich fruits. Between 1987 and 1993, the consumption of milk and milk products, in particular, increased in urban areas but decreased in rural ones.

TABLE 9
Trends in per capita food consumption (grams) by urban and rural residence, 1987 and 1993

Food group/sub-group	Rural		Urban	
	1987	1993	1987	1993
Cereals and cereal products	361	350	318	318
Rice and products	317	289	281	273
Maize and products	31	55	11	17
Other cereals and products	13	16	26	28
Starchy roots and tubers	25	21	17	13
Sugars and syrups[1]	22	17	26	20
Fats and oils[2]	12	11	15	14
Fish, meat and poultry	145	133	174	161
Fish and products	109	99	112	97
Meat and products	28	23	52	44
Poultry	8	9	11	19
Eggs	8	9	13	15
Milk and milk products	34	24	56	64
Whole milk	30	22	45	48
Milk products	4	2	11	16
Dried beans, nuts and seeds[3]	9	8	11	11
Vegetables	104	102	91	86
Green leafy, yellow vegetables	32	34	25	25
Other vegetables	72	68	66	61
Fruits	115	84	123	93
Vitamin C-rich foods	31	26	44	39
Other fruits	84	58	79	54
Miscellaneous	27	16	24	23
Beverages[4]	13	6	10	11
Condiments	11	9	11	9
Others	3	1	3	2
Total (g)	863	786	869	819

Sample sizes: 1987, 3 200; 1993, 4 050.
[1] Includes soft drinks (sugar content), sherbet and similar preparations.
[2] Includes grated coconut and coconut milk (fat).
[3] Includes mung beans, soybeans, peanuts and other dried beans, nuts.
[4] Includes coffee, tuba (local wine), alcoholic beverages and others.
Numbers may not add up to totals owing to rounding off.
Sources: NNS, 1987; 1993.

The food intake in rural areas has followed the same trend as that in urban areas. As in urban areas, the consumption of rice and rice products, starchy roots and tubers, and fruits decreased in rural areas between 1987 and 1993, while that of other cereals and cereal products increased. Urban patterns of food consumption are reflected significantly in the diets of the rural population for various reasons, including the influence of urban migrants on the families they leave behind, improved transport and communications between urban and rural areas, and the increasing availability of processed foods in rural markets. It should be noted that reduced intakes were reported for nearly all of the food groups in terms of weight and total dietary energy intake, in both urban and rural areas between 1987 and 1993; this is shown in the national data in Table 4.

In terms of adequacy of energy and nutrients in the diet, urban and rural households did not differ. In 1993, both had inadequate intakes of energy and nutrients, except protein in urban and rural areas and vitamin A in urban areas only. Per capita vitamin A intake was more than 100 percent adequate in urban households, but only 74 percent in rural ones.

TABLE 10
Trends in per capita nutrient intakes and percentage adequacy, by urban and rural residence, 1987 and 1993

Nutrients	Rural		Urban	
	1987[1]	1993[2]	1987[1]	1993[2]
Energy				
Intake (kcal)	1 748	1 696	1 761	1 673
% adequacy	87.2	88.6	86.9	87.0
Protein				
Intake (g)	49.1	49.1	50.7	50.8
% adequacy	97.6	104.9	99.0	107.6
Iron				
Intake (mg)	10.5	9.9	10.9	10.2
% adequacy	91.3	64.3	91.6	64.6
Vitamin A				
Intake (ug RE)	357.5	327.9	440.4	457.0
% adequacy	70.3	73.8	84.9	102.7
Calcium				
Intake (g)	0.43	0.39	0.42	0.39
% adequacy	76.8	66.1	76.4	67.2
Thiamine				
Intake (mg)	0.65	0.65	0.73	0.70
% adequacy	63.7	66.3	70.9	71.4
Riboflavin				
Intake (mg)	0.52	0.51	0.62	0.61
% adequacy	51.0	52.0	60.2	61.6
Niacin				
Intake (mg)	16.1	15.8	16.6	16.5
% adequacy	118.4	86.3	121.2	89.7
Ascorbic acid				
Intake (mg)	54.7	48.7	51.8	44.6
% adequacy	82.0	76.6	76.5	69.7

Sample sizes: 1987, 3 200; 1993, 4 050.
[1] 1976 RDA for Philippines (Annex 1).
[2] 1989 RDA for Philippines (Annex 2).
Sources: NNS, 1987; 1993.

Urban and rural differences are also noted with regard to the contributions of fat, protein and carbohydrate to total dietary energy supply (Table 11). Generally, the contribution of fats to total dietary energy has been higher in urban (about 18 percent in 1987 and 1993) than in rural (13 percent) households, while the latter consume more carbohydrates (75 to 76 percent versus 70 percent of dietary energy).

TABLE 11
Trends in percentage proportions of per capita dietary energy from fat, protein and carbohydrates, by urban and rural residence, 1987 and 1993

	Total dietary energy intake (kcal)		% dietary energy from fat		% dietary energy from protein		% dietary energy from carbohydrates	
	1987	1993	1987	1993	1987	1993	1987	1993
Urban	1 761	1 673	18.4	18	11.3	12.3	70.2	69.7
Rural	1 748	1 696	13.0	12.9	10.8	11.7	76.2	75.4

Sample sizes: 1987, 3 200; 1993, 4 050.
Sources: NNS, 1987; 1993.

The urban–rural disaggregation of the 2003 NNS data is not yet available, but regionally disaggregated data on food intake (Annex 8) support the urban–rural differences in diet patterns that were noted from the earlier surveys. In very urban areas such as Metro Manila, the consumption of other cereals and cereal products, fats and oils, meats and meat products, and milk and milk products continues to be higher, while that of vegetables is lower than in other regions with varying extents of urbanization. Apart from Metro Manila, the regions with the highest proportion of urban population (specifically, Central Luzon and Calabarzon, which are at least 60 percent urban) have higher consumption of other cereals and cereal products, meats and meat products, eggs, and milk and milk products than the least urbanized regions (Cagayan Valley and Eastern Visayas, which are only 19 to 22 percent urban). Central Luzon and Calabarzon have lower intakes of starchy roots and tubers and vegetables than most of the other less urbanized regions.

Dietary changes in the Philippines in the past 25 years have followed much the same pattern as those described in the nutrition transition literature of, for example, Shetty and Gopalan (1998) and Popkin (1994). The Philippine diet has become more energy-dense, with a greater proportion of energy from fat. Important changes in the types of food in the diet include:

- increasing intake of other cereals and cereal products, including breads and other bakery products and different forms of noodles and pasta;
- increasing intakes of sugars and syrups, fats and oils, and animal food sources such as meat, poultry, eggs and dairy products;
- decreasing intakes of fruit, vegetables, and starchy roots and tubers.

There are noticeable differences between the consumption patterns of urban and rural groups. In particular, urban residents are showing a strong trend towards consumption of non-traditional staples and animal source foods, accompanied by a declining intake of fruits and vegetables.

In general, the overall adequacy of the Philippine diet has improved, as illustrated by the increasing adequacy of energy and most micronutrients. There are, however, some declining trends in adequate intakes of iron and vitamin C. The latter is most probably associated with a steep drop in consumption of vitamin C-rich fruits, while the decline in iron intake is more difficult to understand, but most likely involves a combination of increasing requirements from the updated Philippine RENIs and decreasing amounts of iron considered to be bioavailable.

Food and nutrient intake of preschool-age children

Infant and young child feeding practices in the Philippines have been shown to be inadequate. The prevalence of breastfeeding was 87 to 89 percent between 1993 and 2003

(Philippines National Demographic and Health Survey, 2003; NNS, 2003), but the mean duration of breastfeeding in 2003 was only 5.6 months (NNS, 2003). In the same year, the prevalence of exclusive breastfeeding was only 41.7 percent among infants under two months of age, and 33.4 percent among those aged two to three months; at four to five months of age, only 11.5 percent of infants were still exclusively breastfed (NNS, 2003).

There is a dearth of published national data on the food intake of Philippine preschool children. Unpublished reports on the food intake of non-breastfeeding preschool-age children from the 1978, 1982, 1993 and 2003 NNS imply that the food intake of preschool children in general has been inadequate in energy and the essential nutrients, except protein. Although, rice, milk and milk products, fish, meat and poultry, and fruits have been the major contributors to preschool children's dietary patterns, intakes have apparently been inadequate to meet those recommended for several essential nutrients, particularly iron, vitamin A and calcium. The consequences of inadequate food and nutrient intakes among children are reflected in their poor nutritional status, which is described in the following sections.

TABLE 12
Trends in mean per capita food consumption (grams) in preschool-age children, 1978 to 2003

Food group/sub-group	1978[a]	1982[a]	1993[b]	2003[c]
Cereals and cereal products	-	-	163	166
Rice and products	88	101	121	122
Maize and products	-	-	15	17
Other cereals and products	-	-	27	27
Fats and oils[1]	n	5	2	6
Fish, meat and poultry	71	82	85	95
Eggs	7	8	8	8
Milk and milk products	88	109	111	179
Vegetables	28	29	22	23
Fruits	77	72	70	31
Other food groups	103[5]	90[5]		
Starchy roots and tubers	-	-	11	8
Dried beans, nuts and seeds[2]	-	-	6	4
Sugars and syrups[3]	-	-	12	15
Miscellaneous[4]	-	-	10	27
Total intake (g)	462	496	500	506

Sample sizes: 1978, 2 800; 1982, 2 280; 1993, 4 050.
[1] Includes grated coconut and coconut milk (fat).
[2] Includes mung beans, soybeans, peanuts and other dried beans, nuts.
[3] Includes soft drinks (sugar content), sherbet and similar preparations.
[4] Includes beverages, condiments and others.
[5] Includes maize and maize products, other cereals, starchy roots and tubers, dried beans, nuts and seeds, sugars, and miscellaneous (beverages, condiments and others).
[a] Six months to four years of age.
[b] Three to 59 months of age (unpublished).
[c] Six months to five years of age.
– = less than 0.5 g.
Numbers may not add up to totals owing to rounding off.
Sources: NNS, 1978; 1982; 1993.

TABLE 13
Trends in mean per capita energy and nutrient intakes and percentage adequacy in preschool-age children, 1978 to 1993

Nutrient	1978[1a]	1982[1a]	1993[2b]	2003[3c]
Energy				
Intake (kcal)	742	873	887	980
% adequacy	53.8	63.3	68.0	83.0
Protein				
Intake (g)	23.8	27.3	28.8	31.5
% adequacy	87.2	100	105.9	102.8
Iron				
Intake (mg)	4.5	5.4	6.0	6.2
% adequacy	67.2	80.6	63.6	72.7
Vitamin A				
Intake (ug RE)	-	-	234.3	315.9
% adequacy	-	-	66.3	79.0
Calcium				
Intake (g)	0.28	0.29	0.27	0.37
% adequacy		58.0	47.6	73.4
Thiamine				
Intake (mg)	0.43	0.47	0.43	0.65
% adequacy		65.3	63.0	123.2
Riboflavin				
Intake (mg)	0.41	0.44	0.41	0.74
% adequacy		61.1	61.8	142.3
Niacin				
Intake (mg)	6.4	8.2	8.6	10.4
% adequacy		87.2	66.6	163.8
Ascorbic acid				
Intake (mg)	29.4	28.9	25.0	31.7
% adequacy		77.1	68.5	105.5

Sample sizes: 1978, 2 800; 1982, 2 280; 1993, 4 050; 2003, 5 514.
[1] 1976 RDA for Philippines (Annex 1).
[2] 1989 RDA for Philippines (Annex 2).
[3] 2002 RENI for Philippines (Annex 3).
[a] Six months to four years of age, non-breastfeeding.
[b] Three to 59 months of age, non-breastfeeding.
[c] Six months to five years of age, non-breastfeeding.
Sources: NNS, 1978; 1982; 1993; 2003.

CHANGES IN NUTRITIONAL STATUS

Data on the nutritional status of the Philippine population come from the NNS rounds in 1993, 1998 and 2003 and the Regional Updating of the Nutritional Status of Children in 1989/1990, 1992, 1996 and 2001.

Trends in the nutritional status of children aged 0 to ten years

Undernutrition among children continues to be a public health problem. In 2003, underweight and stunting still affected three out of every ten children aged 0 to 5.9 years (Figure 8) and six to 10.9 years (Figure 9). According to 2003 population projections based on 2000 census data from the National Statistics Office, there are 3.2 million underweight children aged 0 to 5.9 years, and 2.4 million aged six to 10.9 years; for stunting the respective figures are 3.4 million and 3.3 million.

However, there was declining prevalence of undernutrition – underweight and stunting – in both age groups between 1989/1990 and 2003. Within this period, the proportion of underweight children aged 0 to five years declined by 7.6 percentage points, from 34.5 to 26.9 percent (an average reduction of 0.58 percentage points a year); among six- to ten-year-old children, the prevalence of underweight dropped by 8.6 percentage points, from 34.2 to 25.6 percent (an average 0.66 percentage points a year). Stunting among 0- to five- and six- to ten-year-old children also declined by 10.0 (0.77 a year) and 9.0 (0.69 a year) percentage points, respectively. Meanwhile, the prevalence of acute malnutrition (wasting) among children aged 0 to five years has not improved, and increased from 5.0 percent in 1989/1990 to 5.3 percent in 2003.

FIGURE 8
**Trends in the prevalence of malnutrition among children aged 0 to 5.9 years,
1989/1990 to 2003**

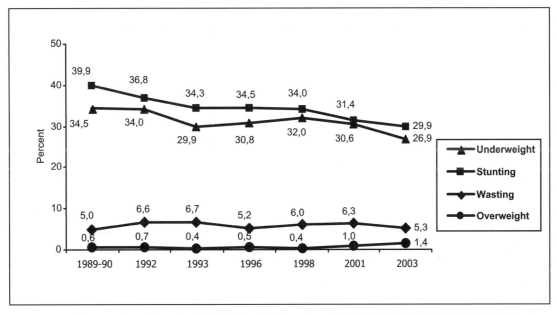

Sample sizes: 1989/1990, 8 008; 1992, 7 243; 1993, 24 000 household members; 1996, 10 385; 1998, 28 698; 2001, 10 634; 2003, 4 110.
References: International Reference Standard/NCHS Growth Reference: underweight = weight-for-age < -2SD;
wasting = weight-for-height < -2SD; stunting = height-for-age < -2SD; overweight-for-age = weight-for-age > 2SD.
Sources: NNS, 1993; 1998; 2003; Regional Updating of the Nutritional Status of Children, 1989/1990; 1992; 1996; 2001.

FIGURE 9
**Trends in the prevalence of malnutrition among children aged six to 10.9 years,
1989/1990 to 2003**

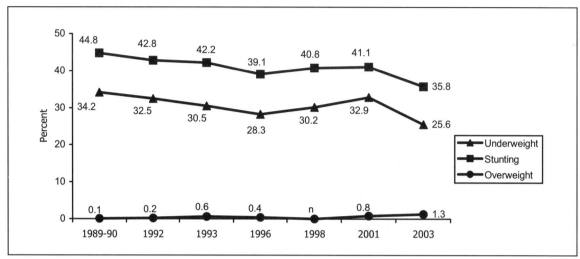

Sample sizes: 1989/1990, 4 306; 1993, 5 636; 1993, 24 000 household members; 1996, 15 530; 1998, 3 040; 2001, 1 791; 2003, 3 436.
References: International Reference Standard/NCHS Growth Reference: underweight = weight-for-age < -2SD;
wasting = weight-for-height < -2SD; stunting = height-for-age < -2SD; overweight-for-age = weight-for-age > 2SD.
Sources: NNS, 1993; 1998; 2003; Regional Updating of the Nutritional Status of Children, 1989/1990; 1992; 1996; 2001.

The average annual percentage reduction of 0.58 percent is not sufficient to meet the
MDG target of reducing the proportion of underweight-for-age children under five years of
age to 17.25 percent by 2015. There are geographical (regional) disparities in the nutritional
status of children, and measures to reduce the prevalence of undernutrition will have to be
strengthened in the regions where the problem is greatest. The proportions of underweight-for-
age children are higher in the Administrative Region of Muslim Mindanao (34 percent) – one of
the poorest in the country – and Mimaropa region (34.2 percent) in Southern Luzon than in
Metro Manila (17.8 percent), Central Luzon (21.7 percent) and the Cordillera Administrative
Region (16.3 percent).

Meanwhile, although overweight-for-age affects smaller proportions of children (1.4
and 1.3 percent, respectively, in the 0 to 5.9 years and the six to 10.9 years age groups), it
has increased significantly between 1998 and 2003. The prevalence of overweight among
both age groups in 1989/1990 and 1998 was unchanged, but in 2003 it had increased nearly
threefold among children aged 0 to 5.9 years and more than tenfold among those aged six
to 10.9 years compared with 1998 levels.

Trends in the nutritional status of 11- to 19-year-olds
In 2003, the proportion of underweight among adolescents aged 11 to 12 years was nearly
the same as that among children up to ten years of age – about three out of ten (25.9
percent). Underweight among those aged 11 to 19 years decreased between 1993 and 2003
for both males and females, but the decrease among females was twice that among males,
particularly after 1998. On the other hand, overweight increased, affecting 4.2 percent of
11- to 12-year-olds, and 3.4 percent of 13- to 19-year-olds in the same year. The
prevalence of overweight among these groups has increased steadily, with larger
percentage increases among females than males.

TABLE 14
Trends in the prevalence of underweight and overweight among 11- to 19-year-olds

Gender/age group	Underweight			Overweight		
	1993	1998	2003	1993	1998	2003
	% prevalence					
Male						
11–12 years	32.1	37.3	31.0	2.6	1.8	4.9
13–19 years	28.8	31.8	17.0	2.5	1.0	2.9
All males	29.8	33.1	20.5	2.6	1.2	3.4
Female						
11–12 years	36.3	36.5	20.6	1.5	3.2	3.4
13–19 years	29.7	32.0	6.4	2.5	5.2	3.9
All females	30.7	33.1	10.1	2.2	4.7	3.8
Male and female						
11–12 years	34.0	37.0	25.9	2.2	2.5	4.2
13–19 years	28.7	31.9	12.0	2.5	3.1	3.4
All adolescents	**30.2**	**33.1**	**15.5**	**2.4**	**2.9**	**3.6**

Sample sizes: 1993, 24 000 household members; 1998, 6 079; 2003, 4 860.
References (Must, Dallal and Dietz, 1991): underweight = < 5 percentile of BMI-for-age; overweight = > 85 percentile of BMI-for-age.
Sources: NNS, 1993; 1998; 2003.

Trends in the nutritional status of adults

In 2003, 12.3 percent of adults were affected by undernutrition (BMI < 18.5). Based on the WHO cut-off for a healthy adult population in which only 3 to 5 percent have BMI below 18.5 (WHO, 1995), adult undernutrition in the Philippines is a problem that needs to be addressed. On the other hand, 24 percent of adults are overweight or obese, with more females (27.3 percent) than males (20.9 percent) affected (overweight = BMI of 25 to < 30; obese = BMI ≥ 30). Although progress in reducing underweight has been slow (about 10 percent over ten years), prevalence of BMI > 25 has been increasing steadily by 20 percent in each five-year interval from 1993 to 2003. The BMI distribution of the population has shifted slightly to the right over the past five years (Figure 10).

TABLE 15
Prevalence of underweight and overweight among adults, 1993 to 2003

Gender/age group	Underweight			Overweight/obese		
	1993	1998	2003	1993	1998	2003
	% Prevalence					
Male	11.5	11.1	10.6	14.4	17.0	20.9
Female	16.1	15.4	14.2	18.6	23.3	27.3
Male and female						
20–39 years	11.0	11.2	10.6	14.4	18.5	20.6
40–59 years	14.5	12.0	10.4	23.2	25.3	30.8
60 years and over	29.1	25.4	23.4	11.4	14.6	19.1
All	13.9	13.2	12.3	16.6	20.2	24.0

Sample sizes: 1993, 24 000 household members; 1998, 9 299; 2003, 11 696.
References: Underweight/chronic energy deficiency (CED) = BMI < 18.5; overweight/obese = BMI ≥ 25.
Sources: NNS, 1993; 1998; 2003.

FIGURE 10
Changes in distribution of adult BMI, 1998 to 2003

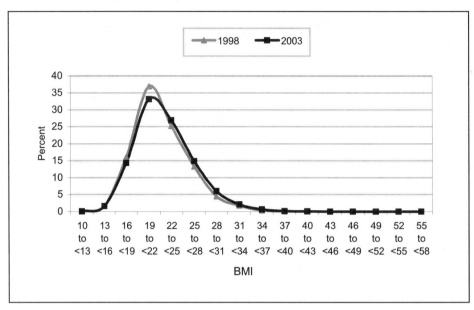

Using the BMI cut-off points recommended by the WHO expert consultation to determine public health and clinical action in relation to cardiovascular disease (CVD) (i.e., BMI 23 to 27.4 = moderate risk; BMI ≥ 27.5 = high to very high risk), the proportion of Philippine adults with moderate to very high risk of co-morbidities related to CVD reaches even more significant proportions than even the overweight or obesity figures imply (Table 16).

TABLE 16
Distribution of adults by cut-off points for determining risk of co-morbidities of CVD based on BMI

Age group (years)	CED (< 18.5)	Low risk (18.5 to < 23.0)	Moderate risk (23.0 to ≤ 27.4)	High risk (≥ 27.5)
20–39	10.6	53.0	27.4	9.0
40–59	10.4	40.6	34.8	14.1
60 and over	23.6	43.7	24.2	8.5
All	12.4	47.4	29.5	10.7

Sample size: 2003, 11 696.
Reference (WHO Expert Consultation, 2004): CED = BMI < 18.5; low risk = BMI 18.5 to < 23.0; moderate risk = BMI 23.0 to ≤ 27.4; high risk = BMI ≥ 27.5.
Source: NNS, 2003.

The problem of overnutrition among adults is further highlighted when waist-to-hip ratio (WHR) and waist circumference (WC) are used. WC reflects intra-abdominal fat mass, while WHR is an index of abdominal fat distribution. Both are indicators of android obesity, which is a risk factor for CVD. The 2003 statistics reflect an overnutrition problem of public health concern, especially among female adults (Tables 17 and 18). Using WHR, android obesity affects one in every two women (54.8 percent) 20 years of age and over; this figure is 38.7 percent higher than the 1998 level. Using WC, android obesity in women increased even more rapidly, by 70 percent (from 10.7 to 18.3 percent) between 1998 and 2003.

TABLE 17
Trends in prevalence of high WHR among adults, 1998 and 2003

Gender	Age group (years)	1998	2003
		% prevalence	
Male	20–29	3.0	6.0
	30–39		11.7
	40–49	12.8	15.1
	50–59		18.8
	60–69	6.8	20.8
	70 +		13.7
	All	7.9	12.1
Female	20–29	36.3	38.7
	30–39		49.6
	40–49	45.8	66.2
	50–59		70.0
	60–69	38.6	64.4
	70 +		62.0
	All	39.5	54.8

Sample sizes: 1998, 9 299; 2003, 4 753.
Reference: male, WHR $\geq$ 1.0; female, WHR $\geq$ 0.85.
Sources: NNS, 1998; 2003.

TABLE 18
Trends in the prevalence of high WC among adults, 1998 and 2003

Gender	Age group (years)	1998	2003
		% prevalence	
Male	20–29	1.7	2.1
	30–39		2.7
	40–49	5.1	4.5
	50–59		4.9
	60–69	1.8	3.3
	70 +		1.0
	All	2.7	3.1
Female	20–29	10.0	10.2
	30–39		10.7
	40–49	11.7	23.8
	50–59		34.8
	60–69	11.5	22.9
	70 +		21.5
	All	10.7	18.3

Sample sizes: 1998, 9 299; 2003, 4 753.
Reference: male, WC $\geq$ 102 cm; female, WC $\geq$ 88 cm.
Sources: NNS, 1998; 2003.

Micronutrient status of population groups
Trends in iron deficiency
Anaemia among infants aged six months to less than one year increased alarmingly from 49.2 percent in 1993 to 66 percent in 2003. Although anaemia was not of public health magnitude among children aged one to five years when aggregated as a group, 53 percent of children aged 12 to 23 months were found to be anaemic in 2003. Pregnant women and

lactating mothers also had anaemia prevalence that was higher than the public health cut-off of 40 percent, a situation that did not change in the ten years from 1993 to 2003.

The unabated problem of anaemia among young children and pregnant and lactating women is partly attributed to continuing inadequate iron intakes. Low birth weight also contributes to the risk of anaemia during early childhood, because low-birth-weight infants are born with low iron stores, which consequently become depleted early. Philippine data in the *State of the world's children* (UNICEF, 2003) placed the prevalence of low birth weight over the period 1998 to 2003 at 20 percent. Among pregnant and lactating women, dietary iron intakes are very low – 28.8 and 33.4 percent, respectively, of those recommended (NNS, 2003). The government is addressing iron deficiency anaemia (IDA) through an iron supplementation programme for pregnant women. However, as the trends show (Figure 11), this supplementation has not been successful because the iron supplements need to be taken daily and their distribution – when supplies are available – depends on pregnant women making regular visits to health centres.

FIGURE 11
Prevalence of anaemia by age/physiologic group, 1993 to 2003

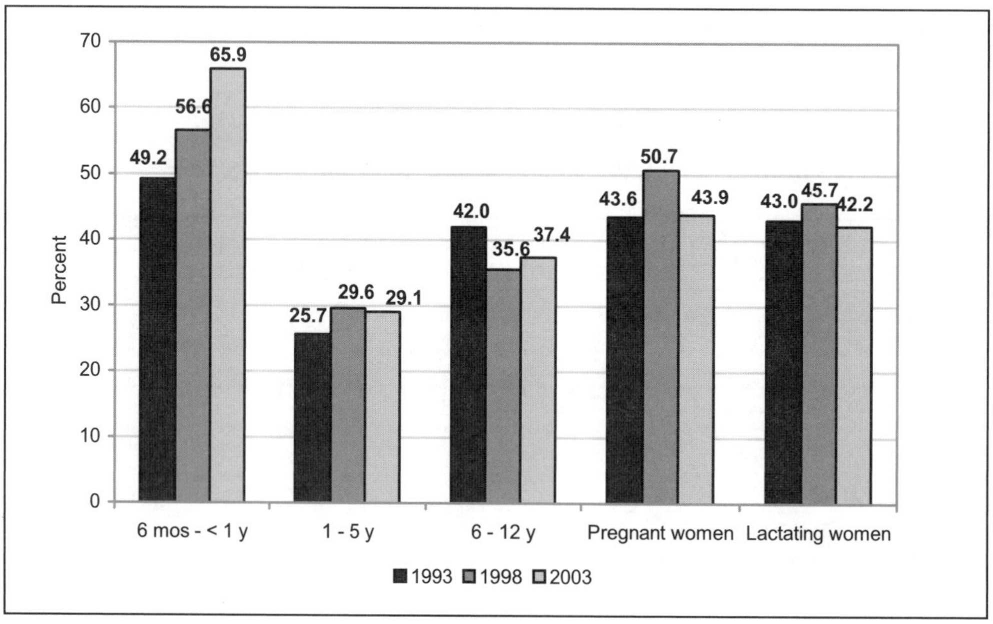

Sample sizes: 6 months to < 1 year – 1993, 400; 1998, 2 790; 2003, 329; 1 to 5 years – 1993, 3 859, 1998, 12 089; 2003, 3 291; 6 to 12 years – 1993, 2 135; 1998, 3 069; 2003, 4 647; pregnant – 1993, 782; 1998, 3 103; 2003, 586; lactating – 1993, 1 043; 1998, 3 260; 2003, 1 190.
Reference (WHO): children 6 months to 6 years, 11.0g/dl; children 6.1 to 14 years, 12.0g/dl; pregnant women, 11.0 g/dl; lactating women, 12.0g/dl.
Sources: NNS, 1993; 1998; 2003.

Trends in vitamin A deficiency

As with anaemia, vitamin A deficiency (VAD) – defined as serum retinol (SR) < 20 µg/dl – is a lingering public health problem that has been affecting more than the public health cut-off of 15 percent of children aged six to 59 months and pregnant and lactating women over the last ten years. The data on VAD from the 2003 NNS reveal that the prevalence among children aged six to 59 months increased from 35 percent in 1993 and 38 percent in 1998 to 40.1 percent. The proportion of children with severe VAD (SR < 10 µg/dl) was 8.5 percent, which is not significantly different from the 8.2 percent of 1998. The prevalence of VAD among lactating women increased from 16.5 percent in 1998 to 20.1 percent in

2003. Referring back to dietary data presented in the previous section, it is clear that the vitamin A intake of preschool children (Table 13) was inadequate. The poor micronutrient status of pregnant and lactating women also explains in part why the prevalence of VAD in young children remains high, in spite of an ongoing national programme of twice-yearly vitamin A supplementation, which was started in 1993.

FIGURE 12
Prevalence of VAD by age/physiologic group, 1993 to 1998

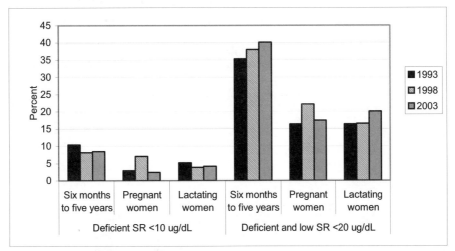

Sample sizes: 6 months to 5 years – 1993, 5 073; 1998, 14 291; pregnant – 1993, 765; 1998, 2 963; lactating – 1993, 1 051; 1999, 3 165.
Reference: deficient = SR < 10 ug/dl; deficient and low = SR < 20 ug/dl.
Sources: NNS, 1993, 1998.

Trends in iodine deficiency

In 1998, iodine deficiency was recognized as a mildly severe public health problem based on International Council for Control of Iodine Deficiency Disorders (ICCIDD) epidemiological criteria (i.e., median urinary iodine excretion [UIE] of between 50 to 99 µg/l among children aged six to 12 years). In that year, the median UIE level among Philippine children aged six to 12 years was 71 µg/L, and 36 percent of them had levels of less than 50 µg/l. In 2003, a significant improvement in the iodine status was noted. The median UIE among six- to 12-year-old children had increased to 201 µg/l, and the proportion of children with UIE levels less than 50 µg/l was down to 11 percent.

TABLE 19
Iodine status of selected population groups, 1998 and 2003

Group	Median UIE (µg/l)		Prevalence (%) of iodine deficiency (UIE < 50 µg/l)	
	1998	**2003**	**1998**	**2003**
6–12 years	71	201	35.8	11.0
Pregnant		142		18.0
Lactating		111		23.7

Sample sizes: 6 months to 12 years – 1998, 10 616; 2003, 4 665; pregnant – 2003, 583; lactating – 2003, 1 184.
Reference: UIE < 50 ug/l.
Sources: NNS, 1998; 2003.

Much of the dramatic improvement in iodine status has been attributed to the Salt Iodization Programme, and the increasing availability and consumption of processed foods among this age group of children in particular. These foods include processed foods and instant noodles that use iodized salt as mandated by the Salt Iodization Programme (described later in this case study). From the distribution of UIE values among six- to 12-year-old children shown in Figure 13 it can be noted that a high proportion (34.3 percent) of the children have UIE values ≥ 250 µg/l, and 14.3 percent have UIE ≥ 300 µg/l. These values correspond to more than adequate and possible excess in iodine intake, respectively (WHO/UNICEF/ICCIDD, 2001), which makes it even more important that compliance with recommended iodine levels in salt is ensured at production and retail sites.

FIGURE 13
Frequency distribution of UIE values of children aged six to 12 years, 1998 and 2003

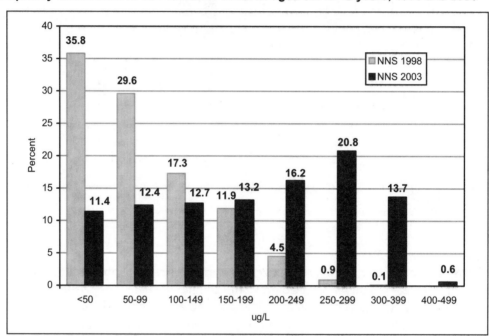

A high proportion of lactating women (23.7 percent) continue to have low UIE (< 50 µg/l), and the challenge of eliminating iodine deficiency in this population group remains. Differences in diet provide a plausible explanation for why this group is generally more iodine deficient than children, even when they come from the same households; processed foods, including instant noodles, snack foods and processed meats, are more commonly consumed by children than lactating women.

TRENDS IN PREVALENCE OF DIET-RELATED CVD RISK FACTORS
NNS reports increasing prevalence of nutrition-related risk factors for CVD among Philippine adults aged 20 years and over. These include overweight and obesity, as discussed earlier, as well as hypertension, diabetes and some indicators of dyslipidaemia.

Hypertension
In NNS 2003, 22.5 percent of Philippine adults were diagnosed as hypertensive, based on blood pressure (BP) (systolic BP > 140 mm Hg, or diastolic BP > 90 mm Hg) – a

significant increase from the 21 percent of 1998. The figures among middle-aged and elderly adults were even higher, ranging from 26.4 percent among those aged 40 to 49 years, to 40.2 percent among those aged 50 to 59 years, 45.8 percent in the 60 to 69 years age group, and 56 percent among people aged 70 years and over.

TABLE 20
Trends in the prevalence of hypertension among adults aged 20 years and over, 1998 and 2003

Age group (years)	1998	2003
	% prevalence	
20–29	11.3	8.8
30–39		14.1
40–49	29.0	26.4
50–59		40.2
60–69	44.3	45.8
70 +		56.0
All	**21.0**	**22.5**

Sample sizes: 1998, 9 299 ; 2003 – 20 to 39 years, 1402 ; 40 to 59 years, 1 021; ≥ 60 years, 2 330.
Reference: systolic BP > 140 mm Hg; diastolic BP > 90 mm Hg.
Source: NNS, 1998; 2003.

Dyslipidaemia

The prevalence of hypercholesterolaemia among Philippine adults in 2003 was 8.5 percent, which is more than twice the rate of 4 percent in 1998. There was a significant increase in the prevalence of hypercholesterolaemia over this period, particularly among middle-aged and older adults, among whom the condition remained significantly more prevalent (at 10 to 20 percent and 15 percent, respectively) than it did in younger adults.

The prevalence of elevated LDL-cholesterol among Philippine adults in 2003 was 3.7 percent, which is significantly higher than (nearly double) the 1998 rate of 2 percent. Over the five-year period, the prevalence of elevated LDL-cholesterol increased significantly among middle-aged and elderly adults.

The increasing trend in hypercholesterolaemia and elevated LDL-cholesterol may be associated with increased consumption of animal-based foods, particularly meats and possibly fats and oils, as well as the decreasing fruit and vegetable consumption as discussed earlier. There is no evidence to suggest increases in the prevalence of low HDL-cholesterol (< 35 mg/dl), which was 3.5 percent in 2003. However, using the cut-off of < 40 mg/dl, 54.2 percent of Philippine adults in NNS 2003 had predisposition to low HDL. Low HDL is associated with low consumption of fruits and vegetables, low physical activity and smoking. In NNS 2003, 62 percent of Philippine adults reported being physically inactive, 35 percent were current smokers, and 10 percent were former smokers.

TABLE 21
Trends in dyslipidaemia among adults aged 20 years and over, 1998 and 2003

Age group (years)	Elevated total cholesterol[1]		Elevated LDL-cholesterol[2]		Low HDL-cholesterol[3]	Elevated triglycerides[3]	
	1998	2003	1998	2003	2003	1998	2003
20–29	3.0	3.3	1.7	1.5	2.9	0.4	0.4
30–39		6.0		2.1	3.2		0.4
40–49	5.8	9.6	2.5	4.5	4.9	1.4	1.3
50–59		19.9		8.3	3.8		1.2
60–69	4.1	15.6	2.3	7.4	2.9	0.4	0.8
70 +		15.4		7.0	4.2		1.1
All	4.0	8.5	2.0	3.7	3.5	0.8	0.7

Sample sizes: 1998, 9 299; 2003 – 20 to 39 years, 1 402; 40 to 59 years, 1 021; ≥ 60 years, 2 330.
[1] Elevated total cholesterol = ≥ 240 mg/dl.
[2] Elevated LDL-cholesterol = > 190 mg/dl.
[3] Low HDL-cholesterol = < 35 mg/dl.
[4] Elevated triglycerides = ≥ 400 mg/dl.
Source: NNS, 1998; 2003.

There is also no evidence of an increasing prevalence of elevated triglycerides that could be associated with the increasing consumption of fats and oils (most of which is coconut oil) in Philippine households. Overall, fewer than 1 percent (0.7 percent) of Philippine adults had elevated triglycerides, which was slightly lower than the 1998 rate (0.8 percent).

In a study on hypertension among Philippine adults, which used data from NNS 1998, Duante *et al.* (2001) identified triglyceride level as one of the significant risk factors for hypertension, but there was no attendant increase in triglycerides with the increased prevalence of hypertension between 1998 and 2003. However, disaggregating the data by age group reveals increasing prevalence of elevated triglycerides among the elderly, rising from only 0.4 percent in 1998 to 0.8 percent among 60- to 69-year-olds and 1.1 percent among those aged 70 years and over in 2003. These groups also had the highest prevalence of hypertension.

Diabetes

The Philippine data show no evidence of a trend towards increasing prevalence of diabetes mellitus; this is surprising given that obesity increased significantly. The proportion of Philippine adults with diabetes mellitus was 3.9 percent in 1998, and 3.4 percent in 2003. However, the proportion of Philippine adults with impaired fasting blood glucose (FBG) – a prediabetic condition that increases the risk of diabetes – rose from 2.5 percent in 1998 to 3.2 percent in 2003 (FBS = 100 – 125 mg/dl).

TABLE 22
Trends in the prevalence of impaired FBG and diabetes mellitus among adults aged 20 years and over, 1998 and 2003

Age group (years)	1998		2003	
	% prevalence			
	Impaired FBG[1]	Diabetes mellitus	Impaired FBG[2]	Diabetes mellitus
20–29	1.9	2.6	1.2	0.7
30–39			2.1	2.0
40–49	3.1	5.4	5.0	4.9
50–59			5.7	8.9
60–69	3.2	6.2	5.6	6.3
70 +			6.2	5.1
All	2.5	3.9	3.2	3.4

Sample sizes: 1998, 9 299; 2003 – 20 to 39 years, 1 402; 40 to 59 years, 1 021; ≥ 60 years, 2 330.
Diabetes mellitus = FBS ≥ 126 mg/dl.
[1] FBS = 110 – 125 mg/dl.
[2] FBS = 100 – 125 mg/dl.
Source: NNS, 1998; 2003.

TRENDS IN MORTALITY FROM ALL CAUSES

Over the last 30 years, mortality from infections (including pneumonias, tuberculosis and bronchitis), other infectious diseases (such as gastroenteritis and colitis, diarrhoea and measles), tetanus, avitaminosis and other nutritional deficiencies has been declining significantly. In 1970, the reported deaths from pneumonia were 118 per 100 000 population, which dropped to 42.7 per 100 000 in 2000. Pneumonia was the leading cause of death in the Philippines in 1970 and until about 1985. Tuberculosis and other infectious diseases were the second and third leading causes of death, with 80 and 63 deaths per 100 000, respectively, in 1970; deaths due to all forms of tuberculosis were down to 36 per 100 000 by 2000. Meanwhile, the pattern regarding deaths from NCDs, such as diseases of the heart (including coronary artery disease and heart failure), diseases of the vascular system (e.g. strokes) and various cancers, has exhibited a significantly increasing trend in the last 30 years. This trend may be associated with changes in food consumption over the past 25 years, including increasing energy density with greater proportions of fat in total energy, and declining intakes of fruits, vegetables and traditional foods. It is also associated with the high prevalence of smoking. NNS 2003 revealed that 35 percent of Philippine adults were current, and 10 percent former, smokers. Diseases of the heart overtook other infectious diseases to become the third leading cause of death by 1975; they overtook tuberculosis as the second leading cause of death by 1980, and pneumonia as the number one cause of death by 1990. In 2000, diseases of the heart (at 79 deaths per 100 000 population), diseases of the vascular system (63 deaths) and various cancers (48 deaths) ranked first, second and fourth, respectively, as leading causes of deaths in the Philippines. Environment and other lifestyle-related diseases (including chronic obstructive pulmonary diseases, other respiratory diseases and diabetes) have emerged as a leading cause of mortality since 1995, and ranked as the third leading cause of death in 2000.

FIGURE 14
Mortality trends by cause of death, 1970 to 2000

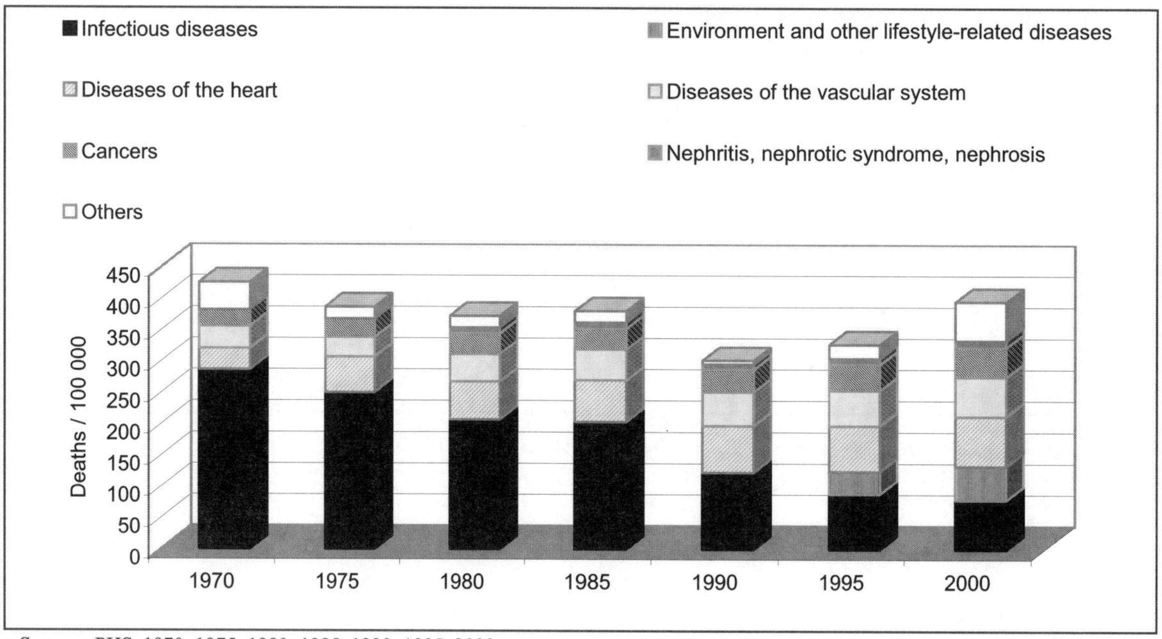

Sources: PHS, 1970; 1975; 1980; 1985; 1990; 1995; 2000.

NATIONAL NUTRITION POLICIES, STRATEGIES AND PROGRAMMES

The Philippines' nutrition policies, strategies and programmes are reflected in the Medium-Term Philippine Plan of Action for Nutrition (MTPPAN), which is formulated every five to six years by the National Nutrition Council (NNC), whose members include representations from various government agencies (e.g., the Departments of Health, Agriculture, Education, Social Welfare, Science and Technology, Interior and Local Government, and Budget and Management) and non-governmental organizations (NGOs). The MTPPAN is the government's blueprint for action to address the nutrition problems identified from NNS. The MTPPAN for 2005 to 2010 specifically aims to reduce underweight among children aged 0 to five years to levels based on the MDG target of 17.2 percent by 2015. This calls for accelerating the reduction rate of child undernutrition from the 0.58 percentage points a year (ppy) of 1998 to 2003, to no less than 0.81 ppy for 2005 to 2010 (NNC, 2005). The 2005 to 2010 MTPPAN also aims to reduce stunting and micronutrient deficiencies, particularly nutritional anaemia and VAD, among this group of children. Its other aims include reducing the following: underweight and stunting among children aged six to ten years; low birth weight; chronic energy deficiency among pregnant women; and micronutrient deficiencies among children aged six to 12 years and pregnant women. Targets are based on the reduction rates that were achieved in previous periods, or on the minimum prevalence for public health significance (e.g., 15 percent for VAD and 20 percent for iodine deficiency).

With regard to NCDs, the 2005 to 2010 MTPPAN will contribute to the achievement of targets that were identified by the National Coalition on the Prevention and Control of Non-Communicable Diseases, including reducing by 30 percent the prevalence of smoking, physical inactivity, hypertension, high FBG, obesity and total cholesterol among adults, and increasing the per capita intake of vegetables (NNC, 2005).

TABLE 23
MTPPAN targets for 2005 to 2010

	2005	2010	Estimated % reduction[1]
Prevalence of underweight among children 0–5 years old	25.88	21.58	16.62
Prevalence of underweight among children 6–10 years old	25.54	22.64	11.4
Prevalence of stunting among children 0–5 years old	28.96	25.36	12.4
Prevalence of stunting among children 6–10 years old	34.78	30.48	12.4
Prevalence of chronic energy deficiency among pregnant women	24.96	20.86	16.4
Prevalence of IDA among infants	59.20	41.70	29.6
Prevalence of IDA among children 1–5 years old	25.10	15.10	39.8
Prevalence of IDA among children 6–12 years old	34.00	25.50	25.0
Prevalence of IDA among pregnant women	43.30	42.10	2.8
Prevalence of VAD among children 6 months to 5 years old	32.90	15.00	54.7
Prevalence of VAD among pregnant women	15.62	10.92	30.1
Prevalence of VAD among lactating women	18.64	15.00	19.5
Prevalence of iodine deficiency among lactating women	22.64	20.00	11.7
Prevalence of current smoking among adult males	49.5	34.7	30%
Prevalence of current smoking among adolescent females	10.6	7.5	30%
Per capita total vegetable intake (g/day)	123.2	160.2	
Prevalence of hypertension among adult males	19.8	13.9	30%
Prevalence of adults with high FBG	3.0	2.1	30%
Prevalence of central obesity (WHR) among females	48.2	33.8	30%
Prevalence of high total serum cholesterol among adult males	7.5	5.2	30%

[1] Computed by subtracting the 2010 target from the 2005 estimated baseline, and dividing by the 2005 estimated baseline.

In spite of its apparently uneven targets for under- and overnutrition, the 2005 to 2010 MTPPAN clearly recognizes and addresses undernutrition as a public health problem among children, and pregnant and lactating women; it also recognizes and addresses nutritional factors associated with overnutrition and risks of NCDs among adults. This can be inferred from the plan's adoption of the life cycle approach, which recognizes that intergenerational consequences of undernutrition start from poor nutrition during pre-pregnancy and adolescence, and include the contribution of foetal undernutrition to adult chronic diseases (Aggett and Schofield, 2000).

The MTPPAN promotes the programmes described in the following paragraphs. Each of these programmes has the potential to address the double burden or coexistence of under- and overnutrition in households and communities, whether implicitly as in the case of micronutrient supplementation and food fortification, or explicitly as with home and community food production and nutrition education.

Home, school and community food production

This programme involves kitchen gardens and small animal raising activities to increase the supply of inexpensive, nutrient-rich sources of energy, protein, vitamin A and iron, as well as dietary fibre, in households. It has the potential to increase home and community production of fresh fruits and vegetables, which can improve the quality of diets for both under- and overweight individuals, while increasing intakes of essential micronutrients (Hawkes *et al.*, 2005). The MTPPAN document makes explicit reference to the role of home and community gardens in increasing the intakes of essential micronutrients and dietary fibre, thereby addressing both undernutrition and the nutrition-related risk factors for CVD, hypercholesterolaemia, elevated LDL-cholesterol levels and certain cancers.

Nutrition education

This programme aims to promote desirable food, health and nutrition practices and lifestyle behaviours to ensure nutritional well-being, and addresses both under- and overnutrition. The intervention uses the Nutritional Guidelines for the Philippines (see Annex 4) as its framework, and follows the life cycle approach by targeting preschool children, schoolchildren, pre-adolescents, teenagers, pregnant and lactating women, and mothers and care providers. Promotion of the Nutritional Guidelines for the Philippines aims to address undernutrition by emphasizing the importance of exclusive breastfeeding, appropriate complementary feeding, consumption of a variety of foods, growth monitoring, and positive health-seeking behaviours. It also aims to address overweight and obesity and other diet and lifestyle factors associated with NCDs by, for example, limiting the consumption of fatty and salty foods, sugars and alcoholic beverages, increasing physical activity and avoiding smoking.

In addition, there are ongoing efforts to incorporate modules into the curricula of public and private schools; these are designed to increase physical activity and healthy lifestyles among schoolchildren. The National Coalition on the Prevention and Control of Non-Communicable Diseases and the Department of Health are carrying out other initiatives, including campaigns for healthy lifestyle in the workplace, communities and restaurants.

Food fortification

To address the persistent problem of micronutrient deficiencies, the Philippines has enacted two laws on food fortification to ensure adequate intakes of vitamin A, iron and iodine among all sectors of the population. These laws include the mandatory fortification of staples such as rice with iron, sugar and cooking oil with vitamin A, and wheat flour with iron and vitamin A, which were introduced in 2000, and the iodization of salt, which was introduced in 1995. The programme also promotes voluntary micronutrient fortification of other processed foods. Under this scheme, the Department of Health awards a Sangkap Pinoy Seal of approval, which the manufacturer puts on to the food label indicating that the food contains the recommended amount and type of fortification. Currently, 142 processed foods on the market carry the Sangkap Pinoy Seal.

However, there has been resistance to the law on mandatory fortification of rice, sugar and cooking oil on the part of manufacturers who object to having to bear the additional costs involved. Legislative consultations with various interest groups, including manufacturers and the public, are being carried out to identify how best to address the concerns of both groups.

Micronutrient supplementation

Similar to food fortification, the micronutrient supplementation programme aims to reduce micronutrient deficiencies. This programme includes universal vitamin A supplementation for all children six months to six years of age and for lactating women, and targeted supplementation to selected populations, particularly iron for infants and young children, pregnant and lactating women and adolescent females, and iodine for schoolchildren and women of child-bearing age in high-risk areas.

Between 1999 and 2003, the vitamin A supplementation programme reached 23 726 215 children, or 92.8 percent of those in the target 12 to 83 months age group, and 3 503 315 or 73.9 percent of nursing women. Over the same period, iron supplementation was provided to 12 979 689 (85.7 percent) pregnant and lactating women, 3 097 116 (80.3 percent) preschool-age children, 1 577 618 (73.3 percent) infants and 3 367 795 (83.2 percent) schoolchildren through the local health system (NNC, 2005). The outreach for iodine supplementation has been far lower, covering 56.2 percent of targeted women and 74.4 percent of targeted schoolchildren.

Clearly, the country's nutrient supplementation and food fortification programmes, except perhaps salt iodization, have not yet had the desired impact on the micronutrient status of target population groups. The iron supplementation programme has been beset with funding problems and inadequate supplies of iron supplements. The current six-monthly dosing schedule for the universal vitamin A supplementation programme, which started in 1993, may be inadequate for areas with high prevalence of VAD (Pedro *et al.,* 2005; Perlas *et al.,* 1996). It is not clear how the target 55 percent reduction of VAD in children can be achieved through universal six-monthly vitamin A supplementation alone.

Food assistance

This programme serves as a short-term, stop-gap measure to rehabilitate undernourished populations, particularly preschool children, immediately and to prevent undernutrition in areas affected by calamities or emergency situations during the critical periods of complementary feeding for children aged six to 24 months and among women in the second trimester of pregnancy. Food assistance also includes the provision of basic food commodities at subsidized prices to poor households in nutritionally and economically depressed communities, as a contribution to the government's poverty alleviation programme. Also being tested are food-for-work and food-for-school schemes, which entail the provision of basic nutritional food commodities to poor households (NNC, 2005).

Other programmes in the 2005 to 2010 MTPPAN are livelihood assistance; the integration of nutrition concerns into mother-and-child health programmes, including newborn screening, infant and young child feeding, integrated management of childhood illnesses, adolescent health and early childhood care and development; and the provision of safe and potable water supply and environmental sanitation (NNC, 2005).

CONCLUSION

The dietary changes that have occurred in Philippine households in the last 25 years are reflections of the increasing urbanization of the country. Urbanization increased from 37 percent in 1980 to 60 percent in 2000. Urban diets have been associated with increasingly Westernized food habits, such as high-fat diets, processed foods and refined carbohydrates. Data from the Philippines exhibit a pattern of increasing intakes of fats and oils, sugars and syrups, meats and processed meat products, and other cereals and cereal products (including breads and bakery products, noodles, and snack foods made from wheat flour), and declining fruit and vegetable consumption. It is likely that these trends will continue given the escalating urbanization of the Philippine population (the urban proportion is expected to reach 68 percent by 2015), coupled with the effects of increasing globalization such as trade liberalization, which has increased the availability and variety of processed and fast foods, the frequency of eating outside the home, the use of computers and computer games, and the influence of mass media.

Based on national data, the food intake in Philippine households in 2003 represents general improvements in quality and quantity, except with regard to declining fruit and vegetable consumption. The improvements have been in the direction of dietary goals and Philippine nutritional guidelines, including increasing the intakes of animal foods ("to increase good quality proteins and absorbable iron to satisfy nutritional requirements") and fats and oils ("as a remedy to caloric deficiency and to help lower the risk of vitamin A deficiency by facilitating its absorption and utilization"). In terms of the Philippines' progress in achieving the MDGs, in 2003 fewer households had less than 100 percent per capita energy adequacy than in 1993. However, the improvement falls short of the rate necessary to meet the target. In spite of increased consumption of the food sources of iron, calcium and riboflavin, as demonstrated by increasing intake of animal source foods – including meats and dairy – these nutrients remain inadequate.

While the increased intake of animal foods and fats and oils was generally an improvement, there may be a trade-off in terms of increased cholesterol and saturated fats in diets, and increased overweight in children, adolescents and adults when coupled with sedentary lifestyles. Although the data show no evidence of increasing prevalence of low HDL-cholesterol and elevated triglycerides, the trend towards increasing obesity, hypercholesterolaemia and elevated LDL-cholesterol, which are known risk factors for CVD, is alarming. There has been increasing mortality from diseases of the heart and vascular system, which in the last ten years have become the top two leading causes of death in the country. While consumption of animal foods and fats and oils, prevalence of obesity, hypercholesterolaemia and elevated LDL-cholesterol, and mortality from CVD and other NCDs are moving in the same direction, the consumption of fruits and vegetables and other traditional staples such as maize and root crops has steadily declined over time. Among the reasons cited for the low intake of fruits and vegetables are cost or affordability and the declining production of fruits and vegetables, including indigenous produce, for local markets. This trend has been associated with policies on trade liberalization and globalization. It should not be discounted that other lifestyle-related factors, particularly physical inactivity and lack of exercise, stress, smoking and alcohol consumption – which are also known risk factors for obesity, hypertension, CVD and other chronic degenerative diseases – have contributed significantly to the increasing incidence of these lifestyle diseases.

"Unhealthy" or "faulty" diets, i.e., those characterized by high fat, refined carbohydrates and meat, are more likely to occur in certain sectors of the population than others: more among urban than rural dwellers, and more among higher-income than lower-income groups, even within urban areas. "Unhealthy" diets at the other end of the spectrum (i.e., those that are inadequate in energy, protein and many essential nutrients) are more common among lower-income groups. The available data on food consumption and nutritional status show national or regional estimates, and should therefore be disaggregated to ascertain disparities in the dietary patterns and malnutrition across income groups (although these are probably decreasing considering the declining income inequality as measured by the Gini ratio), as well as across age groups.

Although there has been progress in addressing undernutrition in the Philippines, it is still a problem of far greater magnitude than overnutrition is, especially among children. Out of every 100 children aged 0 to five years, 27 are underweight-for-age, 30 are stunted, more than 30 are anaemic, 40 are vitamin-A deficient, and only one is overweight. Out of every 100 children aged six to ten years, 27 are underweight, 37 are stunted, 37 are anaemic, 11 are iodine deficient, and again only one is overweight. The burden of undernutrition is also greater among 11- to 12-year-olds and 13- to 19-year-olds, with six underweight to every one overweight in the former, and four underweight to every one overweight in the latter age group. Among adults, on the other hand, there are twice as many cases of overweight as underweight.

There are indications that the country is facing a double burden of malnutrition, as evidenced by the coexistence at the population level of undernutrition among children and the elderly with overnutrition among adults. The malnutrition double burden within households, e.g., an underweight child and an overweight mother, is also reported to be emerging, with prevalence of 8.2 percent in one poor urban community, rising to about 20 percent in a high-income urban community (Agdeppa, Laña and Barba, 2003). There is increasing scientific evidence to support Barker's hypothesis that chronic diseases such as CVD, type-2 diabetes and hypertension in later life may have their origins in foetal cardiovascular, metabolic and endocrine adaptation to intrauterine growth retardation (Aggett and Schofield, 2000). The prevalence of low birth weight was estimated to be about 9 to 11 percent in the 1990 to 1997 period, rising to about 18 percent in 1995 to 2000 (UNICEF 2000; 2002; de Onis, Blössner and Villar, 1998). Based on this hypothesis, the increasing prevalence of non-communicable or chronic degenerative diseases may be associated with maternal and foetal undernutrition, rather than dietary and lifestyle changes alone. Thus, addressing undernutrition from early life, including pre-pregnancy and maternal undernutrition, will contribute to reducing NCDs in the Philippines. Overnutrition increases with age, so programmes aimed at preventing overweight/obesity and NCDs in later life should start with children, particularly by increasing physical activity and exercise.

The life cycle approach calls for integrated, rather than distinct, intervention programmes that address under- and overnutrition in both communities and households by, for example, increasing fruit and vegetable production and consumption, encouraging the consumption of dried beans, nuts and seeds, marine products and lean meats, and promoting increased physical activity and exercise in children and adults.

REFERENCES

Agdeppa, I.A., Laña, R.D. & Barba, C.V.C. 2003. A case study on dual forms of malnutrition among selected households in District 1, Tondo, Manila. *Asia Pacific J. Clin. Nutr.,* 12(4): 438–446.

Aggett, P.J. & Schofield, L. 2000. Early nutrition and adult health: how strong are the links? *Mal. J. Nutr.,* 6(2): 181–187.

Cerdeña, C.M., Laña, R.D., Molano, W.L., Chavez, M.C. & Nones, C.A. 2002. *Philippine Nutrition Facts and Figures Supplement 1: 2002 Update of the Nutritional Status of 0–10-year-old Filipino Children.* Manila, FNRI-DOST.

Cheong Revelita, Madriaga, J.R., Perlas, L.A., Desnacido, J.A., Marcos, J.M. & Cabrera, M.I.Z. 2001. Prevalence of anemia among Filipinos. *Philippine Journal of Nutrition,* 48(1–2): 45–57.

De Onis, M., Blössner, M. & Villar, J. 1998. Levels and patterns of intrauterine growth retardation in developing countries. *European J. of Clinical Nutrition,* 52(S1): S5–S15.

Department of Health. No date. Field Health Service Information System (FHSIS).

Department of Health. No date. *Health statistics.* Available at www.doh.gov.ph.

Duante, C.A., Velandra, F.V., Orense, C.L. & Tangco, J.B.M. 2001. Correlates of hypertension and android obesity among Filipino adults. *Philippine Journal of Nutrition,* 48(1–2): 81–102.

FAO. 2003. *The state of world food insecurity.* Rome.

Florentino, R.F., Pedro, M.R.A. & Molano, W.L. 1996.The changing dietary intake and food consumption patterns in the Philippines. In *Changing dietary intake and food consumption in Asia and the Pacific.* Tokyo, Asian Productivity Organization.

FNRI-DOST. 1976. *Recommended dietary allowance (RDA) for Philippines.* Manila.

FNRI-DOST. 1989. *Recommended dietary allowance (RDA) for Philippines.* Manila.

FNRI-DOST. 2000. *Nutritional guidelines for Philippines.* Manila.

FNRI-DOST. 2001. *Philippine nutrition facts and figures.* Manila.

FNRI-DOST. 2002a. *Baseline survey and data generation on nutritional status, psychosocial development and care of 0–6 year-old children in ECD provinces (final report).* Manila.

FNRI-DOST. 2002b. *Recommended energy and nutrient intakes (RENI).* Manila.

Hawkes, C., Eckhardt, C., Ruel, M. & Minot, N. 2005. Diet quality, poverty and food policy: A new research agenda for obesity prevention in developing countries. *SCN News,* 29: 20–22.

Kuizon, M.D., Perlas, L.A., Madriaga, J.R., Cheong, R.L., Desnacido, J.A., Marcos, J.M., Fuertes, R.T. & Valdez, D.H. 1993. *Fourth National Nutrition Survey: Philippines, 1993. Part D. Biochemical Nutrition Survey.* Manila, FNRI-DOST.

Madriaga, J.R., Cheong Revelita, Desnacido, J.A., Marcos, J.M., Cabrera, M.I.Z. & Perlas, L.A. 2001. Prevalence of vitamin A deficiency among specific Filipino population groups. *Philippine Journal of Nutrition,* 48(1–2): 29–43.

Madriaga, J.R., Cheong Revelita, Desnacido, J.A., Marcos, J.M., Loyola, A.S., Sison, C.C. & Cabrera, M.I.Z. 2001. Prevalence of iodine deficiency in the Philippines. *Philippine Journal of Nutrition,* 48(1–2): 59–68.

Magbitang, J.A., Tangco, J.B.M., Dela Cruz, E.O., Flores, E.G. & Guanlao, F.E. 1988. Weight for height as measure of nutritional status in Filipino pregnant women. *Public Health Asia Pacific Journal,* 2(2): 96–104.

Must, A., Dallal, G.E. & Dietz, W.H. 1991. Reference data for obesity: 85th and 96th percentiles of body mass index (wt/ht2) – a correction. *American Journal of Clinical Nutrition,* 53: 839–846.

National Statistical Coordination Board. No date. *Poverty statistics.* Available at: www.nscb.gov.ph.

National Statistics Office. 2003. *Philippine National Demographic and Health Survey.* Manila.

NEDA. 2005. Medium Term Philippines Development Plan 2005–2010 (draft). Manila, National Economic Development Authority (NEDA).

NNC. *The Medium-Term Philippine Plan of Action for Nutrition 2005 to 2010.* Manila. (draft)

Pedro, M.R.A., Barba, C.V.C. & Candelaria, L.V. No date. *Globalization, food consumption, health and nutrition in urban areas.* Manila, FNRI-DOST.

Pedro, M.R.A., Madriaga, J.R., Barba, C.V.C., Habito, R.F.C., Gana, A.E., Deitchler, M. & Mason, J.B. 2004. The national vitamin A supplementation and sub-clinical vitamin A deficiency among preschool children in the Philippines. *Food and Nutrition Bulletin,* 25(4): 319–329.

Pedro, M.R.A., Cerdeña, C.M., Constantino, M.A.S., Patalen, M.L.P., Palafox, E.F., Delos Reyes, C.M., Castillo, E.V., De Leon, J.Y. & Barba, C.V.C. 2005. *Sixth National Nutrition Survey: Philippines, 2003. National Food Consumption Survey: Household Level.* Manila, FNRI-DOST.

Pedro, M.R.A., Cerdeña, C.M., Patalen, M.L.P., Nones, C.A., Vargas, M.B., Laña, R.D., Castillo, E.V. & Barba, C.V.C. 2005. *Sixth National Nutrition Survey: Philippines, 2003. Update on the Nutritional Status of Filipinos.* Manila, FNRI-DOST.

Perlas, L.A., Florentino, R.F., Fuertes, R.T., Cheong Revelita, Madriaga, J.R., Desnacido, J.A., Marcos, J.M. & Cabrera, M.I.Z. 1996. Vitamin A status of Filipino preschool children given a massive oral dose. *Southeast Asian Journal of Tropical Medicine,* 27(4): 785–791.

Perlas, L.A., Madriaga JR, Cheong Revelita, Marcos, J.M., Desnacido, J.A., Perez, E.S., Ulanday, J.R.C., Sumayao Jr., R.E., Cabrera, M.I.Z. & Barba, C.V.C. 2005. *Sixth National Nutrition Survey: Philippines, 2003. Biochemical Phase.* Manila, FNRI-DOST.

Popkin, B. 1994. The nutrition transition in low-income countries: an emerging crisis. *Nutrition Reviews,* 52(9).

Population Commission. 2002. *APPC Country Report,* pp. 27–32. Available at www.popcom.gov.ph.

Reyes, C.M. 2003. Country development programming framework for the Philippines: assessment of the social sector. (unpublished paper)

Shetty, P. & Gopalan, C., eds. 1998. *Diet, nutrition and chronic disease: an Asian perspective.* London, Smith-Gordon and Co.

Templo, O.M. 2003. Country development programming framework for the Philippines: Philippine development context and challenges. (unpublished paper)

UNDP. 2004. *Human development report 2004.* New York.

UNICEF. 2000. *The state of the world's children 2000.* New York.

UNICEF. 2002. *Official summary: The state of the world's children 2002.* New York.

UNICEF. 2003. *The state of the world's children 2003.* New York.

UN Population Division. 2004. *World population prospects: The 2004 revision* and *world urbanization prospects.* New York, Department of Economic and Social Affairs of the United Nations Secretariat.

USDA. No date. Nutrient Data Laboratory. Available at: www.nal.usda.gov/fnic/foodcomp/search/.

Velandria, F.V., Duante, C.A., Mendoza, T.S., Mendoza, S.M. & Dela Cruz, E.O. 2001. Prevalence of android obesity among Filipino adults, 20 years and over. *Philippine Journal of Nutrition,* 48(1–2): 69–80.

Villavieja, G.M., Valerio, T.E., Abaya, H.S.P., Angelo, T.N., Cerdeña, C.M. & Domdom, A.C. 1981. *First Nationwide Nutrition Survey: Philippines, 1978. Part A – Food Consumption Survey, 2nd revision.* Manila, FNRI, National Science Development Board.

Villavieja, G.M., Valerio, T.E., Abaya, H.S.P., Cerdeña, C.M. & Domdom, A.C. 1984. *Second Nationwide Nutrition Survey: Philippines, 1982. Part A – Food Consumption Survey.* Manila, FNRI, National Science and Technology Authority.

Villavieja, G.M., Cerdeña, C.M. & Chavez, M.C. 1985. *Dietary assessment of infants and toddlers in the Philippines.* Manila, FNRI, National Science and Technology Authority.

Villavieja, G.M., Valerio, T.E., Cerdeña, C.M., Abaya, H.S.P., Feliciano, E.A., Boquecosa, J.P., Red, E.R., Nones, C.A. & Constantino, A.S. 1989. *Third National Nutrition Survey: Philippines, 1987. Part A – Food Consumption Survey.* Manila, FNRI-DOST.

Villavieja, G.M., Cerdeña, C.M., Molano, W.L., Laña, R.D., Boquecosa, J.P., Raymundo, B.E., Nones, C.A., Abaya, H.S.P., Palafox, E.F., Chavez, M.C., Burayag, G.A., Pine, C.R., Recuenco, J.R.D., Saturno, D.S. & Delos Reyes, C.M. 1997. *Fourth National Nutrition Survey: Philippines, 1993. Part A-Food Consumption Survey.* Manila, FNRI-DOST.

Villavieja, G.M., Molano, W.L., Cerdeña, C.M., Laña, R.D., Constantino, A.S., Tarrayo, M.E.R., Concepcion, D.S., Juguan, J.A. & Sario, I.S. 1997. Fourth National Nutrition Survey, Philippines, 1993. Part B Anthropometric Survey. *Philippine Journal of Nutrition,* 44(1–2): 34–48.

Villavieja, G.M., Laña, R.D., Cerdeña, C.M., Constantino, A.S., Boquecosa, J.P., Chavez, M.C., Palafox, E.F., Nones, C.A., Concepcion, D.S., Tarrayo, M.E.R. & Casio, M.B. 1998. Updating of Nutritional Status of Filipino Children at the Provincial Level. *Philippine Journal of Nutrition,* 48(1–2): 1–14.

Villavieja, G.M., Constantino, A.S., Laña, R.D., Nones, C.A., Nueva España, M.B. & Pine, C.R. 2001. Anthropometric assessment of adolescents, adults, pregnant and lactating women: Philippines, 1998. *Philippine Journal of Nutrition,* 48(1–2): 15–28.

WHO. 1995. *Physical status: the use and interpretation of anthropometry.* Report of a WHO Expert Committee. WHO Technical Report Series No. 854. Geneva.

WHO/FAO. 2003. *Diet, nutrition and the prevention of chronic diseases.* Report of a Joint WHO/FAO Expert Consultation. WHO Technical Report Series No. 916. Geneva.

WHO/UNICEF/ICCIDD. 2001. *Assessment of iodine deficiency disorders and monitoring their elimination.* Geneva. (WHO/NHD/01.1).

ANNEX 1: PHILIPPINE RDAs, 1976

Age group	Weight	Energy	Protein	Calcium	Iron	Vitamin A	Vitamin B12	Thiamine	Ribo-flavin	Niacin	Vitamin C
	kg	kcal	g	g	mg	RE	IU	mg	mg	mg	mg
Males											
20–39 years	56	2 580	63	0.5	10	650	4 500	1.3	1.3	17	75
40–49 years	56	2 450	63	0.5	10	650	4 500	1.2	1.2	16	75
50–59 years	56	2 320	63	0.5	10	650	4 500	1.2	1.2	15	75
60–69 years	56	2 060	63	0.5	10	650	4 500	1.0	1.0	14	75
70 + years	56	1 810	63	0.5	10	650	4 500	0.9	0.9	13	75
Females											
20–39 years	48	1 920	54	0.5	18*	550	3 800	1.0	1.0	13	70
40–49 years	48	1 820	54	0.5	18*	550	3 800	0.9	0.9	13	70
50–59 years	48	1 730	54	0.5	8	550	3 800	0.9	0.9	13	70
60–69 years	48	1 540	54	0.5	8	550	3 800	0.8	0.8	13	70
70 + years	48	1 340	54	0.5	8	550	3 800	0.7	0.7	13	70
Infants, 6–11 months	9	970	25	0.6	9	250	1 800	0.5	0.5	6	30
Children											
1–3 years	13	1 310	26	0.5	6	250	1 800	0.7	0.7	9	35
4–6 years	18	1 640	32	0.5	8	325	2 300	0.8	0.8	11	45
7–9 years	24	1 870	37	0.5	7	400	2 800	0.9	0.9	12	55
Boys											
10–12 years	32	2 270	43	0.7	11	500	3 500	1.1	1.1	15	65
13–15 years	44	2 510	59	0.7	12	550	4 300	1.3	1.3	17	75
16–19 years	55	2 700	67	0.6	13	650	4 500	1.4	1.4	18	90
Girls											
10–12 years	35	2 170	48	0.7	18*	500	3 500	1.1	1.1	14	70
13–15 years	44	2 200	59	0.7	18*	550	4 300	1.1	1.1	15	75
16–19 years	48	2 060	59	0.6	18*	550	4 300	1.0	1.0	14	80

Age group	Weight kg	Energy kcal	Protein g	Calcium g	Iron mg	Vitamin A RE	Vitamin B12 IU	Thiamine mg	Ribo-flavin mg	Niacin mg	Vitamin C mg
Pregnant, 2nd and 3rd trimesters											
13–15 years		2 630	73	1.0	18	625	4 300	1.5	1.5	18	120
16–19 years		2 490	73	1.0	18	625	4 300	1.4	1.4	17	120
20–39 years		2 350	68	1.0	18	575	4 000	1.4	1.4	16	120
40–49 years		2 250	68	1.0	18	575	4 000	1.3	1.3	16	120
Nursing, 1st 6 months											
13–15 years		2 750	87	1.0	18	975	6 800	1.4	1.7	19	120
16–19 years		2 610	87	1.0	18	975	6 800	1.3	1.6	18	120
20–39 years		2 470	82	1.0	18	975	6 800	1.3	1.6	17	120
40–49 years		2 370	82	1.0	18	975	6 800	1.2	1.5	17	120
Nursing, next 6 months											
13–15 years		2 640	75	1.0	18	800	5 600	1.4	1.5	18	120
16–19 years		2 500	75	1.0	18	800	5 600	1.3	1.4	17	120
20–39 years		2 360	70	1.0	18	800	5 600	1.3	1.4	16	120
40–49 years		2 260	70	1.0	18	800	5 600	1.2	1.3	16	120
Per capita/day[1]		**2 016**	**50**	**0.6**	**12**	**520**	**3 612**	**1.0**	**1.0**	**14**	**67**

* It is preferable that these amounts be higher than indicated. Supplemental iron is recommended during pregnancy,
[1] Based on 1977 population structure (low assumption).

ANNEX 2: PHILIPPINE RDAs, 1989

Age group	Weight kg	Energy kcal	Protein g	Vitamin A ug	Vitamin C mg	Thiamine mg	Ribo-flavin mg	Niacin mg	Folate ug	Calcium g	Iron mg	Iodine mg
Infants												
3–< 6 months	6	620	a	325	30	0.3	0.3	5	20	300	10	40
6–< 12 months	9	880	14	325	30	0.4	0.4	8	30	400	15	50
Children												
1–3 years	13	1 350	27	350	35	0.7	0.7	13	40	600	9	55
4–6 years	18	1 600	32	375	45	0.8	0.8	15	60	600	10	65
7–9 years	24	1 740	35	400	55	0.9	0.9	17	80	600	12	70
Males												
10–12 years	32	2 090	45	425	65	1	1	20	100	700	16	85
13–15 years	44	2 340	60	475	75	1.2	1.2	22	140	700	18	105
16–19 years	55	2 580	69	525	90	1.3	1.3	25	170	700	17	120
20–39 years	56	2 570	60	525	75	1.3	1.3	25	170	500	12	120
40–49 years	56	2 440	60	525	75	1.2	1.2	23	170	500	12	120
50–59 years	56	2 320	60	525	75	1.2	1.2	22	170	500	12	120
60–69 years	56	2 090	60	525	75	1	1	20	170	500	12	120
70 + years	56	1 880	60	525	75	0.9	0.9	18	170	500	12	120
Females												
10–12 years	35	1 910	49	400	70	1	1	18	110	700	17	80
13–15 years	44	2 010	56	425	75	1	1	19	140	700	21	100
16–19 years	48	2 020	56	450	80	1	1	19	150	500	25	100
20–39 years	49	1 900	52	450	70	1	1	18	150	500	26	100
40–49 years	49	1 800	52	450	70	0.9	0.9	17	150	500	26	100
50–59 years	49	1 710	52	450	70	0.8	0.8	16	150	500	11	100
60–69 years	49	1 540	52	450	70	0.8	0.8	15	150	500	11	100
70 + years	49	1 390	52	450	70	0.7	0.7	13	150	500	11	100
Pregnant												
1st trimester		0	9	25	10	0	0	0	200	400	41	25
2nd trimester		300	9	25	10	0.3	0.6	3	200	400	41	25
3rd trimester		300	9	25	10	0.3	0.6	3	200	400	41	25
Lactating												
1st 6 months		500	16	325	35	0.4	0.4	5	100	400	23	50
2nd 6 months		500	12	275	30	0.4	0.4	5	100	400	23	50

ANNEX 3: PHILLIPINE RENIs, 2002

Age group	Weight kg	Energy kcal	Protein g	Vitamin A ug	Vitamin C mg	Thiamine mg	Ribo-flavin mg	Niacin mg	Folate ug	Calcium mg	Iron mg	Iodine mg
Infants												
< 3 months		0	0	0	0	0	0	0	0	0	0	0
3–< 6 months	6	560	9	375	30	0.2	0.3	1.5	65	200	0	90
6–< 12 months	9	720	14	400	30	0.4	0.4	4	80	400	10	90
Children												
1–3 years	13	1 070	28	400	30	0.5	0.5	6	160	500	8	90
4–6 years	19	1 410	38	400	30	0.6	0.6	7	200	550	9	90
7–9 years	24	1 600	43	400	35	0.7	0.7	9	300	700	11	120
Males												
10–12 years	34	2 140	54	400	45	0.9	1	12	400	1000	13	120
13–15 years	50	2 800	71	550	65	1.2	1.3	16	400	1000	20	150
16–18 years	58	2 840	73	600	75	1.4	1.5	16	400	1000	14	150
19–29 years	59	2 490	67	550	75	1.2	1.3	16	400	750	12	150
30–49 years	59	2 420	67	550	75	1.2	1.3	16	400	750	12	150
50–64 years	59	2 170	67	550	75	1.2	1.3	16	400	750	12	150
65 + years	59	1 890	67	550	75	1.2	1.3	16	400	800	12	150
Females												
10–12 years	35	1 920	49	400	45	0.9	0.9	12	400	1000	19	120
13–15 years	49	2 250	63	450	65	1	1	14	400	1000	21	150
16–18 years	50	2 050	59	450	70	1.1	1.1	14	400	1000	27	150
19–29 years	51	1 860	58	500	70	1.1	1.1	14	400	750	27	150
30–49 years	51	1 810	58	500	70	1.1	1.1	14	400	750	27	150
50–64 years	51	1 620	58	500	70	1.1	1.1	14	400	800	27	150
65 + years	51	1 410	58	500	70	1.1	1.1	14	400	800	10	150
Pregnant												
1st trimester		0	66	800	80	1.4	1.7	18	600	800	27	200
2nd trimester		300	66	800	80	1.4	1.7	18	600	800	34	200
3rd trimester		300	66	800	80	1.4	1.7	18	600	800	38	200
Lactating												
1st 6 months		500	81	900	105	1.5	1.7	17	500	750	27	200
2nd 6 months		500	76	900	100	1.5	1.7	17	500	750	30	200

ANNEX 4: NUTRITIONAL GUIDELINES FOR THE PHILIPPINES, 2000

1. Eat a variety of foods every day.
2. Breastfeed infants from birth to four to six months, and then give appropriate foods while continuing breastfeeding.
3. Maintain children's normal growth through proper diet, and monitor their growth regularly.
4. Consume fish, lean meat, poultry or dried beans.
5. Eat more vegetables, fruits and root crops.
6. Eat foods cooked in edible/cooking oil daily.
7. Consume milk, milk products and other calcium-rich foods, such as small fish and dark-green leafy vegetables, every day.
8. Use iodized salt, but avoid excessive intake of salty foods.
9. Eat clean and safe food.
10. For a healthy lifestyle and good nutrition, exercise regularly, do not smoke and avoid drinking alcoholic beverages.

ANNEX 5: TRENDS IN PERCENTAGE CONTRIBUTION OF FOOD GROUPS TO TOTAL DIETARY ENERGY INTAKE (KCAL), 1978 TO 2003

Food group/sub-group	% distribution				
	1978	1982	1987	1993	2003
Energy giving foods					
Cereals and cereal products	69.7	69.8	69.2	71.0	67.5
Rice and products	58.2	57.1	58.3	56.4	52.8
Maize and products	7.6	7.2	4.7	6.8	5.2
Other cereals and products	3.9	5.5	6.2	7.8	9.5
Starchy roots and tubers	2.2	2.3	1.3	1.0	1.2
Sugars and syrups[1]	3.7	4.5	4.8	4.2	4.4
Fats and oils[2]	4.9	6.2	6.3	5.9	5.9
Body building foods					
Fish, meat and poultry	7.5	8.6	9.5	9.5	12.0
Fish and products	3.8	3.6	4.0	3.7	3.4
Meat and products	3.2	4.3	4.9	4.9	7.4
Poultry	0.5	0.6	0.6	1.0	1.2
Eggs	0.6	0.7	0.8	1.0	1.0
Milk and milk products	5.2	1.5	1.3	1.4	1.4
Whole milk				1.3	1.2
Milk products				0.1	0.2
Dried beans, nuts and seeds[3]	1.1	1.3	1.3	1.3	1.1
Regulating foods					
Vegetables	1.9	1.6		1.5	1.7
Green leafy and yellow vegetables	0.5	0.5	0.4	0.4	0.5
Other vegetables	1.4	1.1	3.4[a]	1.1	1.2
Fruits	2.5	2.3		2.1	1.6
Vitamin C-rich foods	0.8	0.6	0.7	0.5	0.2
Other fruits	1.7	1.7		1.7	1.4
Miscellaneous	0.6	1.0	1.0	1.1	2.2
Beverages[4]					1.6
Condiments					0.4
Others					0.2
Total kcal	**1 804**	**1 808**	**1 753**	**1 684**	**1 887**

Sample sizes: 1978, 2 800; 1982, 2 280; 1987, 3 200; 1993, 4 050; 2003, 5 514.
[1] Includes soft drinks (sugar content), sherbet and similar preparations.
[2] Includes grated coconut and coconut milk (fat).
[3] Includes mung beans, soybeans, peanuts and other dried beans, nuts.
[4] Includes coffee, tuba (local wine), alcoholic beverages and others.
[a] Includes other fruits and other vegetables.
Numbers may not add up to totals owing to rounding off.
Sources: NNS, 1978; 1982; 1987; 1993; 2003.

ANNEX 6: TRENDS IN MEAN PER CAPITA IRON INTAKE (MG) BY FOOD GROUP, 1978 TO 2003

Food group/sub-group	Consumption (mg)				
	1978	1982	1987	1993	2003
Energy giving foods					
Cereals and cereal products	4.7	4.6	4.5	4.1	4.6
Rice and products	3.8	3.4	3.3	2.7	2.8
Maize and products	0.3	0.4	0.2	0.3	0.2
Other cereals and products	0.7	0.9	1.0	1.2	1.5
Starchy roots and tubers	0.3	0.3	0.2	0.2	0.2
Sugars and syrups[1]	0.1	0.0	0.0	0.0	0.1
Fats and oils[2]	0.1	0.1	0.1	0.1	0.1
Body building foods					
Fish, meat and poultry	2.6	2.6	2.8	2.9	2.2
Fish and products	2.2	2.1	2.1	2.2	1.0
Meat and products	0.3	0.4	0.6	0.6	1.0
Poultry	0.1	0.1	0.1	0.1	0.2
Eggs	0.2	0.2	0.3	0.3	0.3
Milk and milk products	0.1	0.1	0.1	0.1	0.2
Whole milk				0.1	0.2
Milk products				0.1	0.0
Dried beans, nuts and seeds[3]	0.4	0.4	0.4	0.4	0.4
Regulating foods					
Vegetables	1.3	1.2		1.1	1.1
Green leafy and yellow vegetables	0.7	0.7	0.6	0.6	0.5
Other vegetables	0.6	0.5	0.8[a]	0.5	0.5
Fruits	0.5	0.5		0.3	0.2
Vitamin C-rich foods	0.2	0.2	0.2	0.1	0.1
Other fruits	0.3	0.3		0.2	0.2
Miscellaneous	0.7	0.6	0.6	0.6	0.8
Beverages[4]					0.4
Condiments					0.3
Others					0.1
Total mg	**11.0**	**10.8**	**10.7**	**10.1**	**10.0**

Sample sizes: 1978, 2 800; 1982, 2 280; 1987, 3 200; 1993, 4 050; 2003, 5 514.
[1] Includes soft drinks (sugar content), sherbet and similar preparations.
[2] Includes grated coconut and coconut milk (fat).
[3] Includes mung beans, soybeans, peanuts and other dried beans, nuts.
[4] Includes coffee, tuba (local wine), alcoholic beverages and others.
[a] Includes other fruits and other vegetables.
Numbers may not add up to totals owing to rounding off.
Sources: NNS, 1978; 1982; 1987; 1993; 2003.

ANNEX 7: TRENDS IN PERCENTAGE CONTRIBUTIONS OF FOOD GROUPS TO IRON INTAKE (MG), 1978 TO 2003

Food group/sub-group	% distribution				
	1978	1982	1987	1993	2003
Energy giving foods					
Cereals and cereal products	42.6	42.8	42.1	40.9	45.7
Rice and products	34.1	31.1	30.4	26.4	28.8
Maize and products	2.4	3.3	2.3	2.7	1.6
Other cereals and products	6.1	8.3	9.4	11.8	15.3
Starchy roots and tubers	3.0	3.0	1.7	1.5	1.7
Sugars and syrups[1]	1.3	0.4	0.4	0.3	0.5
Fats and oils[2]	0.6	0.9	0.8	0.7	0.7
Body building foods					
Fish, meat and poultry	23.8	23.8	25.9	28.4	22.0
Fish and products	20.2	19.0	19.6	21.5	10.0
Meat and products	3.0	3.8	5.4	5.6	10.2
Poultry	0.6	0.9	0.9	1.3	1.8
Eggs	1.8	2.1	2.4	2.9	3.2
Milk and milk products	0.6	0.9	1.2	1.0	1.6
Whole milk				0.9	1.5
Milk products				0.5	0.1
Dried beans, nuts and seeds[3]	3.4	3.7	4.1	4.0	3.9
Regulating foods					
Vegetables	11.7	11.5		11.0	10.5
Green leafy and yellow vegetables	6.7	6.6	5.7	5.7	5.2
Other vegetables	5.0	4.9	7.6[a]	5.3	5.3
Fruits	4.5	4.9		3.2	2.4
Vitamin C-rich foods	2.1	2.4	2.1	0.9	0.5
Other fruits	2.4	2.5		2.3	1.9
Miscellaneous	6.4	5.8	6.0	6.2	7.8
Beverages[4]					4.5
Condiments					2.8
Others					0.5
Total mg	**11.0**	**10.8**	**10.7**	**10.1**	**10.0**

Sample sizes: 1978, 2 800; 1982, 2 280; 1987, 3 200; 1993, 4 050; 2003, 5 514.
[1] Includes soft drinks (sugar content), sherbet and similar preparations.
[2] Includes grated coconut and coconut milk (fat).
[3] Includes mung beans, soybeans, peanuts and other dried beans, nuts.
[4] Includes coffee, tuba (local wine), alcoholic beverages and others.
[a] Includes other fruits and other vegetables.
Numbers may not add up to totals owing to rounding off.
Sources: NNS, 1978; 1982; 1987; 1993; 2003.

ANNEX 8: MEAN DAILY PER CAPITA FOOD CONSUMPTION BY REGION, 2003

Food group/sub-group	Philippines	NCR	Ilocos	CAR	Cagayan Valley	Central Luzon	Cala-barzon	Mima-ropa	Bicol
	Consumption, in grams raw as purchased								
Energy giving foods									
Cereals and cereal products	364	320	377	393	389	363	352	399	361
Rice and products	303	267	350	363	359	325	315	371	296
Maize and products	31	5[a]	1[a]	4[a]	6[a]	4[a]	4[a]	4[a]	27[a]
Other cereals and products	30	47	26	26	24	34	33	24	38
Starchy roots and tubers	19	19[a]	14[a]	34[a]	32[a]	13[a]	10	26[a]	23[a]
Sugars and syrups[1]	24	28	27	25	22	27	24	23	23
Fats and oils[2]	18	29	16[a]	14[a]	16	18	22	17[a]	17
Body building foods									
Fish, meat and poultry	185	226	188	175	149	209	194	167	146
Fish and products	104	94	102	59	69	102	98	96	97
Meat and products	61	102	75	84	54[a]	82	73	59	43[a]
Poultry	20	30[a]	11[a]	3[a]2	26[a]	25	23[a]	12[a]	6[a]
Eggs	13	18	14	10[a]	12	18	15[a]	11	8[a]
Milk and milk products	49	76	42	30[a]	37[a]	65	64	27	29
Whole milk	35	53	37	26[a]	26[a]	40	41	21	24[a]
Milk products	14	23	5	4	11	25	23	6	5
Dried beans, nuts and seeds[3]	10	13[a]	8	18[a]	13	9	8	9[a]	10
Regulating foods									
Vegetables	111	88	171	155	132	99	99	129	118
Green leafy and yellow vegetables	31	22	43	49	46	19	24	22	30
Other vegetables	80	66	128	106	86	80	75	107	88
Fruits	54	60[a]	41[a]	49[a]	22[a]	56	43[a]	87[a]	52[a]
Vitamin C-rich foods	12	15[a]	11[a]	16[a]	7[a]	13[a]	10[a]	16[a]	13[a]
Other fruits	42	45[a]	30[a]	33[a]	15[a]	43[a]	33[a]	71[a]	39[a]
Miscellaneous	39	56[a]	29	26[a]	26[a]	38	50[a]	41[a]	25[a]
Beverages[4]	26	43[a]	16[a]	18[a]	15[a]	20	36[a]	28[a]	14[a]
Condiments	10	10	11	6	9	10	10	10	10
Others	3	3	2	2	2	8	4	3	1
Total food	**886**	**933**	**927**	**929**	**850**	**915**	**881**	**936**	**812**

Food group/sub-group	Western Visayas	Central Visayas	Eastern Visayas	Zamboanga Peninsula	Northern Mindanao	Davao	Sossk-Sargen	Caraga	ARMM
	Consumption, in grams raw as purchased								
Energy giving foods									
Cereals and cereal products	390	350	357	380	404	381	401	385	350
Rice and products	351	187	309	243	252	300	364	308	336
Maize and products	18[a]	136	26[a]	116[a]	133[a]	55[a]	22[a]	54[a]	1[a]
Other cereals and products	21	27	22[a]	21[a]	19	26	15	23	13
Starchy roots and tubers	14[a]	18[a]	18[a]	22[a]	35[a]	30[a]	17[a]	25[a]	29[a]
Sugars and syrups[1]	22	21	20	17	16	28	24	21	21
Fats and oils[2]	11	13	19	13[a]	16	16[a]	11	14[a]	12[a]
Body building foods									
Fish, meat and poultry	200	153	168	138	158	194	170	157	151
Fish and products	140	103	122	108	101	113	117	105	120
Meat and products	43	43[a]	34[a]	21[a]	37	53[a]	39[a]	35[a]	13[a]
Poultry	17[a]	7[a]	12[a]	9[a]	20[a]	28[a]	14[a]	17[a]	18[a]
Eggs	14	12	8[a]	8[a]	10[a]	14	9[a]	10[a]	9[a]
Milk and milk products	49[a]	31[a]	33[a]	21[a]	46	57[a]	32[a]	36[a]	19[a]
Whole milk	35[a]	26[a]	28[a]	20[a]	38	37	21	29	19[a]
Milk products	14[a]	5[a]	5[a]	1[a]	8[a]	20[a]	11[a]	7[a]	0[a]
Dried beans, nuts and seeds[3]	8[a]	11[a]	10	9[a]	13[a]	11	8	9[a]	4[a]
Regulating foods									
Vegetables	127	108	93	84[a]	131	101	139	121	80
Green leafy and yellow vegetables	35	43[a]	20	29[a]	42	39	44	37	19
Other vegetables	92	65	73	55[a]	89	62	95	84	61
Fruits	58[a]	39[a]	44[a]	51[a]	66[a]	98[a]	56	60[a]	38[a]
Vitamin C-rich foods	7[a]	9[a]	4[a]	3[a]	17[a]	24[a]	13[a]	12[a]	4[a]
Other fruits	51[a]	30[a]	40[a]	48[a]	49	74[a]	43	48[a]	34[a]
Miscellaneous	40[a]	30	43[a]	23[a]	38[a]	43[a]	31	48[a]	16[a]
Beverages[4]	28[a]	17[a]	31[a]	9[a]	24[a]	29[a]	18[a]	33[a]	9[a]
Condiments	10	12[a]	11	12	12	12	11	14	6
Others	2[a]	1[a]	1[a]	2[a]	2[a]	2[a]	2[a]	1[a]	1[a]
Total food	**933**	**786**	**813**	**766**	**933**	**973**	**898**	**886**	**729**

Sample size: 5 514.
[1] Includes soft drinks (sugar content), sherbet and similar preparations.
[2] Includes grated coconut and coconut milk (fat).
[3] Includes mung beans, soybeans, peanuts and other dried beans, nuts.
[4] Includes coffee, tuba (local wine), alcoholic beverages and others.
[a] CV ≥ 15 percent.
Numbers may not add up to totals owing to rounding off.
Source: NNS, 2003.

ANNEX 9: MEAN DAILY PER CAPITA ENERGY AND NUTRIENT INTAKES AND PERCENTAGE ADEQUACY BY REGION, 2003

	Region					
	NCR	Ilocos	Cagayan	CAR	Central Luzon	Cala-Barzon
Energy (kcal)						
Intake	1 942	1 944	1 940	2 072	1 955	1 888
RNI	1 955	1 922	1 938	1 971	1 946	1 943
% adequacy	99.4	101.2	100.1	105.1	100.5	97.2
Protein (g)						
Intake	61.4	56.6	53.3	60.4	57.9	56.7
RNI	56.8	56.8	56.9	57.3	56.9	56.9
% adequacy	108.1	99.6	93.5	105.4	101.8	99.7
Iron (mg)						
Intake	11.2	11.0	10.2	11.4	10.6	10.4
RNI	17.3	16.3	16.6	16.8	16.8	17.2
% adequacy	64.6	67.5	61.3	67.8	62.8	60.3
Retinol equivalent (mcg)						
Intake	557.1	524.3	461.1	718.2	374.2	583.5
RNI	499.6	497.8	497.7	497.9	500.0	498.2
% adequacy	111.5	105.3	92.6	144.2	74.8	117.1
Calcium (g)						
Intake	0.46	0.50	0.45	0.47	0.42	0.41
RNI	0.76	0.77	0.77	0.77	0.76	0.77
% adequacy	60.8	65.5	58.5	60.4	55.2	54.1
Thiamine (mg)						
Intake	0.97	0.93	0.89	1.17	0.89	0.91
RNI	1.03	1.03	1.03	1.03	1.03	1.03
% adequacy	93.9	90.3	86.8	113.1	86.6	88.3
Riboflavin (mg)						
Intake	0.84	0.78	0.74	0.88	0.74	0.82
RNI	1.08	1.07	1.07	1.08	1.07	1.07
% adequacy	77.8	73.3	68.7	82.0	69.2	76.3
Niacin (mg)						
Intake	22.4	21.4	20.2	24.7	20.9	21.6
RNI	13.3	13.2	13.3	13.3	13.2	13.3
% adequacy	168.4	161.5	152.2	185.6	157.9	162.5
Ascorbic acid (mg)						
Intake	47.8	45.5	42.9	60.8	42.6	39.5
RNI	62.8	62.2	62.3	62.3	62.3	62.5
% adequacy	76.0	73.1	68.9	97.6	68.3	63.3

Nutrients	Region					
	Mima-Ropa	Bicol	Western Visayas	Central Visayas	Eastern Visayas	Zamboanga Peninsula
Energy (kcal)						
Intake	2 008	1 856	1 936	1 782	1 803	1 762
RNI	1 921	1 924	1 937	1 925	1 912	1 914
% adequacy	104.5	96.5	99.9	92.6	94.3	92.1
Protein (g)						
Intake	54.8	50.6	58.0	51.8	51.6	50.6
RNI	56.0	56.7	56.4	56.4	55.9	56.0
% adequacy	97.8	89.2	102.8	91.8	92.4	90.4
Iron (mg)						
Intake	10.1	9.2	10.5	8.7	8.7	7.9
RNI	16.6	16.5	16.5	16.5	16.1	16.7
% adequacy	61.2	55.9	63.8	52.9	53.9	47.7
Retinol equivalent (mcg)						
Intake	469.5	371.3	426.2	349.1	361.5	337.7
RNI	495.0	500.7	496.1	495.6	491.5	492.1
% adequacy	94.9	74.2	85.9	70.4	73.5	68.6
Calcium (g)						
Intake	0.43	0.40	0.50	0.42	0.41	0.37
RNI	0.76	0.76	0.76	0.77	0.76	0.77
% adequacy	56.5	51.8	65.8	54.4	54.4	48.6
Thiamine (mg)						
Intake	0.88	0.80	1.08	0.79	0.77	0.69
RNI	1.01	1.03	1.02	1.02	1.01	1.01
% adequacy	87.1	77.7	106.2	77.3	76.6	68.0
Riboflavin (mg)						
Intake	0.67	0.62	0.70	0.64	0.61	0.57
RNI	1.05	1.07	1.06	1.06	1.05	1.05
% adequacy	63.8	57.4	65.6	60.1	58.4	54.4
Niacin (mg)						
Intake	21.3	18.3	21.7	16.2	19.4	16.8
RNI	13.0	13.2	13.1	13.1	12.9	13.0
% adequacy	163.5	138.6	165.1	124.1	149.6	129.5
Ascorbic acid (mg)						
Intake	52.8	47.2	45.9	50.1	38.1	37.7
RNI	60.8	62.3	61.6	61.3	60.7	60.7
% adequacy	86.9	75.7	74.4	81.8	62.8	62.1

Nutrients	Region				
	Northern Mindanao	Davao	Soccsk-Sargen	Caraga	ARMM
Energy (kcal)					
Intake	1 955	1 998	1 911	1 898	1 683
RNI	1 994	1 948	1 980	1 898	1 874
% adequacy	98.0	102.6	96.5	100.0	89.8
Protein (g)					
Intake	57.7	59.0	56.8	52.6	47.4
RNI	58.1	56.9	57.2	55.4	53.7
% adequacy	99.3	103.8	99.2	94.9	88.3
Iron (mg)					
Intake	9.9	10.4	9.3	9.8	7.5
RNI	16.6	16.9	16.8	16.2	16.0
% adequacy	59.2	61.3	55.6	60.8	46.8
Retinol equivalent (mcg)					
Intake	399.3	451.5	380.0	597.9	236.2
RNI	505.0	504.1	502.0	495.6	484.7
% adequacy	79.1	89.6	75.7	120.7	48.7
Calcium (g)					
Intake	0.46	0.45	0.41	0.44	0.32
RNI	0.77	0.76	0.77	0.75	0.75
% adequacy	59.6	58.5	53.2	58.1	43.3
Thiamine (mg)					
Intake	0.83	0.87	0.83	0.80	0.59
RNI	1.05	1.03	1.03	1.00	0.97
% adequacy	78.8	84.9	80.9	79.9	61.6
Riboflavin (mg)					
Intake	0.67	0.76	0.66	0.72	0.53
RNI	1.10	1.08	1.08	1.05	1.01
% adequacy	61.2	70.9	61.0	69.2	52.9
Niacin (mg)					
Intake	19.8	21.8	22.3	19.4	19.1
RNI	13.5	13.2	13.3	12.9	12.3
% adequacy	146.6	165.1	167.9	151.1	155.3
Ascorbic acid (mg)					
Intake	62.0	61.8	48.1	52.8	31.8
RNI	63.4	62.4	62.3	60.3	57.7
% adequacy	97.8	99.1	77.3	87.6	55.1

Sample size: 5 514.
Source: NNS, 2003.

ANNEX 10: TRENDS IN LEADING CAUSES OF MORTALITY AND PERCENTAGE OF TOTAL DEATHS, 1970 TO 2000

Cause	1970		1975		1980		1985		1990		1995		2000	
	Rate	% of total	Rate	% of total	Rate	% of total	Rate	% of total	Rate	% of total	Rate	% of total	Rate	% of total
Pneumonias	118.2	17.6	102.0	16.0	93.6	15.2	96.7	15.8	66.3	13.1	49.0	10.4	42.7	8.9
Diseases of the heart	34.0	5.0	56.6	8.9	60.8	9.8	10.8	66.3	74.4	14.7	73.2	15.5	79.1	16.5
Tuberculosis, all forms	80.1	11.9	69.2	10.9	59.6	9.7	57.9	9.5	39.1	7.7	39.4	8.3	36.1	7.5
Diseases of the vascular system	35.8	5.3	31.8	5.0	43.8	7.2	49.7	8.1	54.2	10.7	56.2	11.9	63.2	13.2
Malignant neoplasms	25.7	3.8	29.4	4.6	33.2	5.4	33.2	5.4	35.7	7.1	41.5	8.8	47.7	9.9
Accidents	24.8	3.7	19.1	3.0	18.7	3.0	18.4	3.0	6.4	1.3	23.0	4.9	42.4	8.8
Avitaminosis and other nutritional deficiencies	25.5	3.8	26.0	4.1	15.3	2.5	13.0	2.1	-	-	-	-	-	-
Nephritis, nephrotic syndrome and nephrosis	-	-	-	-	9.3	1.5	10.0	1.6	8.3	1.6	9.6	2.0	10.4	2.2
Other infectious diseases (gastroenteritis and colitis, bronchitis, diarrhoeas, measles)	62.9	9.2	43.0	6.8	38.6	6.2	35.8	5.8	17.6	3.5	-	-	-	-
Lifestyle-related diseases (COPD and allied conditions, other diseases of the respiratory system, diabetes)	-	-	-	-	-	-	-	-	-	-	36.1	7.7	54.7	11.3
Other diseases (ill-defined disease peculiar to early infancy, tetanus, septicaemia)	19.1	2.8	10.0	1.6	-	-	-	-	9.4	1.9	-	-	-	-

Rates are given per 100 000 of population.

Dietary changes and the health transition in South Africa: implications for health policy

N.P. Steyn, D. Bradshaw, R. Norman, J.D. Joubert, M. Schneider and K. Steyn

INTRODUCTION

South Africa is a middle-income country with a variety of living conditions ranging through wealthy and middle-income suburbs, deprived peri-urban areas, rural farms and undeveloped rural areas. Changing social, political and economic factors have resulted in increased urbanization and changes in diet and health behaviours. Estimates for South Africa show that despite the high burden of infectious diseases, non-communicable diseases (NCDs) account for a large proportion of deaths. In 2000, infectious diseases accounted for 44 percent of deaths, and HIV/AIDS alone for 29 percent (Bradshaw *et al.*, 2003). NCDs accounted for 37 percent of deaths; cardiovascular disease (CVD) and diabetes accounting for 19 percent, and cancers for a further 7.5 percent. In contrast, nutritional deficiencies related to undernutrition accounted for 1.2 percent of deaths. As a result of the relatively high burdens of injuries and HIV/AIDS, the burden of disease in South Africa has been described as a "quadruple burden" of conditions related to underdevelopment, emerging chronic diseases related to unhealthy lifestyles, HIV/AIDS, and injuries.

This case study provides data from published research of diet, dietary trends, nutritional status and diet-related chronic diseases in South Africa over recent decades. These are assessed in the context of trends in the communicable disease burden. A review of the changes in diet and the health transition experienced in South Africa could contribute to the development of a national strategy with a strong dietary policy component that would be effective in the long term.

Brief historical background

South Africa has a heterogeneous population of approximately 46 million people of diverse origins. Historically, people of Khoi, San, Bantu, European and Indian descent pioneered the country, and at present more than a million people are from other African countries, Asia, Europe, Australia, New Zealand and the Americas. The rich heritage of South Africa has resulted in vast cultural and ethnic diversity, with 11 official languages and several other indigenous languages and dialects. The largest organized religion is Christianity, and others include Islam, Hinduism and Judaism. In addition, many people follow a "traditionalist" belief system (Department of Health, SAMRC and Measure DHS+, 2002). The 2001 census (Statistics South Africa, 2003) incorporated the following self-classified and self-reported population groups: black/African (79 percent), coloured/mixed origin (8.9 percent), white (9.6 percent) and Asian/Indian (2.5 percent).[1]

---

[1] These population group classifications reflect self-reporting according to groups defined by the Population Registration Act of 1950. This classification highlights issues that reflect the effects of historical disparities, and the authors do not subscribe to it for any other purpose. The terms "black" and "African" are used interchangeably.

Segregation and discrimination had been part of South Africa's history for hundreds of years. Over the last century, the country's people endured complex systems of neo-colonial and Apartheid repression and oppression. In the 1980s, escalating conflict, civil unrest, changes in the ideology of the then-ruling National Party, declining economic growth and international sanctions contributed to the creation of alternative political views. Subsequent negotiations resulted in the country's first democratic elections in April 1994 and the development of a new political dispensation (Blaauw and Gilson, 2001). South Africa is currently undergoing a profound social transition from its segregationist past to a democracy supported by a progressive constitution entrenching extensive human rights and fundamental political freedoms. The country's political past was intertwined with its geographic formation and governing system. Hence, 11 geopolitical areas consisting of the former provinces, four independent states and six self-governing areas have been restructured into nine provinces (Figure 1), and a new governing system has been established at the national, provincial and local levels (Blaauw and Gilson, 2001).

The development challenge faced by South Africa is enormous. While aiming to build a society based on human rights and social justice, the country has to grapple with the legacy of an income distribution that is among the most unequal in the world, combined with high levels of poverty and unemployment. Furthermore, strategies to promote economic growth are likely to reduce the likelihood of eliminating these inequalities in the near future (Terreblanche, 2004).

Demographic and socio-economic indicators

The dietary and individual risk behaviour of people defines their nutritional status, health, growth and development. These do not occur in a vacuum but within a cultural, economic, social and political context, which can either aggravate or promote health (WHO, 2003). As South Africa is undergoing major transformations, it is important to describe some demographic, economic, health and development trends that may play diverse roles in nutrition and health.

Selected demographic indicators

Common to the situation in most sub-Saharan countries, South Africa's demographic and epidemiological data systems have limitations. Determined efforts over the past decade have improved the processes and products of vital registration systems, but sources of complete and reliable vital statistics remain difficult to achieve (Bradshaw *et al.*, 2003). The country's rapidly growing AIDS epidemic has affected many demographic and epidemiological trends in atypical ways that would challenge data systems under even optimal circumstances. The internationally acknowledged model of the Actuarial Society of South Africa (ASSA) has the best potential for the purposes of this case study, which has used the ASSA2002 suite of models when empirical data were not available or reliable. Details of the models and their assumptions are available on the Internet at www.assa.org.za.

FIGURE 1
Current geographic composition of South Africa

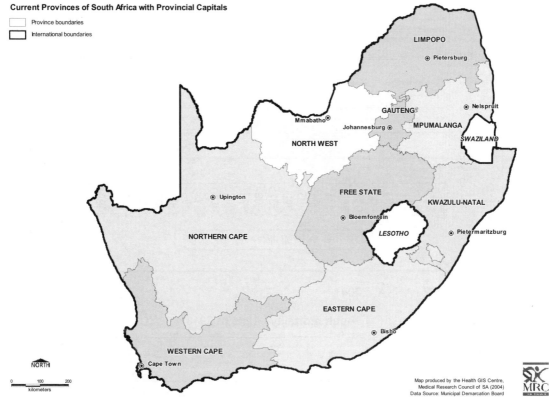

Source: HSRC, 2003.

Life expectancy and adult, child and infant mortality rates: After a steadily increasing average life expectancy at birth throughout the 1980s, the mortality impact of the country's severe AIDS epidemic is evident in the considerable drop in life expectancy in the early 1990s, from 61.6 years in 1992 to 49.7 in 2006, and is also reflected in increased infant and child mortality. The harshness of the impact on women is made clear by the unusually rapid narrowing of the difference between female and male life expectancy, from eight years in the early 1990s to less than four years in 2010 (Figure 2). Both the fall in life expectancy and the change in the sex differential are mirrored in the steeply upward trend of the 45q15, or the probability that a person aged 15 years will not live another 45 years to reach 60 years of age (Figure 3). The infant and child mortality rates do not reflect the country's middle-income economic status, particularly since the AIDS epidemic. However, assuming dedicated efforts to prevent vertical HIV transmission in the model, a recovery to and improvement of pre-AIDS trends in infant and child mortality are projected (Figure 4).

FIGURE 2
Average life expectancy at birth, 1985 to 2010

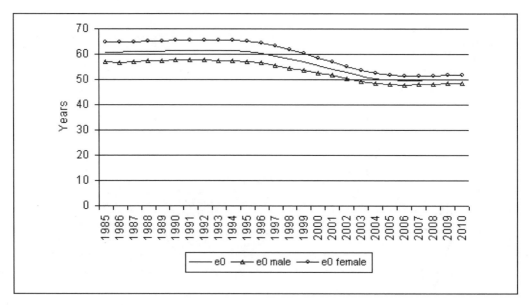

Source: ASSA2002 (ASSA, 2004).

FIGURE 3
Adult mortality,[1] 1985 to 2010

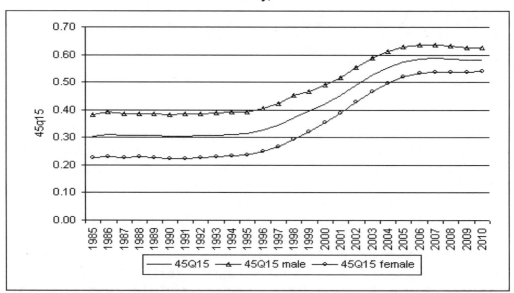

[1] *nqx* represents the proportion of people in a particular cohort who are alive at the beginning of an indicated age interval (*x*) and who will die before reaching the end of that age interval (*x* + *n*). In other words, the *nqx* values stand for the probability that a person at his/her *x*th birthday will die before reaching his/her *x* + *n*th birthday. So, 45q15 represents the probability that people aged 15 years will die before they reach the age of 60 (or 15 + 45). This can also be called "premature adult mortality". The 45q15 is widely used as a demographic indicator of adult mortality.
Source: ASSA2002 (ASSA, 2004).

FIGURE 4
Infant and child mortality rates, 1985 to 2010

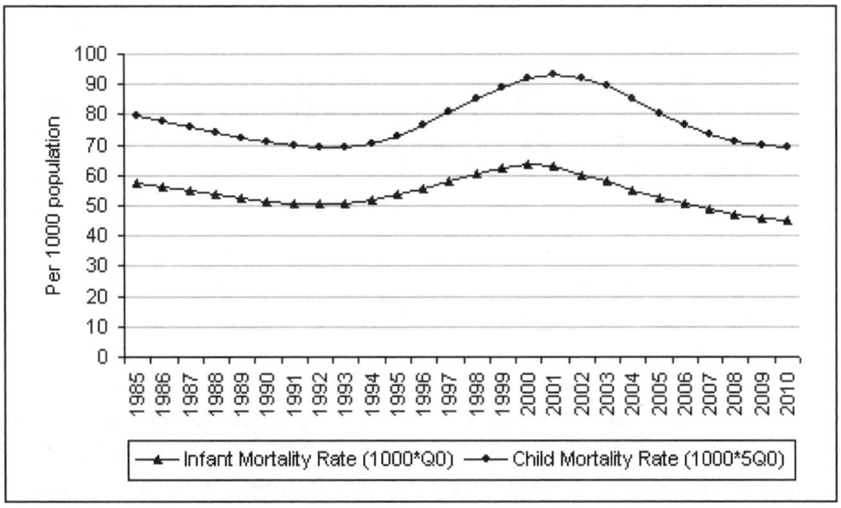

Source: ASSA2002 (ASSA, 2004).

Total population and fertility rates: South Africa's total fertility rate has been declining for several decades, and is currently estimated at 2.6 children born alive per woman during her reproductive lifetime, indicating that the population is well-advanced in its fertility transition (Moultrie and Timæus, 2003). With increasing mortality rates and decreasing fertility and birth rates, the average annual growth rate of the total population is projected to decline dramatically over a short period. These demographic changes reflect an epidemic with a vast impact. Figures 29 and 30, presented in another section of this case study, convey part of the vastness by illustrating the projected numbers of HIV-infected and AIDS-sick people, and showing the huge mortality from AIDS alone compared with that from all other diseases, disabilities and injuries combined.

Urbanization trends: Urbanization and other migration patterns are perceived as important issues in health and nutrition, but relationships and patterns of migration are complex in South Africa, and suitable data sources are very scarce. The 1996 population census provides data on internal migration for the entire population for the first time, but the absence of suitable data prior to this has constrained the analysis of migration data over time (Kok *et al.,* 2003). Urbanization, in particular, has different histories for the country's four main population groups, with the urbanization levels of black South Africans diverging most prominently from those of other groups. Until July 1986 when it was abolished, "influx control" legislation prevented the black population from settling permanently outside the independent and self-governing states. The "group areas" legislation, repealed in June 1990, enforced the resettlement of millions of South Africans, mostly black African people (Gelderblom and Kok, 1994; Kok *et al.,* 2003). These and other political controls and legislation were directed not only towards restricting black migration, but also towards controlling black labour (Terreblanche and Nattrass, 1990). By 2001, almost 90 percent of the white and coloured population and nearly 100 percent of the Indian population were urbanized, compared with about 50 percent of the black population (P. Kok, personal communication, 2004).

Selected socio-economic indicators

Gross domestic product (GDP): Sufficient, safe and varied food supply can prevent under- and overnutrition and reduce the risk of chronic disease. However, there is also evidence that poverty and inequity are part of the root causes of malnutrition (WHO, 2003). South Africa's per capita GDP, corrected for purchasing power parity (PPP) at US$11 240 per year in 2001, placed it among the 50 wealthiest nations in the world (May, 2004). However, in 1993 the World Bank described the country as one of the world's most unequal economies, with a Gini coefficient for income as high as 0.58 (World Bank, cited in May, 2004); this indicator had deteriorated to 0.69 in 2000, making South Africa the third most unequal society in the world (UNDP, 2001). This also suggests that income inequality has worsened nationally, despite official efforts to increase wages at the lower end of the income scale, such as for domestic and farm workers (cf. Department of Labour, 2002).

Figure 5 shows the country's per capita GDP, corrected for PPP, which has increased steadily since the 1980s. However, such macroeconomic indicators conceal important concerns that may affect community or individual nutritional status and well-being. For example, in 1993, 19 million people – almost half of the country's population – were categorized as poor (Klasen, 1997 cited in May, 1998), and 11.5 percent of the population were living on less than PPP$1 per day, while 35.8 percent lived on less than PPP$2 (World Bank, 2000 cited in May, 2004). In a rigorous analysis of poverty and related data, Woolard and Leibbrandt (2001 cited in May, 2004) used 1995 data to indicate that the situation continues to be bleak, with 40 to 50 percent of South Africans categorized as poor, including 25 percent ultra-poor. Although definitions of poverty have been adapted over the years and changes in the incidence and severity of poverty are debated, various studies suggest that poverty levels and the number of people living in poverty have increased over recent years (cf. Budlender, 2000; Statistics South Africa, 2002; Van der Ruit and May, 2003; Meth and Dias, 2004 – all cited in May, 2004).

FIGURE 5
GDP per capita: 1980, 1990 and annual values for 1994 to 2002

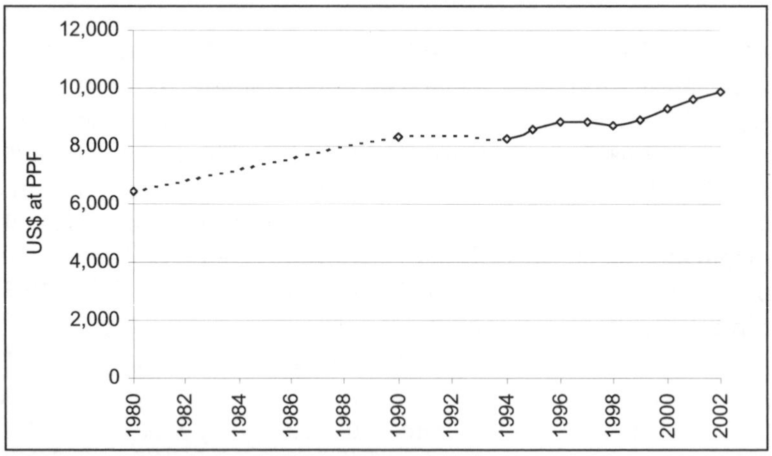

Data points for 1981 to 1989 and 1991 to 1993 are interpolated.
Source: Quatec Dataset in UNDP, 2003.

Unemployment: Differing conceptual, methodological, theoretical and ideological positions can influence the measuring of unemployment, and this seems to be particularly true in South Africa (Archer *et al.,* 1990). However, there is wide consensus that the unemployment rate has increased considerably over the past three decades (Figure 6). Since the mid-1970s, every year there have been fewer wage jobs available than the number of people entering the labour market (Archer *et al.,* 1990). Towards the turn of the century this observation was highlighted by May (1998), who said that the South African economy is creating employment too slowly to make a meaningful impression on unemployment levels. Despite employment creation efforts by the new government, after ten years of democracy the rate of unemployment had risen significantly – whether unemployment be defined broadly or narrowly (HSRC, 2003).

FIGURE 6
Unemployment rates, 1970 to 2002

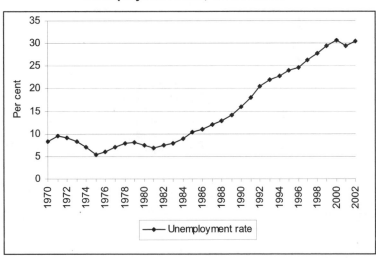

Sources: South African Reserve Bank Quarterly Bulletin 2003, q1; EIU Country Data; World Bank Global Development Indicators; and IMF Financial Statistics – reported in UNDP, 2003.

Housing and sanitation: The environment that people live in has the potential to aggravate or promote their health. Despite improvements over the past decade, almost a third of South Africa's households live in informal and traditional dwellings, about a third have piped water inside their homes, slightly more than half use a flush or chemical toilet, and 14 percent have no toilet. A considerable number of households continue to lack basic services, and much still has to be done to enhance the country's inherited skewed system of access to these services.

Burden of disease

The initial burden of disease study of 2000 (Bradshaw *et al.,* 2003) provides the first set of estimates of the causes of mortality experienced in South Africa. This study made use of several sources of cause of death data, together with the ASSA model to overcome the underregistration of deaths and the misclassification of causes. Figure 7 shows the age distribution of the estimated number of deaths in 2000 by broad cause group. The distinct age pattern of AIDS deaths among children and young adults is clear. Communicable diseases occur across all ages, while injuries affect particularly young adult men. NCDs occur in adult age groups. More such deaths occur under the age of 60, reflecting the age structure of the population. The South African National Burden of Disease Study (SANBDS) estimates that in 2000 NCDs accounted for 37 percent of deaths, followed by HIV/AIDS, which accounted for 30 percent. NCDs accounted for 40 percent of female and 36 percent of male deaths. Stroke is the most common fatal NCD among women, and ischaemic heart disease (IHD) among men. Hypertensive heart disease, diabetes mellitus and chronic obstructive pulmonary disease were also among the leading causes of fatal

NCDs in 2000. These conditions coexist with low birth weight, protein–energy malnutrition and other infectious diseases as leading causes of death.

FIGURE 7
Male and female deaths by age and cause, 2000

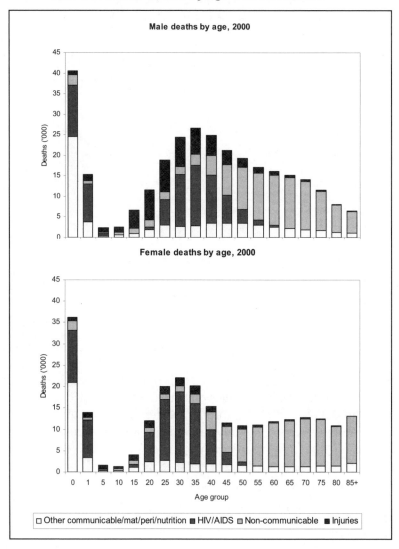

Source: 2000 SANBD in Bradshaw *et al.,* 2003.

DIETARY TRENDS AND ASSOCIATED RISK FACTORS
Changes in total dietary energy, carbohydrate, protein and fat intakes
The food balance sheets for 1962, 1972, 1982, 1992 and 2001 were used to describe trends in per capita consumption and are presented in Annex 1 (FAO, 2004). The contributions of different macronutrients to total energy intake are shown in Figure 8. These ratios have not changed much, even though the available per capita energy supply has increased by more than 300 kcal. It is important to remember that food balance sheets present total amounts of food available (not consumed) and do not account for how commodities are distributed according to region, socio-economic sector, gender or other demographic factor. These

data are regarded as very crude estimates of dietary intake and have only been included because national data on dietary intake surveys are not available prior to 1999.

FIGURE 8
Trends in dietary energy supplies from fat, protein and carbohydrate (CHO), 1962 and 2001

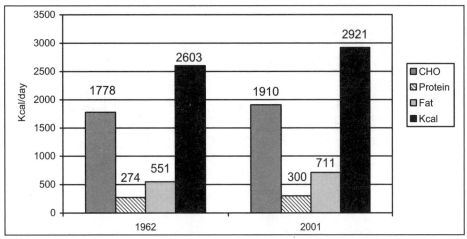

Source: FAO, 2004.

However, certain trends emerge for the 40-year period (Annex 1). The per capita available energy supply increased from 2 603 kcal/day in 1962 to 2 921 kcal in 2001, available protein supplies increased from 68.4 to 75.1 g, fat from 61.2 to 79 g, and available carbohydrate supplies from 445 to 478 g. The implication is that at the national level more food is available to consumers. However, the increase in fat availability per capita may be detrimental to health from a chronic diseases perspective.

The first nationally representative dietary study in South Africa – the National Food Consumption Survey (NFCS) – was undertaken in 1999 (Labadarios *et al.,* 2000). It was a cross-sectional survey of children aged one to nine years, with provincial representation drawing on the 1996 census data. The aim of the survey was to collect baseline data from which to formulate appropriate policy guidelines for food fortification, as well as to develop appropriate nutrition education material for South African children. The final sample comprised 2 894 children, with a response rate of 93 percent. Socio-demographic, dietary and anthropometric data were collected for each participant.

As the NFCS was the first national dietary study in South Africa, it is not possible to compare macronutrients over time in a reliable manner. However, by examining two studies, one in adults and one in schoolchildren, some changes can be deduced. Bourne (1996) examined the macronutrient intake of black adults living in Cape Town (Figure 9). Certain trends are noticeable, for example, the intake of carbohydrate calculated as percentage of total energy intake decreased from 61.4 to 52.8 percent as people spent more of their lives in the city.[2] In contrast, fat intake increased from 23.8 to 31.8 percent according to time spent in the city. Protein intake remained more or less the same over time, although the contribution of animal protein increased, whereas the amount of plant protein decreased. Fibre intake (not shown), also decreased significantly – from 20.7 to 16.7 g – with increased time living in the city.

---

[2] People living in a city all their lives have spent 100 percent in an urban area. Alternatively, people living in rural areas for most of their lives (50 years) with five years in the city have spent only 10 percent of their lives in an urban area.

These changes are all consistent with a population undergoing the nutrition transition, i.e., changes in diet from a traditional high-carbohydrate, high-fibre, low-fat diet to one with higher fat and sugar intakes and lower carbohydrate and fibre intakes (Popkin, 2001).

FIGURE 9

Changes in contributions of macronutrients to total energy intake among black adults (19 to 44 years) according to percentage of time lived in the city (Cape Town)

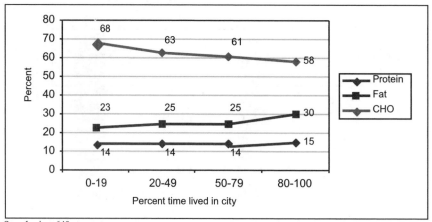

Sample size: 649.
Source: Bourne, 1996.

In urban areas of Gauteng, mean fat intake increased from 17 percent in 1962 to 25.8 percent in 1999, while carbohydrate intake decreased from 72 to 60.3 percent, as shown in Figure 10 (Lubbe, 1973; Labadarios *et al.,* 2000). Some differences between the two studies need to be kept in mind, however. Results from the 1962 study are reported for six- to nine-year-olds, using a modified diet history, while results from 1999 are for one- to nine-year-olds, using a 24-hour recall dietary method. Despite these differences, schoolchildren showed similar patterns of macronutrient intakes to those of adults in the Cape Town study by Bourne (1996). These two studies support the trends that energy and fat intakes have increased since 1962, as shown by the food balance sheets.

FIGURE 10

Macronutrient distribution as percentages of total energy consumed by black schoolchildren in urban areas of Gauteng in 1962 (six to nine years) and 1999 (one to nine years)

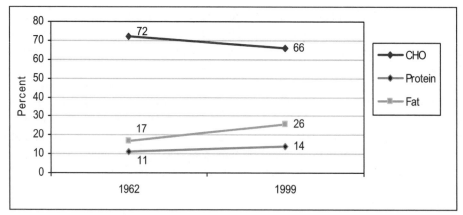

Sample sizes: 1962, 552; 1999, 427.
Sources: 1962 – Lubbe, 1973; 1999 – NFCS, 1999 (Labadarios *et al.,* 2000).

Differences in nutrient intake among ethnic groups and between urban and rural areas

It is important to note that there is a diversity of ethnic and cultural groups in South Africa with different traditional eating patterns. The white population consume a typical Western diet, which has a high fat intake (> 30 percent of total energy), low carbohydrate intake (< 55 percent energy), low fibre and high free sugar intake (> 10 percent energy) (Wolmarans *et al.,* 1989). The Indian and coloured (mixed ancestry) populations have a very similar pattern to this, albeit each group consumes certain foods more commonly (Langenhoven, Steyn and van Eck, 1988). The black African population has two distinct types of eating patterns. The rural population still follows a very traditional diet, which is high in carbohydrates (> 65 percent of total energy), low in fat (< 25 percent total energy), low in sugar (< 10 percent total energy) and moderately high in fibre (Steyn *et al.,* 2001). On the other hand, the urban black African population demonstrates an adoption of the Western diet of the other groups. The carbohydrate (< 65 percent total energy) and fibre intakes of this group are lower, and its fat intake is higher (> 25 percent total energy) (Bourne *et al.,* 1993).

In Figure 11, macronutrient distributions show marked differences among whites, urban blacks and rural blacks. White males (aged 35 to 44 years) have the highest intakes of fat, protein and added sugar and the lowest intake of carbohydrates (Wolmarans *et al.,* 1988). Rural black adults of the same age have the highest intake of carbohydrates and the lowest of protein, fat and added sugar (Steyn *et al.,* 2001). Black urban males lie between the two extremes (Bourne *et al.,* 1993). This figure suggests that there is a diet transition among urban blacks from a traditional rural diet to an urban one that is approaching the completely Westernized diet of the white population. However, it should be remembered that the studies were not undertaken at the same point in time, which may have influenced the results.

FIGURE 11

Macronutrient distribution as percentages of total daily energy among adult white urban (15 to 64 years), black urban (19 to 44 years) and black rural (20 to 65 years) males

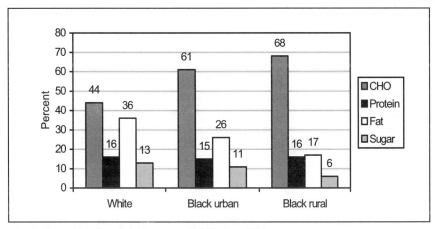

Sample sizes: white urban, 454; black urban, 285; black rural, 74.
Sources: white – Wolmarans *et al.,* 1989; black urban – Bourne *et al.,* 1993; black rural – Steyn *et al.,* 2001.

Table 1 shows the differences in dietary intake among all the main ethnic groups (males) in South Africa, with urban and rural subgroups for blacks (Bourne *et al.,* 1993; Langenhoven, Steyn and van Eck, 1988; Steyn *et al.,* 2001; Vorster *et al.,* 1995; Wolmarans *et al.,* 1988; 1999). These studies were geographically and ethnically representative of the areas where they were undertaken, and can be regarded as a good reflection of the typical diet of each specific group.

The white, Indian and coloured groups have the highest intakes of fats, protein and free sugar, which are not in line with the WHO/FAO (2003) recommendations. Black males in rural areas have the lowest intakes of all types of fat and protein. Urban males, once again, illustrate the nutrition transition that has taken place. Table 2 shows various transitions that have taken place in the black population (MacIntyre *et al.,* 2002).

The urban upper income group has the highest fat and protein intakes as a percentage of energy intake. This group also has the highest cholesterol intake, which is higher than the WHO/FAO (2003) recommendation (< 300 mg/day). At the other end of the scale are rural residents and rural farm workers, who have a prudent diet that is low in fat and high in carbohydrate.

TABLE 1

Comparison of macronutrient mean ranges in six dietary studies in adult males and females

Dietary factor	CORIS white rural n = 1 113 15–64 years	DIKGALE black rural n = 210 20–65 years	VIGHOR white urban n = 317 15–64 years	BRISK black urban n = 983 19–44 years	Indians urban n = 370 15–69 years	CRISIC coloured urban n = 276 20–34 years	WHO goals % energy
Energy (kJ) [1]	6.3–12.7	6.0–6.7	5.9–12.5	5.8–8.5	5–8.5	7.1–10.3	
Energy (kcal)	1 500–3 024	1 434–1 590	1 405–2 976	1 386–2 035	1 190–2 024	1 690–2 452	
Total fat (% E) [2]	34.6–36.5	15.7–17.1	33.3–38.6	23.8–28.3	32.8–36.9	37.3–38	15–30%
SFA (% E) [3]	12.6–13.6	3.7–4.4	12.2–14.6	8.5–9.2	7.0–9.8	11.8–11.9	< 10%
PUFAs (% E) [4]	5.9–7.0	3.7–3.9	5.6–7.8	4.5–7.2	9.5–12.5	9.1–9.2	6–10%
CHO (% E) [5]	44.1–51.5	62.4–70.8	46.9–53.3	59.2–64.3	45.5–53.0	45–46.5	55–75%
Free sugar (% E)	10.8–15.4	5.2–4.2	13.0–18.6	10.7–14.6	10.8–15.8	15–16	< 10%
Protein (% E)	13.8–16.6	14.2–15.6	13.6–16.3	13.1–15.3	11.9–13.8	14.9–15	10–15%
Cholesterol (mg)	243–509	144.9–116.6	140–176 mg /4.2kJ	-	76–117 mg /4.2kJ	290–440	≤ 300 mg/day

[1] kJ = kilojoules.
[2] E = energy.
[3] SFA = saturated fats.
[4] PUFA = poly-unsaturated fats.
[5] CHO = carbohydrate.

Sources: CORIS – Wolmarans *et al.,* 1988; DIKGALE – Steyn *et al.,* 2001; VIGHOR – Vorster *et al.,* 1995; BRISK – Bourne *et al.,* 1993; Indian Study – Wolmarans *et al.,* 1999; CRISIC – Langenhoven, Steyn and van Eck, 1988; WHO/FAO, 2003.

TABLE 2
Distribution of macronutrients in the diet of black South African males (15 to 80 years), by area and income

Dietary factor	Rural Low-income n = 194	Farm workers (rural) low-income n = 109	Urban (informal settlement) low-income n = 128	Urban middle-income n = 229	Urban high-income n = 83	WHO[7] goals % of energy
Energy (kJ)	9.6	8.9	9.3	9.9	9.8	
Energy (kcal)	2 285	2 122	2 222	2 356	2 338	
Total fat (% E)	22.9	22.8	24.3	26.0	30.6	15 - 30%
CHO (% E)	67.4	67.2	65.5	64	57.3	55 - 75%
Protein (% E)	11.6	12.1	12	11.8	13.2	10 - 15%
Cholesterol (mg)	315.6	283	332	377	420	≤ 300 mg /day
Fibre (g)	19.2	15.6	17.4	18.8	19.7	

Sources: MacIntyre *et al.,* 2002; WHO/FAO, 2003.

Changes in intakes of types of food and food groups over time

According to FAO data (Annex 1), cereal availability increased from 169.3 kg per capita per annum in 1962 to 187.8 kg in 2001; as did the availability of starchy roots (from 13 to 29.7 kg), vegetable oils (5.7 to 14.5 kg), fruits (24.1 to 36.0 kg), alcohol (43.8 to 56.8 litres), meat (31.6 to 37.5 kg), eggs (2.5 to 6.1 kg) and fish (5.5 to 7.9 kg). Foods whose per capita availability decreased were sugar and sweeteners (from 39.4 to 32.8 kg), offal (4.5 to 3.8 kg), animal fats (including butter) (3.0 to 0.7 kg) and milk (78.0 to 54.1 kg).

These data reflect a number of scenarios. Availability of staple cereals gradually increased, as did that of other items mentioned in the previous paragraph; these increases account for the overall increase in energy intake. Vegetable oil and meat per capita also increased significantly, which accounts for the large increase in fat and saturated fat intakes. Of concern is the fact that vegetable availability remained constant (at 43.5 to 44.2 kg per annum). Overall fruit and vegetable availability was 185 g/day (excluding starchy roots), which is far less than the recommended intake of 400 g/day (WHO/FAO, 2003). This has serious implications, because low fruit and vegetable intake is a risk factor for many NCDs.

Among black adults, the amounts consumed from different food groups changed with increasing time spent in Cape Town, as shown in Figure 12. Groups for which consumption rose were meat, fruit and vegetables, fats and non-basic foods (such as drinks and sweets), while consumption from the dairy and cereal groups decreased. Similar findings are presented for young females in Figure 13. The higher consumption of sugar-containing food items in urban compared with rural areas is shown in Figure 14.

FIGURE 12

Percentage contributions of different food groups to energy, by time spent in Cape Town by black adults (19 to 44 years)

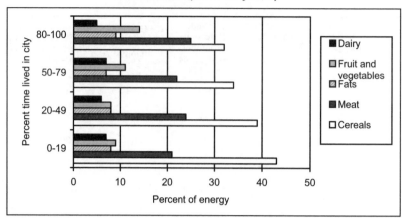

Sample size: 649.
Source: Bourne, 1996.

FIGURE 13

Food consumption of black female university students from urban and rural areas

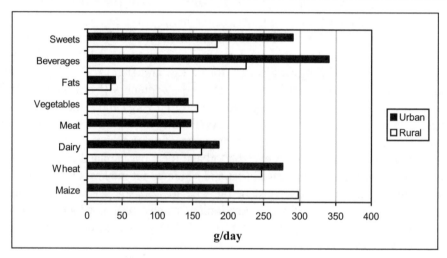

Sample size: 115.
Source: Steyn *et al.*, 2000

FIGURE 14
Percentage consumption of sugar-containing items by children aged six to nine years

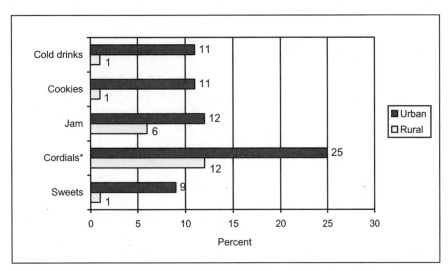

Sample size: 439.
Cordial = a drink made from sweet sucrose concentrate.
Cold drink = soft drink.
Source: NFCS in Labadarios *et al.,* 2000.

Current diet

The results from NFCS provide the first nationally representative dietary data for South Africa. Table 3 indicates the mean nutrient intakes of children and compares them with recommended nutrient intakes (RNI) (FAO/WHO, 2002). Overall, the energy intakes of both rural groups were less than the RNIs, as were the intakes of vitamins A and C, niacin, vitamin B_6 and zinc. For folate and calcium, urban and rural intakes were less than the RNIs. An important aspect of the study was the disparities in intakes between urban and rural areas. For most nutrients, the mean values in urban areas were significantly higher than those in rural ones.

To understand the dynamics of dietary change, the main food groups consumed by South African adults and children in urban and rural areas were examined (Table 4). In lieu of the lacking national data on adults, data from combined databases were summarized using secondary data analyses to show the dietary intakes of adults (Steyn *et al.,* 2001; Nel and Steyn, 2002) and children (aged one to five years) (Labadarios *et al.,* 2000). Although rural dwellers have higher cereal and vegetable intakes, urban adults and children far exceed the rural people's consumption of most other food groups, particularly sugar, meat, vegetable oil, dairy, fruit, roots and tubers and alcohol.

TABLE 3
Mean nutrient intakes of children

Nutrient	Children 1–3 years (n = 1 308)			Children 4–6 years (n = 1 083)		
	Urban	Rural	RSA	Urban	Rural	RSA
#Energy (kJ)	4 403 (2 043)	3 992* (1 790)	4 200 (1 933)	5 614 (2 375)	4 963* (2 283)	5 271* (2 349)
Energy (kcal)	1 048 (486)	950* (426)	1 000 (460)	1 337 (565)	1 182* (544)	1 255* (559)
CHO (g)	154 (72)	151 (71)	152 (72)	192 (80)	193 (91)	193 (86)
#Added sugar (g)	26 (23)	18 (17)	22 (21)	36 (30)	24 (34)	29 (33)
#Protein (g)	33 (18)	29 (17)	31 (18)	43 (21)	36 (19)	39 (21)
Fat (g)	29 (21)	22 (16)	25 (19)	38 (25)	42 (21)	31 (24)
Fibre (g)	9 (6)	10 (7)	9 (6)	13 (7)	13 (8)	13 (8)
#Vitamin A (RE)	463 (943)	252* (349)	359* (723)	544 (1 313)	319* (1 007)	425* (1 167)
#Vitamin C (mg)	41 (96)	20* (36)	31* (73)	36* (65)	29* (78)	33* (72)
Thiamine (mg)	0.6 (0.3)	0.6 (0.3)	0.6 (0.3)	0.7 (0.4)	0.7 (0.4)	0.7 (0.4)
#Riboflavin (mg)	0.8 (0.8)	0.6 (0.6)	0.7 (0.7)	1.0 (1.0)	0.7 (1.0)	0.8 (0.9)
#Niacin (mg)	6.4 (4.7)	4.8* (3.8)	5.6 (4.3)	9 (6.2)	6.3 * (4.4)	7.6 * (5.5)
#Vitamin B6 (mg)	0.6 (0.4)	0.4* (0.3)	0.5 (0.4)	0.8 (0.6)	0.5 * (0.4)	0.6 (0.5)
#Vitamin B 12 (ug)	2.7 (8.4)	1.4 (4.4)	2.1 (6.8)	3.7 (12.1)	2 (10.2)	2.8 (11.2)
#Folate (mg)	102* (81)	86* (84)	94* (83)	161* (119)	127* (111)	143* (116)
#Calcium (mg)	345* (326)	302* (326)	324* (327)	342* (282)	270 * (254)	304* (269)
#Iron (mg)	4.9* (3.6)	4.7* (3.8)	4.8 * (3.7)	6.7 (4.2)	6.1 (4.6)	6.4 (4.5)
#Zinc (mg)	4.5 (2.7)	3.9* (2.5)	4.2 (2.6)	5.9 (3.3)	4.8* (3.1)	5.3 (3.2)

* = mean intake is less than the FAO/WHO (2002) RNI.
\# = significant urban/rural differences (p < 0.01).
Source: Steyn *et al.* in Labadarios *et al.,* 2000

TABLE 4
Adults' and children's consumption, by food group and residence

Food group	Adults and children 10+ years (n = 817)			Children 1–5 years (n = 2 048)		
	RSA g/day	Urban g/day	Rural g/day	RSA g/day	Urban g/day	Rural g/day
Cereals	870	736	1 023	489	433	546
Sugar	76	120	27	65	93	39
Stimulants: tea, coffee	382	390	371	147	143	151
Vegetables	93	85	101	52	45	58
Meat and offal	86	102	67	45	56	34
Vegetable oils	8	11	5	5	6	3
Dairy	73	109	31	124	147	102
Fruit	61	83	36	48	70	27
Eggs	15	16	14	10	12	8
Legumes	35	34	36	17	15	18
Fish	12	14	10	7	8	5.8
Roots and tubers	40	59	19	29	32	27
Nuts and oilseeds	2	2	2	1	2	1
Alcohol	54	67	38	-	-	-
Soups	2.6	4.3	0.6	6	3	9
Condiments	0.5	0.7	0.3	0.2	0.2	0.1
Animal fat	1.0	1.6	0.4	0.1	0.1	0.2

Source: Nel and Steyn, 2002.

Changes in alcohol intake

According to the food balance sheets, per capita alcohol consumption in South Africa increased between 1962 and 2001 (Annex 1). Certain trends are noticeable from two surveys carried out in the 1990s: SADHS in adults (Department of Health, SAMRC and Measure DHS+, 2002) and the Youth Risk Behaviour Study (YRBS) (Reddy *et al.,* 2003) in teenagers (Figure 15). YRBS found that more than 30 percent of teenagers had drunk and/or binged on alcohol in the preceding 30 days. According to SADHS, nearly 30 percent of adult males reported using alcohol excessively, based on the CAGE test (Ewing, 1984), compared with 10 percent of females. High alcohol consumption is a risk factor for chronic diseases such as stroke, diabetes and cancer of the oesophagus, liver and breast, and so needs to be addressed as an underlying determinant in the prevention of NCDs (WHO/FAO, 2003).

FIGURE 15
Prevalence of teenager (13 to 19 years) school attendees reporting drinking alcohol or bingeing in the past month, and prevalence of alcohol-dependent adults

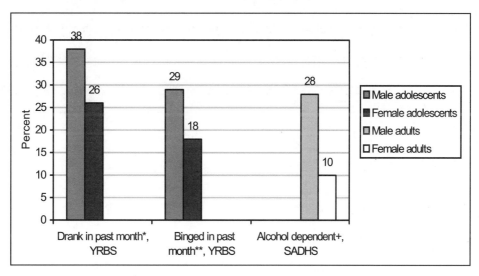

* Consumed an alcoholic drink on one or more days during the previous month.
** Consumed five or more alcoholic drinks on one or more days during the previous month.
+ According to the CAGE questionnaire.
Sources: YRBS; SADHS.

TRENDS IN NUTRITIONAL STATUS
Trends in the prevalence of undernutrition and protein–energy malnutrition

Nationally representative and comparable anthropometric data over time are only available for 1994 and 1999 in children and for 1998 in adults; hence, they do not show long-term trends. In order to obtain longer time trends, smaller localized studies have been used to provide comparisons with the 1994 and 1999 data on children. Data on one localized and two national studies undertaken in South Africa between 1986 and 1999 are shown in Table 5. Given the differences in children's ages, conclusions on trends should be interpreted cautiously. The 1986 study sampled black preschool children on farms in areas other than the "homelands", where the greater part of the black population lived. Consequently, the data are not a true reflection of the actual prevalence of malnutrition, which would have been higher if these areas had been included. Before democratization, the health care services provided to the population in "homelands" were totally insufficient. In 1994, the South African Vitamin A Consultative Group (SAVACG, 1995) undertook a national study of preschool children, and the 1999 NFCS included school-going children. These studies showed similar results, with underweight ranging from 6.9 to 10.7 percent, stunting from 16.1 to 27 percent and wasting from 1.8 to 3.7 percent. Malnutrition prevalence was always higher in rural than urban areas. There appears to be a small improvement in the prevalence of stunting between 1994 and 1999 in these two nationally representative surveys.

Two earlier studies (1969 and 1975) were undertaken as representative studies of the Transvaal, now partly Gauteng (Figure 16). These studies used the Harvard–3rd percentile as an indicator of underweight, while the later studies used the National Center for Health Statistics (NCHS) percentiles, and there are some discrepancies even though the two standards are very similar. There are large decreases in the prevalence of underweight in urban and rural areas until 1994. The smaller increases after 1994 in urban Gauteng are probably because of the large migration into this region following the lifting of migration restrictions.

TABLE 5
Prevalence of low weight-for-height, height-for-age and weight-for-age in children, 1986, 1994 and 1999

	1986 rural 0–59[1] months	1994 urban 6–71 months	1994 rural 6–71 months	1994 RSA 6–71 months	1999 RSA 12–72[1] months
	N = 1 745	n = 4 757	n = 6 062	n = 10 819	n = 2 200
Weight-for-age < -2 SD (NCHS)	8.4	6.9	10.7	9.3	8.8 (9.7)[2]
95% confidence interval	6.8; 9.9	6.0; 7.9	9.6; 11.9	8.5; 10.1	7.6; 10.1
Height-for-age < -2 SD	24.5	16.1	27.0	22.9	19.3 (22.1)[2]
95% confidence interval	19.2; 29.7	14.4; 17.8	24.8; 29.3	21.4; 24.5	17.5; 21.2
Weight-for-height < -2 SD	1.8	2.1	2.8	2.6	3.7 (3.7)[2]
95% confidence interval	1.3; 2.3	1.5; 2.7	2.3; 3.4	2.2; 2.9	3.0; 4.4

[1] Six to 71 months category not available.
[2] 12 to 96 months.
Sources: 1986 – Kustner, 1987; 1994 – SAVACG, 1995; 1999 – Labadarios *et al.*, 2000; Steyn *et al.*, 2005.

FIGURE 16
Prevalence of underweight in black preschool children (under 72 months), 1969, 1975, 1994 and 1999

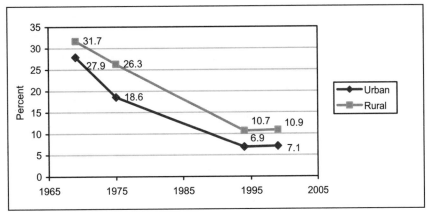

Sample sizes: 1969, 2 073; 1975, 3 655; 1994, 11 238); 1999, 2 200.
Sources: 1969 and 1975 – Richardson, 1977; 1994 – SAVACG, 1995; 1999 NFCS – Labadarios *et al.,* 2000;
Steyn *et al.,* 2005.

Trends in the prevalence of overweight and obesity

The prevalence rates of overweight and obese children at the time of NFCS 1999 are shown in Table 6. There were significant differences between urban and rural areas, among location domains and among age groups. Overweight was highest in formal urban areas and in children aged one to three years. The finding that overweight/obesity was higher in urban areas is an indication that the nutrition transition is under way, and that undernutrition and associated infectious diseases should not be the only health concern among policy-makers. The data show that the prevalence of combined overweight and obesity (17.1 percent) is nearly the same as that for stunting (21.6 percent) (Steyn *et al.,* 2005). Furthermore, stunting was associated with an increased risk (OR = 1.80, CI = 1.48–2.20) of being overweight (BMI ≥ 25) (Steyn *et al.,* 2005). This finding suggests that stunting in childhood predisposes to overweight or obesity when sufficient food becomes available. This poses a threat for the emergence of chronic disease risk factors when stunted children become obese adults.

TABLE 6
Percentages of children with BMI values ≥ 25 and ≥ 30 using the Cole *et al.* (2000) cut-off points

BMI cut-off points	Domain analysis by area of residence*				Domain analysis by urban/rural*		Domain analysis by age group*			All
	Farms	Formal urban	Informal urban	Tribal	Rural	Urban	1–3 years	4–6 years	7–8 years	
	n = 108	n = 946	n = 272	n = 874	n = 982	n = 128	n = 795	n = 861	n = 544	n = 2 200
% ≥ 30 BMI	3.54	6.18	5.89	3.74	3.71	6.11	7.78	3.81	2.98	5.04
Lower 95% CI	0.77	4.40	3.15	2.55	2.64	4.55	6.07	2.50	1.13	4.07
Upper 95% CI	6.30	7.96	8.63	4.93	4.79	7.67	9.49	5.12	4.83	6.02
% ≥ 25 BMI	10.76	20.10	13.41	15.83	15.27	18.61	23.75	15.79	9.53	17.12
Lower 95% CI	6.03	16.01	10.02	13.52	13.15	15.15	20.87	12.84	6.37	15.00
Upper 95% CI	15.50	24.19	16.80	18.14	17.40	22.06	26.62	18.75	12.69	19.23
Chi-square*	p = 0.0066				0.0257		< 0.0001			

* Chi-square p-value for testing for associations, using weighted values, between BMI groupings, area of residence, urban/rural and age groups.
CI= confidence interval. SD = standard deviation.
Source: 1999 NFCS in Steyn *et al.,* 2005.

SADHS (1998) was the first nationally representative health survey in adults aged 15 years and over, so in order to examine trends from previous years and compare with these data it is necessary to evaluate earlier studies that were representative of specific ethnic groups. Interpretation of these data should keep these limitations in mind. The earlier studies include a baseline study in 1979 on coronary heart diseases risk factors in white adults in three towns of the Western Cape Province (CORIS) (Jooste *et al.,* 1988), and similar studies in 1982 in the coloured population (CRISIC) (Steyn *et al.,* 1985), the black population in Cape Town (BRISK) (Steyn *et al.,* 1991) and the Indian population (Seedat *et al.,* 1990).

Figures 17 and 18 show the extent of obesity as a problem in men and women in South Africa. In women, the prevalence of obesity has remained high in all studies since 1979, particularly in black women, who show the highest prevalence. In men there appears to be a large increase in obesity in whites when the 1979 study is compared with that of 1998.

The most recent SADHS data on overweight and obesity in adults indicate that obesity increases with age until about 35 years in both men and women and declines from about 55 years. More than 40 percent of women aged 35 years and over are obese, and more than 20 percent of all women are overweight. For the ethnic groups, obesity is highest in black women and white men. At 12.9 percent and 5.6 percent, respectively, for men and women, the prevalence rate of underweight (BMI < 18.5) in adults is far lower than those of overweight and obesity (Department of Health, SAMRC and Measure DHS+, 2002).

The rising prevalence of obesity in South Africa gives cause for serious concern because of the increased risk of diabetes and CVD (WHO/FAO, 2003). These diseases have direct costs, which may be as high as 6.8 percent of total health care costs, as well as indirect costs, such as workdays lost, doctor visits, impaired quality of life and premature mortality (WHO/FAO, 2003).

The data presented in this section of the case study illustrate that both over- and undernutrition exist in South Africa, with the extremes being most clearly seen among the black population.

FIGURE 17
The prevalence of obesity (BMI ≥ 30) in women, 1979 to 1998

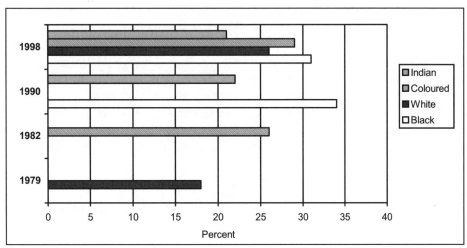

Sample sizes : 1979, 3 831; 1982, 498; 1990, 544); 1998, 7 970.
Sources: 1979 – Jooste *et al.,* 1988; 1982 – Steyn *et al.,* 1985; 1990 – Seedat *et al.,* 1990; Steyn *et al.,* 1991; 1998 – Department of Health, SAMRC and Measure DHS+, 2002.

FIGURE 18
The prevalence of obesity (BMI ≥ 30) in men, 1979 to 1998

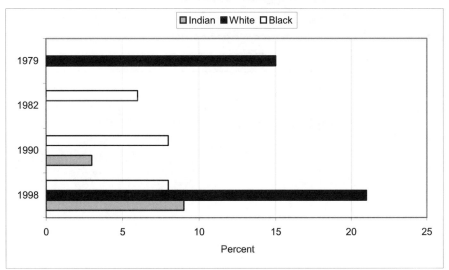

Sample sizes: 1979, 3 357; 1982, 478; 1990, 442; 1998, 5 558.
Sources: 1979 – Jooste *et al.,* 1988; 1982 – Steyn *et al.,* 1985; 1990 – Seedat *et al.,* 1990; Steyn *et al.,* 1991; 1998 – Department of Health, SAMRC and Measure DHS+, 2002.

Trends in micronutrient status

The nationally representative SAVACG survey in 1994 examined, among other factors, the vitamin A and iron status of children aged 0 to five years (SAVACG, 1995). This was the first study to examine micronutrients in children at the national level. Micronutrient intakes of children will be measured again in 2005.

About 3 percent (Figure 19) of the sampled children showed serum vitamin A deficiency (VAD) (serum retinol < 10 ug/dl), while 33 percent were marginally deficient (serum retinol < 20 ug/dl) (SAVACG, 1995). Children in the 36 to 47 months age group were the most affected, with 11 percent having haemoglobin concentrations of less than 11 g/dl and 25 percent with low iron stores (ferritin < 12 ug/dl) (Figure 20). The mandatory fortification of maize and wheat with vitamin A, iron and other micronutrients since 2003 is expected to decrease these micronutrient deficiencies in South African children in the future.

Results from an iodine deficiency survey in 1998 in primary schoolchildren show that within provinces between 0 and 42 percent of schools had children who were iodine deficient (Immelman, Towindo and Kalk, 2000) (Figure 21). Schools in rural areas of Mpumalanga and Limpopo provinces were most affected. The survey also found that mandatory salt iodization since 1995 had considerably improved the iodine status of children. However, there are still some minor weaknesses in the national salt iodization programme, such as the use of non-iodized salt in 6.5 percent of households and the under- or non-iodization of a substantial percentage of household salt.

FIGURE 19
Vitamin A status of children aged six to 71 months, 1994

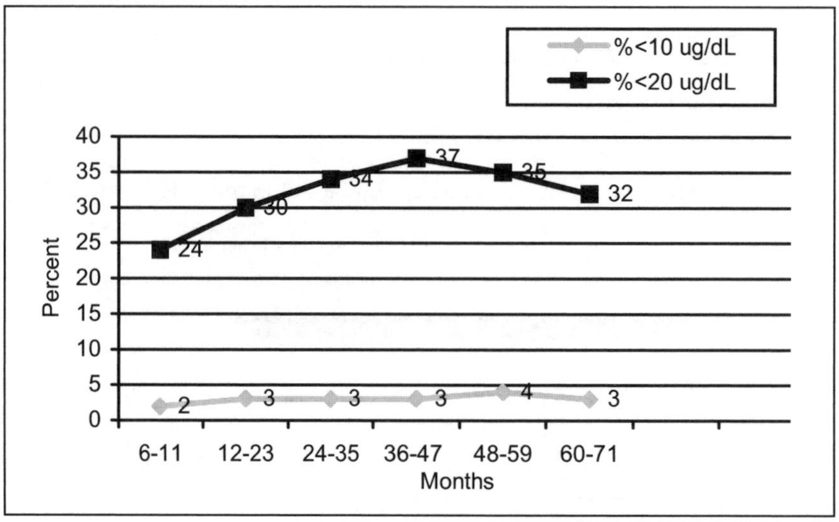

Sample size: 4 283.
Source: SAVACG, 1995.

FIGURE 20
Iron status of children aged six to 71 months, 1994

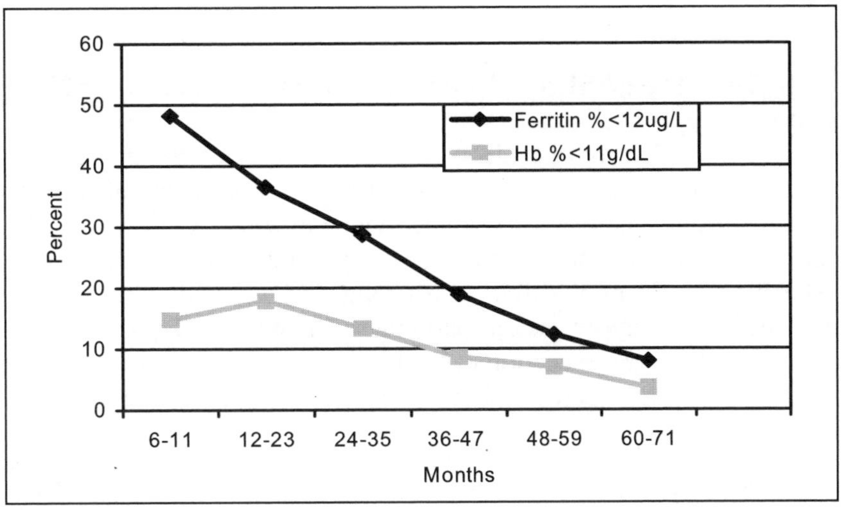

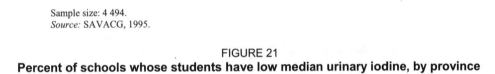

Sample size: 4 494.
Source: SAVACG, 1995.

FIGURE 21
Percent of schools whose students have low median urinary iodine, by province

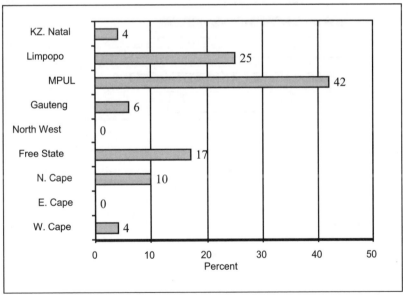

Sample size: 179 schools.
Source: Immelman, Towindo and Kalk, 2000.

Micronutrient deficiencies continue to contribute to the burden of mortality in South Africa. Preliminary results of a study to assess the burden attributable to selected nutritional deficiencies estimate that in 2000 nearly 3 000 deaths to diarrhoea in children aged 0 to four years were attributed to VAD. Furthermore, about 200 maternal deaths were attributed to VAD in pregnant women, while more than 3 500 perinatal deaths and about 180 maternal deaths (0.7 percent of total deaths) were attributed to iron deficiency anaemia (IDA) (Nojilana *et al.,* in press).

No national data on biochemical deficiencies among adults are available. However, numerous localized studies have shown high prevalence of iron deficiency in women (Kruger *et al.,* 1994;

Dannhauser *et al.,* 1999) and of VAD, particularly in HIV-infected adults (Kennedy-Oji *et al.,* 2001; Visser *et al.,* 2003).

OTHER CHRONIC DISEASES AND ASSOCIATED LIFESTYLE RISK FACTORS
Physical inactivity

There is a paucity of data on the physical activity levels of South Africans, making it difficult to show trends over time. Figure 22 shows current levels of inactivity in South African teenagers from a national survey undertaken in 2002 (Reddy *et al.,* 2003). Overall, coloured girls have the highest levels of inactivity, with nearly 60 percent doing little or nothing. The high levels of inactivity go a long way to explaining the high levels of overweight, obesity and hypertension, particularly in women. Figure 23 reports data on inactivity in adults. With the exception of the black population, the prevalence of inactivity was very high (more than 90 percent), both at work and during leisure time.

FIGURE 22
Percentages of 13- to 19-year-olds reporting insufficient or no physical activity at work,*
2002

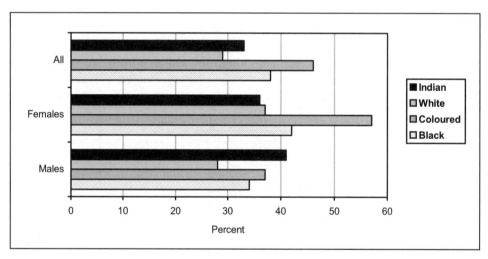

Sample size: 10 100.
* Insufficient or no physical activity means the person did not participate in vigorous or moderate activity that would have been sufficient for a health benefit over the previous seven days.
Source: YRBS, 2002 in Reddy *et al.,* 2003.

FIGURE 23
Percentages of 15- to 64-year-olds reporting insufficient or no physical activity at work (< 32 300 kJ/wk) and during leisure times (< 8 400 kJ/wk)

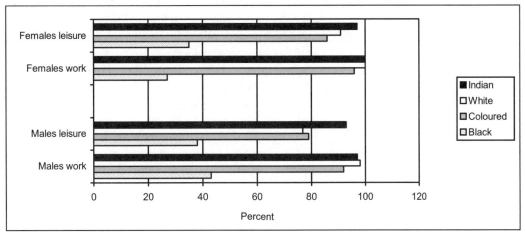

Sample sizes: white, 7 188; coloured, 976; black, 986; Indian, 778
Sources: white – CORIS in Rossouw *et al.,* 1983; coloured – CRISIC in Steyn *et al.,* 1985; black – BRISK in Steyn *et al.,* 1991; Indian – Seedat *et al.,* 1990.

All these studies identified physical activity patterns by means of questionnaires. The measurement of physical activity by questionnaires is challenging in large epidemiological studies. Consequently, the patterns shown here must be interpreted with caution, but the overall trends suggest that the Indian and white populations are the most inactive at work and leisure, while the black population is the least inactive.

Tobacco intake

Tobacco consumption patterns in South Africa between 1990 and 2004 illustrate the impact of an aggressive tobacco control policy that was phased in during this period. The policy had two distinct aspects: tobacco control legislation and rapidly increasing excise taxes. Major legislative milestones include the Tobacco Controls Act, which was passed in 1993 and introduced health warnings on cigarette packets and advertisements. The act was amended in 1999 with the banning of all advertisements and prohibitions on smoking in all indoor public areas and on selling tobacco products to minors. In 1994, the government announced the phasing in of an increased excise tax, which added 50 percent to the retail price of tobacco. This resulted in a real increase of 256 percent in the excise tax per pack of cigarettes between 1994 and 2004; the real price of cigarettes increased by 127 percent over the same period. WHO's Tobacco Framework Convention has been ratified by South Africa and a sufficient number of Member States to require all countries to comply with these laws. South Africa is currently expanding its tobacco control legislation to ensure compliance (Van Walbeek, 2005).

In 1992, Martin, Steyn and Yach reported that 31.5 percent of South Africans smoked. The prevalence rate peaked at 34 percent in 1995, as recorded by Reddy *et al.* (1998), declining steadily thereafter to reach 24 percent in 2003. The average number of cigarettes per smoker per year decreased from 229 packs in 1993 to 163 in 2003. Africans, males, young adults and poorer people experienced the most rapid decreases in smoking prevalence, while the decrease was less pronounced among whites, females and older and more affluent people.

Despite these positive trends, the prevalence of tobacco smoking is still high, particularly among youth. A recent survey found that the prevalence of cigarette smoking (daily and occasionally) was higher in 14-year-old adolescent males than females (21.5 versus 15.7 percent)

(Reddy *et al.,* 2003). At 16 years of age, 30.4 percent of males were already smoking cigarettes, rising to 38 percent in 18-year-old males.

In 1998, SADHS found that more than 39 percent of African, white, coloured and Indian adult males (15 years and over) smoked daily or occasionally, with the lowest prevalence in rural black males (37 percent). In rural areas, only 4 percent of black females smoked daily, compared with 6 percent in urban areas. The overall prevalence of daily smoking for females was lowest in the black population (5 percent) and highest among whites (27 percent) (Department of Health, SAMRC and Measure DHS+, 2002). Because tobacco use is a risk factor for heart disease and lung cancer, which are serious contributors to both morbidity and mortality in South Africa, it calls for preventive measures, particularly among youth. The finding that nearly one-third of 16-year-old males are current smokers is a serious concern. Figure 24 shows the prevalence of smoking in adult males for 1984 and 1998. The highest prevalence rates were in whites and Indians. Despite the finding that smoking prevalence peaked in 1995 (Reddy *et al.,* 1998), it is still considerably higher than it was in 1984.

FIGURE 24
Prevalence of smoking in adult males by population group, 1984 and 1998

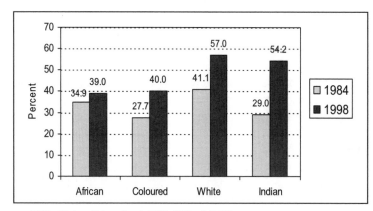

Sources: 1984 – Yach and Townshend, 1988; 1998 – SADHS.

Hypercholesterolaemia

No national surveys on serum cholesterol levels have been conducted. Figure 25 presents the results from four studies undertaken in different ethnic groups in localized settings. White men had the highest mean total cholesterol values, and black men the lowest. Indian and coloured men had similar mean values to those of white men, albeit slightly lower. With the exception of black men, all were found to have mean values above the recommended limit of 5.2 mmol/l. Hence, high serum cholesterol was a strong risk factor for CHD in South African men who are not black. These studies were conducted in the late 1970s and early 1980s, and it is not possible to say what trends and changes have taken place in the cholesterol values of black males since then.

FIGURE 25
Mean total serum cholesterol values (mmol/l) in adult males, by age and ethnic group

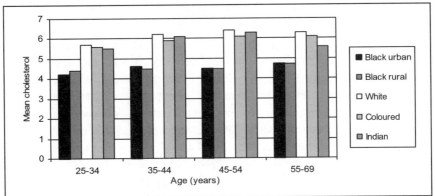

Sources: black – Norman *et al.*, unpublished data, 2005; white – CORIS in Rossouw *et al.*, 1983; coloured – CRISIC in Steyn *et al.*, 1985; Indian – Seedat *et al.*, 1990.

Hypertension

SADHS was the first national survey to measure blood pressure of adults, and its findings are presented in Figure 26. The lowest prevalence of hypertension (BP > 140/90 mmHg) was found in black men (20.2 percent) and the highest in white men (38 percent). Coloured and white women and Indian men also had very high prevalence, at close to 30 percent. Of great concern, however, are the levels of hypertension control, namely control of those who have hypertension (BP > 140/90 mmHg). The highest levels of control were found in white women and Indians, and the lowest in black men and coloured women. Fewer than 10 percent of the latter were found to be controlled. The high levels of hypertension illustrated in Figure 26, together with the high prevalence rates of obesity, tobacco use (shown earlier) and hypercholesterolaemia help to explain the high prevalence of CVD in adults.

FIGURE 26
Prevalence of hypertension (BP > 140/90 mmHg) in adults, 1998

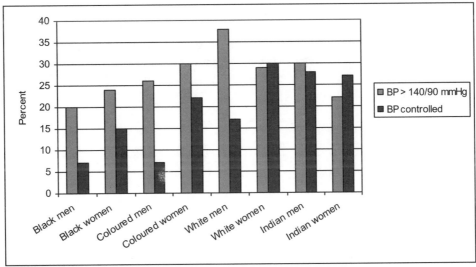

Sample size: 2 049.
BP controlled = among those with hypertension, BP is < 140/90 mmHg, i.e. controlled.
Source: SADHS.

Cardiovascular diseases and diabetes

The poor quality of historical cause of death data makes it very difficult to assess trends in mortality. Bradshaw *et al. (*1995) calculated age-standardized deaths rates by population group for 1985, based on the deaths reported for the years 1984 to 1986 relative to population estimates for 1985. Rates for blacks were calculated for urban areas only because there was high underregistration of deaths for blacks in rural areas. These are compared with estimated death rates for 2000 (Bradshaw *et al.,* 2004). Figure 27 shows age-standardized mortality rates for IHD, stroke, hypertensive heart disease and diabetes in 1984 to 1986 compared with 2000, by population group. These comparisons must be interpreted carefully as the estimates for 2000 have been adjusted for misclassification and underregistration of deaths, but those for 1984 to 1986 have not. The increase in IHD across all groups is likely to be a result of the adjustment for misclassification of ill-defined cardiac causes in 2000. From Figure 27, it appears that hypertensive disease and stroke increased dramatically in the black population. Diabetes mortality increased in all ethnic groups, but most in the black population. The increased rates in the black population may be an artefact of the adjustment for underregistration of deaths in the 2000 estimate.

IHD was the main cause of mortality among CVDs and diabetes in white males between 1949 and 1985 (Bradshaw *et al.,* 1995). IHD mortality increased from 260 per 100 00 in 1949 to more than 300 per 100 000 between 1964 and 1979. It subsequently decreased from 312 per

100 000 in 1978 to 139 in 1989 (Walker, Adam and Küstner, 1993). IHD was also the main cause of CVD mortality in white females, although the rates were about half those of males.

IHD was the main cause of mortality among CVDs and diabetes in coloured males until 1969, when it was replaced by stroke (Bradshaw *et al.,* 1995). There was a very large increase in mortality from IHD between 1958 and 1969; it then remained stable at about 150 per 100 000 until 1985. Stroke was the major cause of mortality in coloured females. Mortality from diabetes increased fourfold, from ten in 1949 to 40 in 1984.

IHD was the major cause of mortality from CVDs and diabetes in Indian males between 1949 and 1985, followed by stroke and diabetes (Bradshaw *et al.,* 1995). During this period the mortality rates remained fairly constant, except that IHD increased to more than 250 per 100 000 and diabetes to more than 70 in 1985. Stroke was the major cause of mortality in Indian females. There was also a dramatic increase in the mortality rate from diabetes, from about 20 per 100 000 in 1949 to 70 in 1984.

These data seem to suggest that both IHD and stroke have high mortality rates and that hypertensive heart disease and diabetes may have been growing. IHD is particularly high for whites and Indians, while hypertensive heart disease and stroke are highest among the black population group.

FIGURE 27
Age-standardized mortality rates from hypertensive heart disease, stroke, IHD and diabetes, per 100 000 population, 1985 and 2000

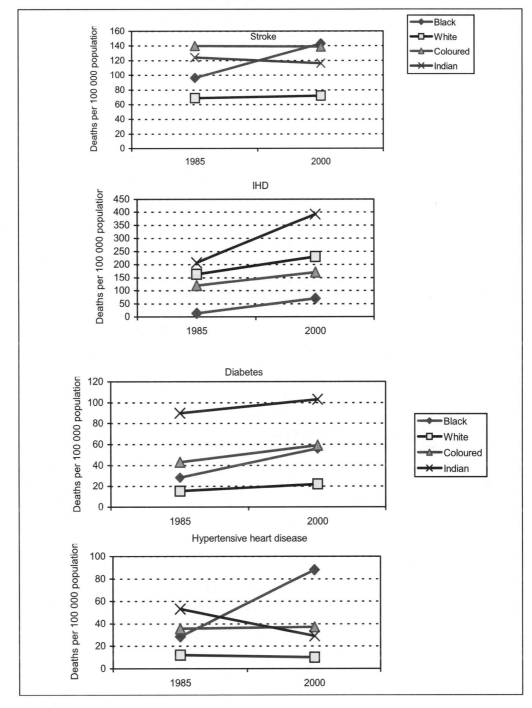

Note: 2000 figures are adjusted for misclassification and underregistration of deaths, but not 1985 figures. 1985 figures for blacks are for urban blacks only.
Sources: 1985 – Bradshaw *et al.,* 1995; 2000 – Bradshaw *et al.,* 2003.

Cancers

In 2000, the South African National Burden of Disease Study (SANBDS) found that cancers as a group (the malignant neoplasms category) accounted for 41 691 deaths (7.5

percent of all deaths), ranking them the fourth leading cause of death for all people and the second leading cause of death for people aged 60 years and over (Bradshaw *et al.,* 2003). In males, trachea/bronchi/lung (also referred to as lung) cancer accounted for 22.5 percent of all cancer deaths, followed by oesophageal cancer (17.2 percent). Among the top causes of cancer deaths in females were cancer of the cervix (17.9 percent), breast (15.7 percent) and lung (10.9 percent).

Lung cancer

There have been marked increases in mortality rates for lung cancer among males of all population groups, with those among whites increasing almost threefold between 1949 and 1979, while those among coloured males increased even more dramatically. Smaller increases are seen among females. In 1984, 34.5 percent of all white deaths could be attributed to smoking-related diseases, compared with 24.5 percent for Indians, 14.5 percent for coloureds and 3.9 percent for blacks (Yach and Townshend, 1988).

From 1984 to 1986 the age-standardized mortality for lung cancer was highest in coloured urban males (88.4/100 000), followed by white urban males (48.7/100 000), black urban males (27.9/100 000) and Indian urban males (21.8/100 000) (Bradshaw *et al.,* 1995). National age-standardized death rates for 2000 (not disaggregated by urban/rural residence) showed that coloured males had the highest rates (82.1/100 000), followed by white males (54.3/100 000). In 2000, the age-standardized death rates of black males and females were 33.4 and 6.0 per 100 000, respectively (Bradshaw *et al.,* 2003).

The differences in smoking rates among the population groups at different stages of the tobacco epidemic, as well as the gender differences, are reflected in the age-specific death rates for lung cancer. (It is important to note, however, that these death rates reflect exposure to tobacco in the past.) In the older age groups, black men had lower rates than coloured and white men, but the lung cancer death rates in black males in the 35 to 44 years and 45 to 54 years age groups were higher than those in the white population. This, however, is not seen in black women, who have lower lung cancer death rates at all ages.

Oesophageal cancer

In South Africa, the incidence of oesophageal cancer has been increasing since the 1950s, with the risk being much higher than the national average for those living in the Eastern Cape, particularly in rural areas of the former Transkei "homeland". Since the mid-1980s, the incidence of oesophageal cancer has decreased, as shown by a declining proportion of oesophageal cancers over time in the National Cancer Registry. The reasons for these secular trends remain uncertain.

There are marked differences among population groups, with the highest incidence rates in the African population. The National Cancer Registry recorded a shift from oesophageal cancer as the leading cancer among African males in 1995, to prostate cancer in 1996 to 1999. Oesophageal cancer then became the second leading cancer in African males (with an age-standardized incidence rate [ASR] of 14.1/100 000), who had a lifetime risk of developing oesophageal cancer of 1 in 59.0 in 1999. Among African females (with an ASR 7.0/100 000), oesophageal cancer was the third leading cancer (after cervical and breast cancers), and the lifetime risk was 1 in 113 (Mqoqi *et al.,* 2004).

Because of its poor prognosis, oesophageal cancer contributes significantly to cancer mortality. In South Africa, it was the second leading cause of cancer deaths in males (17.2 percent of all male cancer deaths) and the fourth leading cause in females (10 percent). It was the leading cause of male cancer deaths in the African population (age-standardized mortality rate 43.5/100 000) and the second leading cause – after cervical cancer – in African females

(16.5/100 000), with relatively young age groups affected and rates increasing steadily from the 35 to 44 years age group (Bradshaw *et al.,* 2003).

The main risk factors for oesophageal cancer are tobacco use and alcohol consumption, and the joint effect of these is multiplicative (Tuyns, Pequinot and Jensen, 1979; Day, 1984; IARC, 1988). Other possible risk factors include poor socio-economic conditions, poor nutritional intake and a diet lacking in vitamins A and C, riboflavin, nicotinic acid, magnesium and zinc (Cook-Mozaffari *et al.,* 1979; Van Rensburg, 1981). Contamination of maize with *Fusarium verticillioides* (previously known as *Fusarium moniliforme*) and the consequent ingestion of mycotoxins (possibly fumonisins) produced by this fungus may also play a role.

Breast cancer
In South Africa from 1984 to 1986, breast cancer age-standardized mortality rates were highest among coloured urban females (26.4/100 000) (Figure 28), followed closely by whites (26.0/100 000) and then urban Indians (14.6/100 000); black urban females had the lowest rates (9.6/100 000) (Bradshaw *et al.,* 1995). In 2000, the age-standardized mortality rates appeared to have increased since 1984 to 1986, although the 2000 national rates were not available by urban/rural residence, and the rate in urban females was probably higher than the national average. As before, the age-standardized death rates for white females were almost threefold those of blacks: whites had the highest rates (33.0/100 000), followed closely by coloureds (31.0/100 000) and Indians (27.4/100 000); black females had the lowest rates (12.1/100 000) (Bradshaw *et al.,* 2003).

However, the age-specific death rates indicate that black females aged 35 to 44 years have very similar rates to those in the corresponding white, coloured and Indian population groups, and it is only in the older age groups that black females have far lower rates. This pattern is also evident in terms of incidence.

FIGURE 28
Age-standardized mortality rates for females from breast cancer, 1985 and 2000

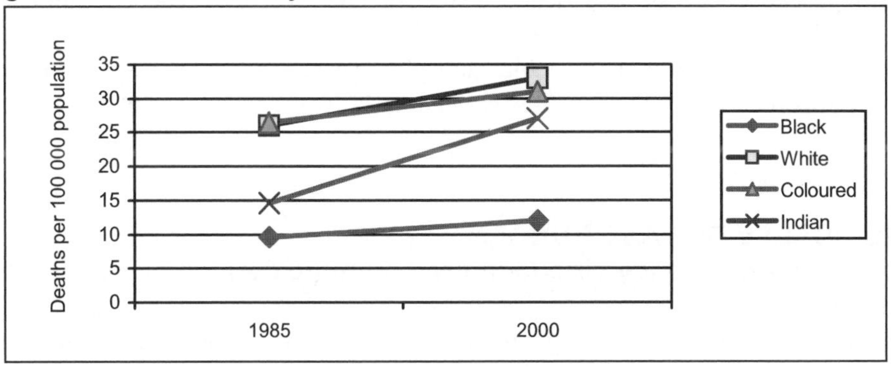

Note: 2000 figures are adjusted for misclassification and underregistration of deaths, but not 1985 figures. 1985 figures for blacks are for urban blacks only.
Sources: 1985 – Bradshaw *et al.,* 1995; 2000 – Bradshaw *et al.,* 2003.

Black females consistently also had the lowest breast cancer incidence rates. In 1999, the national ASR in blacks was 18.4 per 100 000, compared with 76.5 for coloured and white females (Mqoqi *et al.,* 2004). The differences in rates are more pronounced in older age groups; in the younger age groups, the incidence rates in black females are closer to those of white and coloured females.

The risk of breast cancer is clearly associated with high socio-economic status, and women with higher education or income are at higher risk (Parkin *et al.,* 2003). These differences may be because of differences in the distribution of risk factors among social classes, such as reproductive factors and other known risk factors for breast cancer, including alcohol, diet, smoking, body weight, physical activity and genetic factors. Increased body weight has been found to increase the risk of breast cancer, whereas physical activity has been found to be beneficial in reducing the breast cancer risk at all ages.

Colorectal cancer

Cancers of the colon and rectum are the second most common malignancy in affluent societies, but are rarer in developing countries. In South Africa, colorectal cancer was the sixth leading cancer among males (5.3 percent) and the fifth among females (6.6 percent) in terms of deaths (Bradshaw *et al.,* 2003). In 1999, colorectal cancer comprised 3.7 percent of all cancer cases in males and 3.4 percent in females, ranking third and fifth in females and males, respectively. The ASR for colorectal cancer in women was 6.6 per 100 000, while males had a higher rate of 9.7 (Mqoqi *et al.,* 2004).

Colorectal cancer was the second leading cause of cancer deaths in the South African white population. The age-standardized death rate was more than five times greater in this population (21.1/100 000) than in the black population (4.1/100 000). Colorectal cancer incidence rates were also highest among white males and females. In 1999, colorectal cancer was the second leading cancer in white males and females in terms of incidence. Coloured males and females had the second highest rates, followed by Indian males and females, with the lowest rates reported in black males and females. The rates in white males (ASR of 25.4/100 000) are more than eight times those found in black males (3.0/100 000), while those in white females (17.5/100 000) are about seven times those in black females (2.3/100 000) (Mqoqi *et al.,* 2004).

Age-specific incidence rates by population group suggest an increased risk in younger black South Africans, probably caused by changing lifestyle and diet, resulting in a reduction in the incidence gap observed in elderly South Africans. Although there is an almost tenfold difference in incidence among the older age groups (75 years and over), at younger ages the incidence rates among the black, white and coloured population groups are almost the same.

A diet high in energy (calories), rich in animal fat and poor in vegetables, fruit and fibre is associated with increased risk. Smoking, meat and alcohol consumption are known risk factors, while consumption of fruit and vegetables and physical activity are known to be protective. Hence, the importance of a healthy lifestyle cannot be overemphasized in the prevention of cancers.

COMMUNICABLE DISEASE BURDEN
Human immunodeficiency virus/acquired immune deficiency syndrome (HIV/AIDS)

The prevalence of HIV among pregnant women attending public sector clinics has been surveyed annually to monitor trends. The surveys show that prevalence has increased from 0.8 percent in 1990 to 27.9 percent in 2003, reflecting a remarkable spread of the epidemic within a decade (Figure 29). It is estimated that in 2004, about 12 percent of the total population was infected with the virus (Dorrington *et al.,* 2004), and that by 2000 HIV/AIDS had become the biggest single cause of death in South Africa (Dorrington *et al.,* 2004).

Prior to 2004, AIDS treatment was available only in the private sector, which restricted its use to people with medical insurance or sufficient money to pay for costly medication. In 2004, the government adopted a treatment five-year plan to roll-out anti-retroviral therapy in the public sector with the aim of meeting at least 80 percent of the need. The ASSA2002 model shows that in 2004 approximately 5 million people were HIV-positive, and 500 000 were AIDS-sick.

Allowing for the impact of the treatment intervention, the number of infected people is projected to peak in 2013 and then decrease slowly, while the number of AIDS-sick people increases slowly. It is further predicted that in 2015 the number of AIDS-sick people will be about three-quarters of a million, with a projected 5.4 million-plus HIV-positive people. Currently, about 10 percent of HIV-positive people are AIDS-sick, and this will rise to just less than 13 percent.

Figure 30 shows that the projected total number of deaths increased as a result of the gradual increase in non-AIDS deaths and the rapid increase in AIDS deaths during the late 1990s. In 2004, the model estimates 389 000 non-AIDS deaths and 311 000 AIDS deaths. The total deaths in 2004 were 701 000, i.e., about 44 percent of total deaths were AIDS deaths. The proportion of AIDS deaths to total deaths is fairly constant over the time span depicted in Figure 30.

FIGURE 29
Prevalence of HIV as determined by antenatal surveys, 1990 to 2002

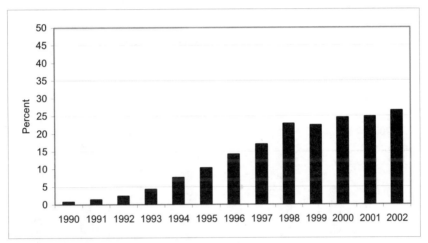

Source: Health Systems Trust, 2004.

FIGURE 30
Projected annual numbers of AIDS and non-AIDS deaths, 1985 to 2025

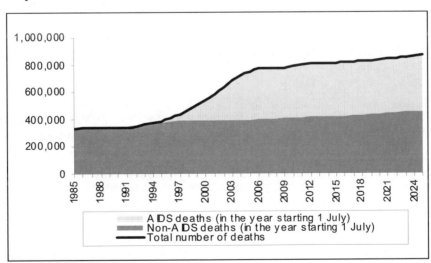

Source: ASSA2002 (ASSA, 2004).

Tuberculosis

Tuberculosis (TB) has been an important disease in South Africa for many years, affecting workers, particularly miners, and poor communities. Despite national treatment programmes, TB has been among the leading causes of death, accounting for more than 5 percent of all deaths in 2000. This has been exacerbated by the HIV/AIDS epidemic, with TB being the common opportunistic infection among HIV-positive people.

In 2002, there were an estimated 243 000 cases of TB in South Africa, making it the country with the seventh highest number of TB cases. The number of TB cases, as well as the number of new smear cases, nearly doubled between 1996 and 2002 (Figure 31). The rise in the number of reported TB cases since the inception of the National TB Control Programme in 1996 reflects a real increase in the number of cases, as well as improved case detection and reporting. The real increase in the number of cases is largely because of the rising prevalence of HIV. HIV infection is now the main single risk factor for TB, and in 2003/2004 more than half the smear-positive TB patients were HIV-positive.

FIGURE 31
Numbers of TB, pulmonary TB and new smear cases reported, 1996 to 2000

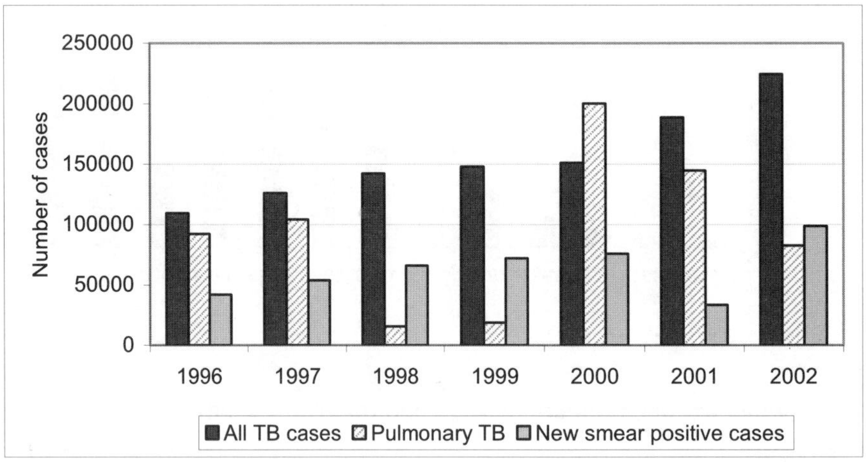

Reproduced by permission of Health Systems Trust. Originally published in Bamford, L., Loveday, M. & Verkuijl, S. 2004. Tuberculosis. *In* P. Ijumba, C. Day, and A. Ntuli, eds. *South African Health Review 2003/04.* Durban, Health Systems Trust.

Malaria

Malaria affects only the northern and northeastern regions of South Africa. Systematic control efforts introduced in the late 1940s and good access to treatment have generally kept the disease in check. In contrast to most other countries in sub-Saharan Africa, malaria is not a major cause of death in South Africa.

For the period 1976 to 1995, annual reported malaria cases ranged from 2 000 to 13 000 per year. In 1996, slightly more than 27 000 cases were reported, rising to more than 60 000 in 2000. The number of notified malaria cases decreased considerably thereafter (Figure 32). The malaria vectors' resistance to existing pesticides, as well as antimalarial drug resistance, in part caused the dramatic increases in numbers of cases and deaths from malaria. Changes in the drugs and insecticide used contributed to the subsequent significant decrease in malaria morbidity and mortality in South Africa in subsequent years.

FIGURE 32
Annual notified malaria cases and deaths, 1971 to June 2003

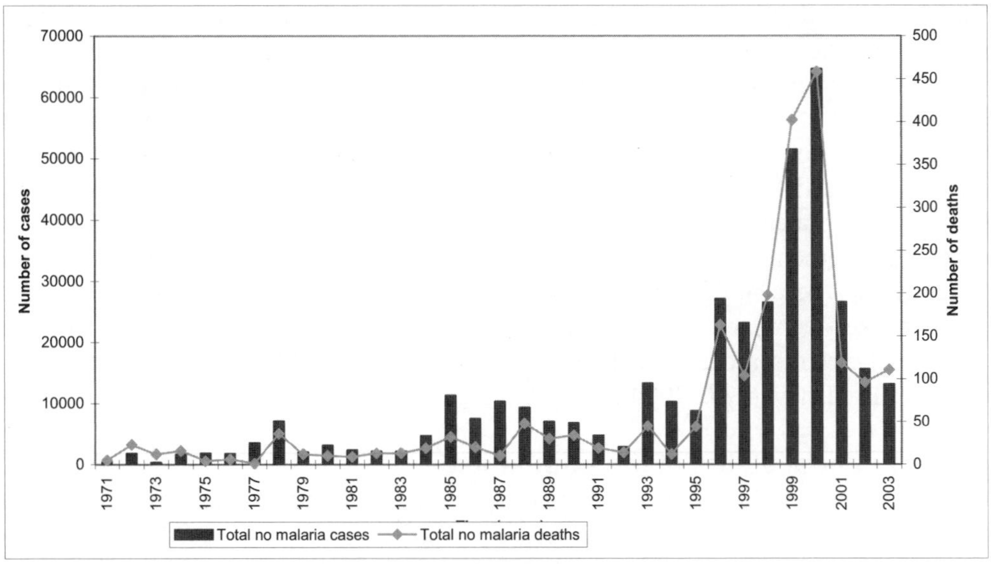

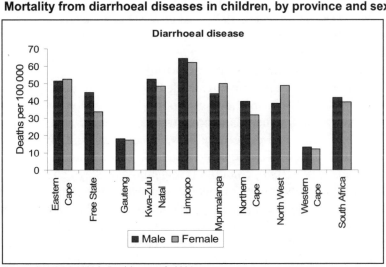

Reproduced by permission of Health Systems Trust. Originally published in Moonasar, D., Johnson, C.L., Maloba, B.,
Kruger, P., le Grange, K., Mthembu,J. & van den Ende, J. 2004. Malaria. *In* P. Ijumba, C. Day, and A. Ntuli, eds.
South African Health Review 2003/04. Durban, Health Systems Trust.

Diarrhoeal disease

SANBD found that diarrhoea accounted for nearly 3 percent of all deaths in South Africa
in 2000. However, death rates for diarrhoeal disease vary by province, ranging from 12 per
100 000 in the Western Cape to more than 60 in Limpopo Province (Figure 33). The
average rates for South Africa are about 42 per 100 000 for males and slightly fewer for
females. Clearly, in some provinces deaths from diarrhoea still make a significant
contribution, affecting infants, children and the elderly in particular. Serious cholera
outbreaks have occurred in recent years, affecting areas where there are poor water
supplies and no sanitation. However, the case fatality rates during these outbreaks have
been remarkably low.

FIGURE 33
Mortality from diarrhoeal diseases in children, by province and sex

Source: SANBDS 2000 in Bradshaw *et al.,* 2004.

SUMMARY
Current burden of disease
The data presented show that South Africa has a quadruple burden of disease: 1) continuation of the infectious diseases associated with underdevelopment, poverty and undernutrition; 2) an emerging epidemic of chronic diseases linked to overnutrition and Western types of diet and lifestyle; 3) the explosive HIV/AIDS epidemic; and 4) the continued burden of injury-related deaths. In 2000, NCDs accounted for 37 percent of deaths, and HIV/AIDS and infectious diseases together for 44 percent (Bradshaw *et al.,* 2003). CVD and diabetes together accounted for 19 percent of total deaths, and cancers for a further 7.5 percent. In contrast, nutritional deficiencies related to undernutrition accounted for 1.2 percent of deaths. In terms of mortality from chronic diseases, in 2000 IHD and stroke accounted for 123 and 124 per 100 000 deaths, respectively, while hypertensive heart disease and diabetes accounted for 68 and 54 per 100 000 deaths, respectively (Bradshaw *et al.,* 2004).

Current nutritional status of the population
Undernutrition and its associated outcomes of stunting and underweight are still prevalent in children. In 1999, 22 percent of children aged one to nine years in South Africa were stunted, and 10 percent were underweight-for-age (Labadarios *et al.,* 2000). However, at the same time, 17 percent of children were overweight and obese (BMI ≥ 25) (Steyn *et al.,* 2005). In adults the prevalence of obesity (BMI ≥ 30) was very high in 1998, particularly in women, among whom it ranged from 21 to 31 percent in different population groups (Department of Health, SAMRC and Measure DHS+, 2002). In white males, the prevalence of obesity was 21 percent, while it was less than 10 percent in the other population groups; the prevalence of overweight (BMI ≥ 25) was 20 percent in all males. Underweight (BMI < 18.5) was less than 6 percent in the adult female population and 13 percent in males (Department of Health, SAMRC and Measure DHS+, 2002). Hence, both under- and overnutrition coexist in South Africa, and sometimes even in the same household, where a child is stunted and a parent/carer overweight or obese.

Micronutrient deficiencies are also still prevalent in children; in 1994, 39 percent of 0- to five-year-olds were marginally vitamin-A deficient and 25 percent had low iron stores (SAVACG, 1995). Iodine deficiency was still found to be prevalent in some provinces in 1998 (Immelman, Towindo and Kalk, 2000). No national data on biochemical deficiencies are available for adults, but numerous localized studies have shown high prevalence of iron deficiency in women (Kruger *et al.,* 1994; Dannhauser *et al.,* 1999) and of VAD, particularly in HIV-infected adults (Kennedy-Oji *et al.,* 2001; Visser *et al.,* 2003).

Current dietary intake patterns of the population
National dietary intake data are only available for children aged one to nine years (Labadarios *et al.,* 2000). The main findings from NFCS 1999 were that many children were deficient in energy and numerous micronutrients (vitamins A and C, niacin, vitamin B6, calcium, iron and zinc), and deficiency prevalence rates were always higher in rural areas. A few localized surveys provide some trends on dietary intake in adults. Studies in the white (Wolmarans *et al.,* 1988), coloured (Langenhoven, Steyn and van Eck, 1988) and Indian (Wolmarans *et al.,* 1999) populations showed that mean carbohydrate intakes were less than 55 percent of total energy, mean fat intakes more than 30 percent, and added (free) sugar intakes more than 10 percent. Rural blacks (Steyn *et al.,* 2001) had a prudent diet with a mean fat intake of less than 20 percent of total energy, carbohydrate intake of more than 60 percent and free sugar intake of less than 10 percent. Urban blacks, on the

other hand, had mean intakes that lay between the extremes of the Western diet and the rural prudent diet (Bourne *et al.,* 1993; Steyn *et al.,* 2001). In the urban upper-income black group (MacIntyre *et al.,* 2002) mean fat intake was more than 30 percent of total energy. Studies on dietary trends in urban blacks showed that the mean intake of fat increased from 24 to 32 percent of total energy among those aged 19 to 44 years as the time they spent in the city increased, while mean carbohydrate intakes decreased from 61 to 53 percent (Bourne, 1996). These trends are typical of the nutrition transition that is taking place.

CURRENT POLICIES AND STRATEGIES FOR ADDRESSING NUTRITION PROBLEMS IN SOUTH AFRICA
Programmes to improve protein-calorie malnutrition and undernutrition
Since the inauguration of the democratic government in 1994, the nutritional status of children has received a great deal of attention from the new government, which made child nutrition one of the cornerstones of its Reconstruction and Development Programme. A great deal of focus was placed on the high prevalence of stunting and underweight found in preschool children, as reported by SAVACG (1995). The Nutrition Directorate of the Department of Health subsequently developed an Integrated Nutrition Programme for South Africa in an attempt to deal with some of the critical issues related to undernutrition and infectious diseases (Department of Health, 1998). As part of this strategy, certain focus areas were devoted to improving the nutritional status of children and decreasing the prevalence of PEM nationally (Nutrition Directorate, 2001).

The most crucial focus area of this strategy is contributing to household food security with the objective of alleviating short-term hunger among primary schoolchildren. A school feeding programme was introduced into schools with needy learners in 1994 and about 5 million learners a year benefit annually from this. Despite many initial problems, a qualitative survey has indicated that the programme makes a major social contribution to schools in terms of difficult-to-measure qualities such as children being more alert and benefiting intellectually (McCoy, 1997).

Additionally, there are three more focus areas in the Integrated Nutrition Programme aimed at dealing with the development and consequences of undernutrition. These are: 1) disease-specific nutrition support, treatment and counselling; 2) growth monitoring and promotion; and 3) promotion of breastfeeding. These are implemented at the primary health care level, where infants and children are brought for routine immunizations and pregnant women come for antenatal and post-natal care. The main objectives of health policy-makers are to reduce the prevalence of low birth weight from 8.3 percent nationally and to reduce the prevalence of stunting and underweight in children from 21.6 and 10.3 percent, respectively, in 1999 to 18 and 8 percent, respectively, in 2007 (Nutrition Directorate, 2001).

Another aspect of dealing with undernutrition and dietary deficiencies has been the development and promotion of food-based dietary guidelines in South Africa. The Nutrition Directorate has adopted 11 guidelines, which were developed by a national working group (Love *et al.,* 2001) to promote healthy eating habits in the child and adult populations. Paediatric guidelines to be introduced in the near future are currently being tested.

HIV/AIDS is another focus area to receive much support in terms of promoting nutrition. Recently, the Nutrition Directorate has implemented an intervention programme aimed at people with TB and/or HIV/AIDS. The objective of this strategy is to provide an energy-dense meal and micronutrient supplements to people who qualify for the scheme. Nutritional guidelines are already available for such patients (Nutrition Directorate, personal communication, 2005).

Programmes to improve micronutrient status

The Department of Health has been successful regarding the implementation of fortification schemes to eliminate micronutrient deficiencies in the South African population. The iodization of salt became compulsory in 1995, and the fortification of maize and wheat flour in October 2003. The latter have to be fortified so as to deliver 33 percent of the RDA per serving at the point of consumption (National Food Fortification Task Group, 1998; 2002). The fortificants added are vitamin A, thiamine, riboflavin, niacin, folic acid, vitamin B6, iron and zinc. Nutrition support for women and children is provided by health care workers at primary care facilities and includes vitamin A and iron supplementation and health promotion aimed at improving diets (Nutrition Directorate, 2001). Adoption of the food-based dietary guidelines will also contribute to eliminating micronutrient deficiencies because one of the guidelines encourages dietary diversity and increased consumption of fruit and vegetables (Love *et al.*, 2001).

Programmes to prevent and manage nutrition-related chronic diseases

The Global Strategy on Diet, Physical Activity and Health has clearly indicated that every government has a primary steering and stewardship role in initiating and developing its own national strategy for the prevention and management of chronic diseases through a strategy for diet, physical activity and health. National circumstances determine the priorities in the development of such strategies (WHO, 2004).

In 1996 the Department of Health instituted the Directorate of Chronic Diseases, Disabilities and Geriatrics, and the first director was appointed. This marked the start of a period during which NCDs were prioritized at national- and provincial-level departments of health. For the first time, provinces appointed people responsible for NCDs; this can be seen as a milestone in the organization of long-term care delivery in the South African health system (C. Kotzenberg, personal communication, 2005).

In support of this initiative, the Department of Health has embarked on a surveillance programme, incorporating health indicators such as BMI, physical inactivity and blood pressure. A nationally representative survey (SADHS) was undertaken in 1998 and repeated in 2003/2004, in order to provide a way of monitoring secular trends for these health indicators in response to the national health strategy.

The Nutrition Directorate has also supported the development of strategies for nutrition-related chronic diseases. In the late 1990s, the department initiated a consultative process to develop a series of guidelines for the prevention and management of NCDs (separate guidelines are available for the prevention and management of diabetes, hypertension, hyperlipidaemia and overweight). In this regard it has set strategic objectives aimed at reducing the prevalence rates of obesity from 9.3 percent in males and 30.1 percent in females in 2000 to 7 and 25 percent, respectively (Nutrition Directorate, 2001). To date, however, there is no clear indication of how these targets will be achieved in terms of strategies at the primary care level.

There are also initiatives within the Ministries of Sport (Sport and Recreation South Africa) and Education, which provide a policy and programme framework that supports the strategic priorities for health care. Sport and Recreation South Africa is responsible for devising and implementing sport and recreation policy in South Africa, specifically targeting increased mass participation and sports development. This mandate is reflected in the theme of the ministerial White Paper on Sport and Recreation in South Africa, which is "getting the nation to play".

The Directorates of Health Promotion and Chronic Diseases have also recognized the need to encourage physical activity, in particular among older adults, and have initiated guidelines for promoting "active ageing" (1999). More recently, in November 2004, the Directorate of Health Promotion in the Department of Health launched an intersectoral strategy aimed at promoting healthy lifestyles and change from risky behaviour, particularly among youth. This forms part of a plan for comprehensive health care in South Africa, and is one of the strategic priorities for the period 2004 to 2009 (Nutrition Directorate, 2001).

Future policy needs to address the nutrition transition

The rising prevalence of obesity in South Africa gives cause for grave concern because of the increased risk of diabetes and CVD (WHO/FAO, 2003). As well as direct costs, which may be as high as 6.8 percent of total health care costs, there are also indirect costs such as workdays lost, doctor visits, impaired quality of life and premature mortality (WHO/FAO 2003). Over the last three decades, many chronic diseases have featured significantly in terms of overall morbidity and mortality. This is particularly so for IHD, hypertensive disease, stroke, diabetes, chronic obstructive pulmonary diseases, lung, oesophageal, breast and colorectal cancers.

In addition, communicable diseases are still major causes of mortality and morbidity in South Africa, and should remain priorities on the health agenda. The death rates from infectious diseases such as HIV/AIDS, TB and diarrhoeal disease are still high, and in the case of HIV and TB increasing. In addition, both under- and overnutrition are coexisting. It is important that health care policy-makers do not neglect any of these areas of concern and, despite the immediate pressure for relief against infectious diseases, the government should also be looking for long-term solutions for chronic diseases. The first step in this regard will be prevention, and it is most feasible that prevention efforts should be aimed mainly at children.

Children are important targets for health interventions. It is increasingly recognized that the occurrence of adult chronic diseases is influenced by factors operating throughout the life course (Kuh and Schlomo, 2004). Increased risk may start in infancy, or even before birth, and continues to be influenced by health-related behaviours during childhood. Hence, future policies should focus on inculcating healthy behaviours in children, where feasible. Some recommendations for policies that can be adopted and implemented are presented in the following paragraphs.

Fiscal policies and levies

Swinburn *et al.* (2004) highlighted the importance of introducing fiscal policies that influence the food supply in order to ensure that the population has access to safe and affordable foods that discourage the intake of high-fat/-sugar products. Another option in this regard would be for the government to introduce small levies on certain high-fat/-sugar foods, including such items as soft drinks and crisps.

School-based intervention programmes

Schools are an established setting for health promotion activities and have the advantage of influencing health-related beliefs and behaviours early in the "health career" so that they become established as adult patterns. Children in schools also represent a large population who are present and accessible over prolonged periods in a setting that is relatively sheltered and where education and learning are the norm. Influencing children in their formative years is a potential mechanism for influencing the emerging culture and health beliefs of society.

An additional potential benefit of school-based health promotion is that by improving the health of schoolchildren, educational performance and learning may be enhanced. A large body of evidence indicates that positive educational outcomes are closely linked to good health in schoolchildren. These positive outcomes include classroom performance, school attendance, participation in school activities and student attitudes (Symons *et al.,* 1997).

The importance of school health promotion programmes for the prevention of chronic diseases was underlined in a recent scientific statement by the American Heart Association (Hayman *et al.*, 2004), which recommended that: "All schools should implement: evidence-based, comprehensive, age-appropriate curricula about cardiovascular health, methods for improving health behaviours, and the reduction of CVD risk; and age-appropriate and culturally sensitive curricula on changing students' patterns of dietary intake, physical activity, and smoking behaviours." An intervention programme to prevent smoking in adolescents is currently being tested at some schools in South Africa (P. Reddy, personal communication, 2005). It is hoped that this may lead to the introduction of similar strategies aimed at diet and physical activity.

Food labelling and claims

Food labelling is currently being revised by the Department of Health, and new regulations are expected for the end of 2005 (Booyzen, Directorate of Food Control, personal communication, 2005). These new regulations are more informative than the present ones, and will provide consumers with detailed nutrition information. In future, consumers will be able to determine whether the products they purchase and consume comply with recommendations for a healthy diet, particularly in terms of fats, free sugars and sodium. Furthermore, the regulatory framework will minimize misleading food, health and nutrition claims. However, consumers need to be educated about these regulations and about how to select healthy foods accordingly. Clearly, the Nutrition Directorate of the Department of Health, together with the Directorate of Food Control, will need to plan and implement specific strategies to do this.

Marketing and advertising standards

To date there have been no regulations regarding the marketing of energy-dense foods to children. Ideally it is hoped that in the near future there will be bans on the television advertising of energy-dense, high-fat and high-sugar foods to young children, particularly because this has been shown to be an effective way of persuading children to make undesirable and unhealthy choices (Swinburn *et al.*, 2004).

Policies aimed at improving the environment

Intersectoral action is required in order to modify the environment so that physical activity and a healthy diet are promoted and enhanced in schools, workplaces and communities. This should include limiting the exposure of young children to heavy marketing of energy-dense, micronutrient-poor foods, which can be done by introducing school policies that prohibit the presence of vending machines and unhealthy food sales in schools, crèches and after-school centres. Furthermore, it is essential that food items that are included in the primary school meal programme are healthy. It is also important to ensure that children have safe and adequate space at school and in the community for playing sports and games that promote physical activity. The onus rests with employers to make workplaces encouraging of physical activity and to provide healthy foods and meals.

Nutrition health logos

In South Africa the Heart Foundation and the Cancer Association provide their logos to food products that meet certain specified health and nutrition standards. In doing so, these associations are raising the awareness of consumers and manufacturers about the value of using healthy foods. The Department of Health should encourage this trend in an effort to persuade the food industry of the benefits of producing healthier food and meal options.

Nutrition education programmes at primary health care facilities

It is important that the food-based dietary guidelines initiated by the Nutrition Directorate be given priority as a tool for nutrition education, and be incorporated into primary health care programmes and school curricula. As these guidelines also cater for overnutrition and promote healthy eating habits for all South Africans, they need to be implemented by all departments and district health authorities, with an important emphasis on avoiding both over- and undernutrition.

Furthermore, it has been found that health professionals working at the primary care level have inadequate knowledge about nutrition and lifestyle modification regarding NCDs; their basic training therefore needs to be updated in this regard (Talip *et al.,* unpublished data, 2005).

CONCLUSIONS

The following important findings regarding nutrition and chronic diseases need to be kept high on the health agenda. First, it should be recognized that malnutrition (both under- and overnutrition) is prevalent in all ethnic groups in South Africa, and poor diet – together with other unhealthy behaviours – leads to the development of a substantial (and growing) burden of chronic diseases. Second, it should be recognized that many children and adults in South Africa have unhealthy lifestyles with high intakes of energy, total fat and added sugar, and low intakes of fruit and vegetables. Many people are inactive, smoke cigarettes and have high intakes of alcohol. In order to reduce the burden of chronic diseases over the next few decades these unhealthy behaviours need to be addressed now.

REFERENCES

Archer, S., Bromberger, N., Nattrass, N. & Oldham, G. 1990. Unemployment and labour market issues – A beginner's guide. *In* N. Nattrass and E. Ardington, eds. *The political economy of South Africa.* Cape Town, Oxford University Press.

ASSA. 2004. ASSA AIDS and Demographic Models: AASA2002. AIDS Committee of ASSA. Available at: www.assa.org.za/. Actuarial Society of South Africa.

Blaauw, D. & Gilson, L. 2001. *Health and poverty reduction policies in South Africa.* Johannesburg, Centre for Health Policy.

Bourne, L.T. 1996. *Dietary intake in an urban African population in South Africa – with special reference to the nutrition transition.* University of Cape Town. (Ph.D. thesis)

Bourne, L.T., Langenhoven, M.L., Steyn, K., Jooste, P.L., Laubscher, J.A. & van der Vyver, E. 1993. Nutrient intake in the urban African population of the Cape Peninsula, South Africa. The Brisk study. *Cent. Afr. J. Medical,* 39(12): 238–247.

Bradshaw, D., Dorrington, R.E. & Sitas, F. 1992. The level of mortality in South Africa in 1985 – what does it tell us about health? *S. Afr. Med. J.,* 82: 237–240.

Bradshaw, D., Bourne, D., Schneider, M. & Sayed, R. 1995. Mortality patterns of chronic diseases of lifestyle in South Africa. *In* J. Fourie and K. Steyn, eds. *Chronic diseases of lifestyle in South Africa,* pp. 5–23. MRC Technical Report. Cape Town, SAMRC.

Bradshaw, D., Groenewald, P., Laubscher, R., Nannan, N., Nojilana, B., Norman, R., Pieterse, D. & Schneider, M. 2003. Initial burden of disease estimates for South Africa, 2000. *S. Afr. Med. J.,* 93(9): 682–688.

Bradshaw, D., Nannan, N., Laubscher, R., Groenewald, P., Joubert, J., Nojilana, B., Norman, R., Pieterse, D. & Schneider, M. 2004. *South African National Burden of Disease Study, 2000: Estimates of Provincial Mortality.* Tygerberg, SAMRC.

Cole, T.J., Bellizzi, M.C., Flegal, K.M. & Dietz, W.H. 2000. Establishing a standard definition for child overweight and obesity worldwide: international survey. *BMJ,* 320: 1240–1243.

Cook-Mozaffari, P., Azordegan, F., Day, N.E., Ressicaud, A., Sabai, C. & Aramesh, B. 1979. Oesophageal cancer studies in the Caspian Littoral of Iran: Results of a case-control study. *Br. J. Cancer,* 39: 293.

Dannhauser, A., Bam, R., Joubert, G. *et al.* 1999. Iron status of pregnant women attending the antenatal clinic at Pelonomi Hospital, Bloemfontein. *S. Afr. J. Clin. Nutr.,* 12: 8–16.

Day, N.E. 1984. The geographic pathology of cancer of the oesophagus. *Br. Med. Bull.,* 40: 329–334.

Department of Health. 1998. *Integrated Nutrition Programme for South Africa. Summary of broad guidelines for implementation.* Pretoria.

Department of Health, SAMRC & Measure DHS+. 2002. *South Africa Demographic and Health Survey 1998.* Full report. Available at: www.doh.gov.za/facts/sadhs-f.html and www.doh.gov.za/facts/1998/sadhs98/.

Department of Labour. 2002. *Sectoral Determination 7: Domestic Worker Section of the Basic Conditions of Employment Act, No. 75 of 1997.* Government Gazette No. 23732. Pretoria.

Dorrington, R.E., Bradshaw, D., Johnson, L, & Budlender, D. 2004. *The demographic impact of HIV/AIDS in South Africa. National indicators for 2004.* Cape Town, Centre for Actuarial Research, SAMRC and ASSA.

Ewing, J.A. 1984. Detecting alcoholism. The CAGE questionnaire. *JAMA,* 252: 1905–1907.

FAO. 2004. *Food balance sheets.* Available at: www.fao.org/faostat.

FAO/WHO. 2002. *Human vitamin and mineral requirements.* Report of a Joint FAO/WHO Expert Consultation. Rome.

Gelderblom, D. & Kok, P. 1994. *Urbanisation: South Africa's challenge. Volume 1: Dynamics.* Pretoria, HSRC Publishers.

Hayman, L.L., Williams, C.L., Daniels, S.R., Steinberger, J., Paridon, S., Dennison, B.A. & McCrindle, B.W. 2004. Cardiovascular health promotion in the schools. AHA Scientific Statement. *Circulation,* 110: 2266–2275.

Health Systems Trust. 2004. *South African Health Review, 2003/4.* Durban.

HSRC. 2003. *Synthesis report on social and economic impacts of government programmes since 1994.* Prepared for the Policy Coordination and Advisory Services, Office of the President. Pretoria, Human Sciences Research Council (HSRC) Publishers.

IARC. 1988. *Alcohol drinking.* IARC Monographs on the Evaluation of the Carcinogenic Risk of Chemicals to Humans No. 44. Lyon, France, WHO, International Agency for Research on Cancer (IARC).

Immelman, R., Towindo, T. & Kalk, W.J. 2000. *Report of the South African Institute for Medical Research (SAIMR) on the Iodine Deficiency Disorder Survey of Primary School Learners for the Department of Health, South Africa.* Johannesburg, SAIMR.

Jooste, P.L., Steenkamp, H.J., Benadé, A.J.S. & Rossouw, J.E. 1988. Prevalence of overweight and obesity and its relation to coronary heart diseases in the CORIS study. *S. Afr. Med. J.,* 74: 101–104.

Kennedy-Oji, C., Coutsoudis, A., Kuhn, L., Pillay, K., Mburu, A., Stein, Z. & Coovadia, H. 2001. Effects of vitamin A supplementation during pregnancy and early lactation on body weight of South African HIV-infected women. *J. Health Popul. Nutr.,* 19(3):167–176.

Kok, P., O'Donovan, M., Bouare, O. & Van Zyl, J. 2003. *Post-apartheid patterns of internal migration in South Africa.* Pretoria, HSRC Publishers.

Kruger, M., Dhansay, M.A., Van Staden, E. *et al.* 1994. Anaemia and iron deficiency in women in the third trimester of pregnancy receiving selective iron supplementation. *S. Afr. J. Food Sci. Nutr.,* 6: 132–137.

Kuh. D.J.L. & Schlomo, B.Y. 2004. *A life course approach to chronic disease epidemiology.* Oxford, UK, Oxford University Press.

Kustner, H.G.V. 1987. First RHOSA Nutrition Study: Anthropometric assessment of nutritional status in black under-fives in rural South Africa. *Epidemiological Comments,* 14(3): 1–32.

Labadarios, D., Steyn, N.P., Maunder, E., MacIntyre, U., Swart, R., Gericke, G., Huskisson, J., Dannhauser, A., Vorster, H.H. & Nesamvuni, E.A. 2000. *The National Food Consumption Survey (NFCS): Children aged 1–9 years, South Africa, 1999.* Pretoria, Department of Health.

Langenhoven, M.L, Steyn, K. & van Eck, M. 1988. The food and meal pattern in Cape Peninsula coloured population. *Ecol. Food Nutr.,* 22: 107–116.

Love, P., Maunder, E., Green, M., Ross, F., Smale-Lovely, J. & Charlton, K. 2001. South African food-based dietary guidelines: Testing of the preliminary guidelines among women in KwaZulu-Natal and the Western Cape. *S. Afr. J. Clin. Nutr.,* 14: 9–19.

Lubbe, A.M. 1973. Nutritional status of Pretoria schoolchildren from four racial groups. *S. Afr. Med. J.,* 47: 679–688.

MacIntyre, U.E., Kruger, H.S., Venter, C.S. & Vorster, H.H. 2002. Dietary intakes of an African population in different stages of transition in the North West Province, South Africa: the THUSA study. *Nutr. Res.,* 22: 239–256.

Martin, G., Steyn, K. & Yach, D. 1992. Beliefs about smoking and health and attitudes toward tobacco control measures. *S. Afr. Med. J.,* 82: 241–245.

May, J. 1998. *Poverty and inequality in South Africa. Summary report.* Available at: www.polity.org.za/html/govdocs/reports/poverty.html.

May, J. 2004. Poverty, social policy and the social wage. Paper presented at a conference on The Politics of Socio-Economic Rights in South Africa: 10 years after Apartheid. Oslo, 8 to 9 June.

McCoy, D. 1997. *An evaluation of the Primary School Nutrition Programme.* Durban, Health Systems Trust.

Mostert, W.P., Hofmeyr, B.E., Oosthuizen, J.S. & Van Zyl, J.A. 1998. *Demography: Textbook for the South African student.* Pretoria, HSRC Publishers.

Moultrie, T.A. & Timæus, I.M. 2003. The South African fertility decline: Evidence from two censuses and a Demographic and Health Survey. *Population Studies,* 57(3): 265–283.

Mqoqi, N.P., Kellett, P., Madhoo, J. & Sitas, F. 2004. *Cancer in South Africa: Incidence of histologically diagnosed cancer in South Africa, 1996–1997.* Johannesburg, National Cancer Registry Report, National Health Laboratory Service.

National Food Fortification Task Group. 1998 and 2002. Reports. Pretoria, Department of Health.

Nel, J.H. & Steyn, N.P. 2002. *Report on South Africa food consumption studies undertaken amongst different population groups (1983–2000): Average intakes of foods most commonly consumed.* Available at: www.sahealthinfo.org/nutrition/scientific.htm.

Nojilana, B., Norman, R., van Blerk, L. & Dhansay, A. in press. Estimating the burden of vitamin A deficiency in South Africa.

Nutrition Directorate. 2001. *Integrated Nutrition Programme Strategic Plan 2001/02 to 2006/7.* Pretoria, Department of Health, Nutrition and Provincial Nutrition Units.

Parkin, D.M., Ferlay, J., Hamdi-Chériff, M., Sitas, F., Thomas, J.O., Wabinga, H. & Whelan, S.L. 2003. *Cancer in Africa: Epidemiology and prevention.* IARC Scientific Publication No.153. Lyon, France, IARC Press.

Popkin, B.M. 2001. The nutrition transition and obesity in the developing world. *J. Nutr.,* 131(3): 871S–873S.

Reddy, S.P., Panday, S., Swart, D., Jinabhai, C.C., Amosun, S.L., James, S., Monyeki, K.D., Stevens, G., Morejele, N., Kambaran, N.S., Omardien, R.G. & Van den Borne, H.W. 2003. *The 1st South African National Youth Risk Behaviour Survey 2002.* Cape Town, SAMRC.

302

Dietary changes and the health transition in South Africa: implications for health policy

Reddy, P., Meyer-Weitz Abedian, I., Steyn, K. & Swart, D. 1998. *Implementable strategies to strengthen comprehensive tobacco control in South Africa: Towards an optimal policy intervention mix.* MRC Policy Brief. Cape Town, SAMRC.

Richardson, B.D. 1977. Underweight – a nutritional risk. *S. Afr. Med. J.,* 51: 42–48.

Rossouw, J.E., du Plessis, J.P., Benadé, A.J.S., Jordaan, P.C., Kotze, J.P., Jooste, P.L. & Ferreira, J.J. 1983. Coronary risk factor screening in three rural communities. *S. Afr. Med. J.,* 64: 430–436.

SAVACG. 1995. *Children aged 6–71 months in South Africa, 1994: Their anthropometric, vitamin A, iron and immunization coverage status.* Stellenbosch, University of Stellenbosch and South African Vitamin A Consultative Group (SAVACG).

Seedat, Y.K., Mayet, F.G.H., Khan, S., Somer, S.R. & Joubert, G. 1990. Risk factors for coronary heart diseases in the Indians in Durban. *S. Afr. Med. J.,* 78: 447–454.

Statistics South Africa. 2003. *Census 2001: Census in brief.* Report No. 03-02-03 (2001). Pretoria.

Steyn, K., Jooste, P., Langenhoven, M.L., Benadé, A.J., Rossouw, J.E., Steyn, M., Jordaan, P.C. & Parry, C.D. 1985. Coronary risk factors in the coloured population of the Cape Peninsula. *S. Afr. Med. J.,* 67: 619–625.

Steyn, K., Jooste, P.L., Bourne, L., Fourie, J., Badenhorst, C.J., Bourne, D.E., Langenhoven, M.L., Lombard, C.J., Truter, H., Katzenellenbogen, J., Marais, M. & Oelofse, A. 1991. Risk factors for coronary heart diseases in the black population of the Cape Peninsula. *S. Afr. Med. J.,* 79: 480–485.

Steyn, N.P., Senekal, M., Brits, S. & Nel, J.H. 2000. Urban and rural differences in dietary intake, weight status and nutrition knowledge of black female students. *Asia Pacific J. Clin. Nutr.,* 9(1): 11–16.

Steyn, N.P., Burger, S., Monyeki, K.D., Alberts, M. & Nthangeni, G. 2001. Variation in dietary intake of the adult population of Dikgale. *S. Afr. J. Clin. Nutr.,* 14(4): 140–145.

Steyn, N.P., Labadarios, D., Maunder, E., Nel, J. & Lombard C. 2005. Secondary anthropometric data analysis of the National Food Consumption Survey in South Africa: The double burden. *Nutrition,* 21: 4–13.

Swinburn, B.A., Caterson, I., Seidell, J.C. & James, W.P.T. 2004. Diet, nutrition and the prevention of excess weight gain and obesity. *PHN,* 7(1A): 123–146.

Symons, C., Cincelli, B., James, T.C. & Groff, P. 1997. Bridging student health risks and academic achievement through comprehensive school health programs. *Journal of School Health,* 6: 220–227.

Terreblanche, S. 2004. *A history of inequality in South Africa, 1652–2002.* Pietermaritzburg, University of Natal Press and KMM Review Publishing Company.

Terreblanche, S. & Nattrass, N. 1990. A periodization of the political economy from 1910. *In* N. Nattrass and E. Ardington, eds. *The political economy of South Africa.* Cape Town, Oxford University Press.

Tuyns, A.J., Pequinot, G. & Jensen, D.M. 1979. Role of diet, alcohol and tobacco in oesophageal cancer, as illustrated by two contrasting high-incidence areas in the North of Iran and West of France. *Front. Gastrointest. Res.,* 4: 101–110.

UNDP. 2001. *Human Development Report 2001.* New York.

UNDP. 2003. *South Africa Human Development Report 2003. The challenge of sustainable development in South Africa: unlocking people's creativity.* Cape Town, Oxford University Press.

Van Rensburg, S.J. 1981. Epidemiologic and dietary evidence for specific nutritional predisposition to oesophageal cancer. *J. Natl. Cancer Inst.,* 67: 243.

Van Walbeek, C. 2005. *The economics of tobacco control in South Africa.* Cape Town, University of Cape Town, Department of Economics. (Ph.D. thesis)

Visser, M.E., Maartens, G., Kossew, G. & Hussey, G.D. 2003. Plasma vitamin A and zinc levels in HIV-infected adults in Cape Town, South Africa. *Br. J. Nutr.,* 89(4): 475–482.

Vorster, H.H., Oosthuizen, W., Steyn, H.S., Van der Merwe, A.M. & Kotze, J.P. 1995. Nutrient intakes of white South Africans – a cause for concern: The VIGHOR Study. *S. Afr. J. Food Sci. Nutr.,* 7(3): 119–126.

Walker, A.R.P., Adam, A. & Küstner, H.G.V. 1993. Changes in total death rate and in ischaemic heart disease death rate in interethnic South African populations, 1978–1989. *S. Afr. Med. J.,* 83: 602–605.

WHO. 2003. *The World Health Report 2002. Reducing risks, promoting healthy life.* WHO Technical Report Series No. 916. Geneva.

WHO. 2004. *Global strategy on diet, physical activity and health.* Fifty-Seventh World Health Assembly. Agenda item 12.6, 17 April. Geneva.

WHO/FAO. 2003. *Diet, nutrition and the prevention of chronic diseases.* Report of a Joint WHO/FAO Expert Consultation. WHO Technical Report Series No. 910. Geneva.

Wolmarans, P., Langenhoven, M.L., Benadé, A.J.S., Swanepoel, A.S.P., Kotze, T.J.W. & Rossouw, J.E. 1988. Intake of macronutrients and their relationship with total cholesterol and high-density lipoprotein cholesterol. The Coronary Risk Factor Study, 1979. *S. Afr. Med. J.,* 73(9): 12–15.

Wolmarans, P., Langenhoven, M.L., van Eck, M. & Swanepoel, A.S.P. 1989. The contribution of different food groups to the energy, fat and fibre intake of the Coronary Risk Factors Study (CORIS) population. *S. Afr. Med. J.*, 75: 167–171.

Wolmarans, P., Seedat, Y.K., Mayet, F.G.H., Joubert, G. & Wentzel, E. 1999. Dietary intake of Indians living in the metropolitan area of Durban. *Public Health Nutr.*, 2(1): 55–60.

Yach, D. & Townshend, D. 1988. *Smoking and health in South Africa: The need for action.* Centre for Epidemiological Research in Southern Africa Technical Report No. 1. Cape Town, SAMRC.

ANNEX 1: FAO FOOD BALANCE SHEETS FOR SOUTH AFRICA, 1962 TO 2001

Product	1962 kg*	1962 kcal	1962 Pro	1962 Fat	1972 kg*	1972 kcal	1972 Pro	1972 Fat	1982 kg*	1982 kcal	1982 Pro	1982 Fat	1992 kg	1992 kcal	1992 Pro	1992 Fat	2001 kcal	2001 Pro	2001 Fat
Total		2 603	68.4	61.2		2 819	74.6	66.4		2 905	77.1	66.0		2 790	75.3	68.8	2 921	75.1	79.0
Cereal, excluding beer	169.3	1 434	38.7	10.9	173.4	1 467	39.9	10.7	173.4	1 576	43.1	11.1	187.8	1 480	40.0	10.5	1 601	42.6	11.5
Starchy roots	13.2	27	0.5	0.0	22.6	45	0.9	0.1	24.9	50	1.0	0.1	29.7	50	1.0	0.1	58	1.2	0.1
Sugar and sweeteners	39.4	383	0.0		40.5	394	0.0		35.5	386	0.0		32.8	346	0.0		319	0.0	
Pulses	2.5	23	1.5	0.1	3.4	32	2.1	0.1	4.0	29	1.9	0.1	2.8	37	2.4	0.2	25	1.7	0.1
Tree nuts	0.1	0	0.0	0.0	0.1	1	0.0	0.1	0.2	1	0.0	0.1	0.3	1	0.0	0.1	2	0.1	0.2
Oil crops	1.1	12	0.5	1.0	1.5	16	0.6	1.4	1.5	11	0.5	0.8	2.2	14	0.8	1.1	23	1.4	1.8
Vegetable oils	5.7	137	0.0	15.6	7.3	176	0.0	19.9	9.4	183	0.0	20.6	14.5	229	0.0	25.9	352	0.0	39.8
Vegetables	43.5	35	1.6	0.3	46.8	36	1.6	0.3	46.1	39	1.7	0.3	44.2	35	1.5	0.4	36	1.5	0.3
Fruits	24.1	26	0.3	0.2	38.0	41	0.5	0.3	35.4	37	0.4	0.2	36.0	42	0.5	0.2	41	0.5	0.3
Stimulants	1.7	5	0.4	0.3	1.8	6	0.4	0.4	1.1	5	0.3	0.4	1.1	2	0.2	0.1	3	0.2	0.2
Spices	0.4	4	0.1	0.1	0.4	4	0.2	0.1	0.3	4	0.2	0.1	0.2	3	0.1	0.1	2	0.1	0.1
Alcoholic beverages	43.8	84	0.3		79.4	146	0.6		64.4	144	0.6		56.8	132	0.6		104	0.5	
Meat	31.6	202	11.9	16.8	35.4	221	13.3	18.3	43.0	222	14.0	18.0	37.5	246	16.6	19.4	204	14.4	15.8
Offal, edible	4.5	14	2.1	0.5	4.1	13	2.0	0.4	3.9	13	2.0	0.4	3.8	12	1.9	0.4	12	1.9	0.4
Animal fats	3.0	58	0.1	6.6	2.0	40	0.0	4.5	1.2	40	0.0	4.5	0.7	26	0.0	2.9	14	0.0	1.5
Milk	78.0	134	7.0	7.9	94.8	149	8.3	8.2	60.3	134	7.5	7.5	54.1	97	5.3	5.5	85	4.7	4.8
Eggs	2.5	9	0.8	0.7	3.6	14	1.1	1.0	4.7	18	1.4	1.2	6.1	18	1.5	1.3	23	2.0	1.6
Fish	5.5	14	2.5	0.4	7.9	19	3.0	0.7	9.2	15	2.3	0.5	7.9	19	2.9	0.8	16	2.4	0.6

* Divide this amount by 365 to obtain the daily per capita availability.

Trends towards overweight in lower- and middle-income countries: some causes and economic policy options

W. Bruce Traill[1]

ABSTRACT

Urbanization, globalization and economic development have led to dietary and lifestyle changes that encourage the consumption of high-value foods, including processed foods and food consumed outside the home. Together with reduced energy expenditure, this has resulted in growing problems associated with overweight in developing and, particularly, middle-income countries. One issue that has created interest but little analysis is the effect of changes in food supply chains that have been associated with globalization and urbanization – most notably the rapid diffusion of supermarkets in developing countries. There is little empirical evidence, but the increased availability of time-saving convenience products and the reduction brought about by supermarkets in the price of packaged groceries relative to fruit, vegetables and traditional staples would account for some of the switch to a higher energy density of the food consumed. The spread of such companies is an inevitable part of economic development and, rather than set up obstacles to their activities, it is sensible to develop policies that counter any harmful consequences of their presence. In developed countries, such policies generally try to respect individual freedom to make unhealthy as well as healthy choices (except possibly in the case of children), but also recognize that reducing health inequalities and influencing social norms are legitimate activities of government. A package of policy measures is necessary to achieve these objectives; such a package may include information, other communications, education, advertising restrictions, taxes on unhealthy foods or ingredients (commonly known as "fat taxes") and subsidies on healthy foods such as fruit and vegetables (sometimes referred to as "thin subsidies"). Good data and careful monitoring of outcomes are important because the existing base of evidence on the effectiveness of health care interventions to improve diets and health is poor, even in developed countries.

INTRODUCTION

The principal aim of this paper is briefly to present the evidence for the recent nutrition transition (towards overweight in developing countries) and dietary transition (changes in consumption of specific foods), paying particular attention to processed foods and looking at the extent to which these changes are linked to urbanization, globalization, changes in the supply chain and income growth. A second aim is to discuss policy options for countering overweight. Policy options for undernutrition and micronutrient deficiencies are not addressed in this paper as most countries already have measures in place to reduce these forms of malnutrition. Policy effectiveness draws on experience in developed countries with a view to learning what may lie in store for today's middle-income and developing countries, and to suggest policy options for avoiding the harmful effects of the nutrition transition. Careful monitoring and data analysis must play an important role in informing policy.

---

[1] At the time of the seminar, W. Bruce Traill was a consultant with the Global Perspective Studies Unit (ESDG), FAO. He was on leave from the University of Reading, United Kingdom, where he is Professor of Food Economics.

The received wisdom is that economic development, globalization and urbanization are bringing about a nutrition transition in which overnutrition joins undernutrition as a major problem facing developing countries. On the overnutrition side, the explanations –which are expressed clearly in Uustialo, Pietinen and Puska (2002), for example – include the following:

- Globalization leads to exposure to global mass media (linked to increasing TV ownership and viewing) and the heavy advertising of "Western" convenience and fast foods that are higher in sodium, sugar and fat (and generally more calorie-dense) and that are more highly refined than traditional foods.
- Urbanization leads to less strenuous forms of labour and (arguably) leisure, which reduces energy requirements.
- Urbanization leads to higher female labour force participation; the consequent higher opportunity cost of time results in a greater demand for convenience foods, convenient shopping and eating out.
- Technical change and openness to the global economy have made vegetable oils, meat and dairy products far cheaper than in the past, especially relative to incomes, so consumption of these products has grown at the expense of traditional staples, which tend to be more expensive in urban areas.
- Technical change and economies of scale in global food manufacturing and retailing, perhaps linked to global sourcing, make processed food cheaper than in the past and more readily available.
- Rising incomes, especially in urban areas, make overconsumption affordable.
- The increased population density associated with urbanization makes it possible to supply cheap foods for eating outside the home.

Overweight has become common in much of the developing world
Annex 1 shows under- and overweight incidence as calculated by Mendez and Popkin (2004) and the International Obesity Task Force. The following are some of the conclusions with respect to overweight:

- Overweight affects a substantial proportion of the population in almost all countries. Rates in Latin America, North Africa and European transition economies are approaching developed country levels.
- In general, overweight is a greater problem in urban areas, but in richer (and more urbanized) countries, the urban–rural distinction in proportion of overweight is relatively small.
- Generally, women are somewhat more overweight than men in low- and middle-income countries, but in developed countries the situation is reversed.

Overweight and income/socio-economic status
People derive pleasure from food and from their physical appearance and fitness/healthiness. Assuming that everyone has an "ideal" body weight – a weight that they would like to be for reasons of health and/or appearance, and that they would aspire to if it did not cost them anything to achieve in terms of money, effort or foregone pleasure from eating and drinking less than they would like – people whose weight is below their ideal would use some or all of any increase in income to eat more; for such people, weight increases with income and they derive extra utility both from eating and from being closer to their ideal weight. Weight will also be positively related to income for people who are heavier than their ideal weight, as long as the additional pleasure derived from being able to consume more food (and drink) exceeds the loss in utility

from any extra weight they would gain. However, beyond some point, the losses in utility from gaining weight exceed the increases in utility from eating more, and the people affected are no longer prepared to spend more of their incomes on a greater quantity of food. In fact, there are good reasons to expect that as such people's incomes continue to increase they will spend money to be less overweight if they can, by buying more expensive healthy foods, joining gyms, paying for membership of weight-loss groups, etc.

The relationship between income and weight is therefore predicted theoretically to be positive at first, then negative – although most people choose to be somewhat overweight. This relationship is strengthened at the population level if, as is generally accepted, income and education are positively related. In that case, better educated people are likely to have a lower ideal body weight than their less educated compatriots who are not as aware of the health risks of being overweight. The better educated population groups may also be better able to understand nutritional concepts of healthier eating.

The empirical evidence supports this theory. In developed countries, it is accepted that the incidence of overweight is greatest among disadvantaged groups, and this also seems to be the case in middle-income countries. Mendez and Popkin (2004) present evidence that in urban areas of highly urbanized countries, women of low socio-economic status (as measured by education) are more likely to be overweight than those of high socio-economic status, whereas the reverse is true in countries with low urbanization. It seems probable that urbanization in this context is really a proxy for income and socio-economic status (they are all highly correlated). Vio and Albala (2004) claim that in Chile the progressive increase in overweight and obesity is more prevalent in low socio-economic groups. Chopra (2004) reports that in the Western Cape of South Africa, 70 percent of women are overweight, but only about 20 percent perceive themselves as such. Whereas overweight is seen as a sign of wealth and status, most of these women associate underweight with illness, notably HIV/AIDS. However, younger and better educated women are aware of and aspire to the benefits of a slim body. In Brazil, obesity is positively associated with income in the poorer northeast of the country, but negatively associated with it in the richer southeast (Sawaya, Martins and Martins, 2004). Thus, this limited within-country data appear to support the view that as people develop economically and culturally (educationally) beyond a certain point, those with higher socio-economic status, especially the young, aspire to lower body weight, know how to achieve this and are able to modify their diets and lifestyles accordingly.[2] This is also consistent with the findings of a recent cross-country analysis (Ezzati *et al.*, 2005), which suggest that country-wide average BMI peaks for females at about US$12 500 (purchasing power parity [PPP]) and for males at US$17 000 (PPP), in each case thereafter declining as national income rises.

Knowledge of the relationships among income, overweight and consumption of specific foods is important for policy purposes. Certain demographic groups are particularly at risk, and the country-specific nature of these at-risk groups suggests the importance of monitoring both anthropometric and food intake data by income and demographic group. For example, a great deal of attention is paid to the rural–urban divide and the impact of urbanization on overweight and obesity. But if urbanization and income are highly correlated (and they are) studying single-variable relationships between overweight or food consumption in rural and urban areas may fail to uncover the main causes of malnutrition or to identify correctly the at-risk groups in the population. If the data allow, more sophisticated multivariate analysis should include other demographic variables such as

---

[2] It is not inconsistent to observe that overall levels of childhood and adult obesity are increasing in the developed world, over time, but remain at lower levels in higher socio-economic status groups at a particular point in time.

education and age. Such detailed analysis of existing data would enlighten the policy process.

Overweight and the food supply chain

Extending slightly the theoretical model of the last section, it is recognized that people also derive pleasure from their leisure-time activities, and while occasional cooking might be a pleasure, for many people everyday cooking is similar to work and not a chosen leisure-time activity. Recent research in the United States (e.g., Philipson and Posner, 1999; Lakdawalla and Philipson, 2002; Cutler, Glaeser and Shapiro, 2003) suggests that technological change that makes available a huge supply of prepared foods (at affordable prices), which reduce enormously the time cost of food preparation, is a major contributor to obesity. In jointly optimizing their use of money and time, households consume more of these prepared foods at the expense of traditional time-intensive products. As both the time and money costs of food fall, people also consume more in total. Cutler, Glaeser and Shapiro (2003) give the potato chip (French fry) as an example. Previously these were laborious to prepare, requiring the peeling, cutting and deep-frying of potatoes, now they are available ready-prepared and frozen for easy final cooking in the oven or microwave (or fast food restaurant). Consumption has increased dramatically in the United States. While not all examples of technological change in manufacturing produce unhealthy foods (e.g., modified atmosphere-packed vegetables), in general prepared foods are more energy-dense and higher in saturated and trans fats, salt and sugar.

Cutler, Glaeser and Shapiro (2003) go on to show that in the United States declining exercise has had a relatively small impact on increasing overweight since the 1980s, mainly because structural adjustments in the United States economy had largely taken place by then; employment in agriculture or industry that requires physical labour was already at a low level and the move to the cities had largely taken place. Based on a detailed analysis of the United States Department of Agriculture's (USDA) *Continuing surveys of food intake by individuals,* the authors' explanation for the observed weight gain was a (small) increase in average calorie intake. Of particular interest, this increase in intake was not associated with larger portion sizes (which would have resulted in increased intake at lunches and dinners), more frequent eating out or female labour force participation, but with more frequent eating – i.e., snacking between meals. Preparing tasty snacks would traditionally have been highly labour-intensive, now it merely requires opening the cupboard or fridge. Thus, the simple availability of such products (at affordable prices) itself drives consumption.

Developing countries are still in transition from rural agriculture- and heavy industry-based economies towards urban, light industry- and service sector-based ones, so continued reductions in average energy use will occur and contribute to increasing problems associated with overweight. Nevertheless, the increasing availability of low-cost processed foods (including fast foods and soft drinks), which are generally more energy-dense and higher in salt, sugar and saturated and trans-fats than unprocessed alternatives, means that consumers will be likely to add such foods to their shopping baskets.

There is not a great deal of empirical evidence from developing countries, but the tendency towards consumption of snack foods is reported for urban India (Vepa, 2004), where there have also been rapid increases in consumption of biscuits, salted refreshments and prepared sweets (between 1987/1988 and 1999/2000 intakes of these products rose from close to zero to 68, 45 and 13 g per capita per day, respectively). Vepa suggests that processed foods, mainly driven by such snack products, may represent as much as

1 000 kcal in the daily diet of high-income consumers.[3] Vepa's data suggest an expenditure elasticity for processed foods in India of about 1.1, meaning that a 1 percent increase in income leads to a 1.1 percent increase in expenditure on processed food – this is high compared with most foods.[4] A similar exercise for Lima, Peru, using data from a 2000 household survey as presented in Senauer and Goetz (2003), gives the following expenditure elasticities: food and drink away from home 1.13; candy and chocolate 1.10; prepared food consumed at home 0.55; and alcoholic beverages 1.09. As to be expected, given that Peru's PPP income per head is more than US$5 000, which is almost twice India's $2 670, the elasticity for prepared food is somewhat lower. Of interest with respect to Peru are the elasticities greater than 1 for food outside the home, confectionery and alcohol, all of which are calorie-dense.

As well as making available foods that consumers would not otherwise be able to obtain, supermarkets might also make a substantial impact on diets through their effect on relative food prices. The evidence suggests that supermarkets (and convenience stores) have reduced the prices of packaged foods but not fresh produce. Limited evidence from Brazil (quantitative) and elsewhere (anecdotal) suggests that supermarket prices for packaged foods are as much as 40 percent lower than prices in traditional outlets (Farina, 2002). By contrast, fresh fruit and vegetables are more expensive, and in general supermarkets offer less variety than traditional markets (thus fruit and vegetable's share of the market is generally only half that of grocery products) while convenience stores often do not carry fresh fruit and vegetables at all.

As well as their natural advantage over small shops in selling cheaply processed, packaged and bulk foods such as edible oil, grains, noodles and condiments (Hu *et al.,* 2004), supermarkets in China have moved very quickly in the past decade into processed semi-fresh foods such as tofu, dairy products and processed meats. Hu *et al.* (2004) argue that supermarkets have largely driven the rapid expansion in the milk products market.

In order to assess the dietary effects of changes in relative prices it would be necessary to obtain a complete matrix of own- and cross-price demand elasticities. In the absence of such a matrix, assume that packaged grocery prices fall by 20 percent owing to the existence of supermarkets, but other prices remain unchanged. If the price elasticity of demand for packaged groceries is -1 (a reasonable assumption for lower-income countries), consumption would rise by about 20 percent. It is harder to speculate on the quantitative impact on the consumption of other food products such as fresh fruit and vegetables, although the direction would unambiguously be down. Overall, the impact on diet quality is likely to be negative.

Changes in the food supply chain in developing countries

If supermarkets, food manufacturers and fast food outlets are to make cheap processed foods widely available to the public, they must have a substantial presence in a country.

The rapid expansion of supermarkets in developing countries has been most widely written about by Reardon and colleagues in a series of articles (e.g., Reardon and Berdegué, 2002; Reardon and Swinnen, 2004; Weatherspoon and Reardon, 2003; Reardon, Timmer and Berdegué, 2004). The line of argument is that supermarkets are no longer

---

[3] However, for the average consumer these products are not very significant in terms of expenditure. The National Sample Survey (2001) includes a category for "beverages, refreshments etc. (including processed food)", which includes all beverages (tea, coffee, cold drinks, commercially produced beverages), biscuits, confectionery, salted refreshments, sweets, pickles, sauces, jams and jellies and cooked meals obtained on payment. This group represents 7 percent of food expenditure in rural and 13.2 percent in urban India.

[4] Consumption (g/day) for urban India is reported for 12 expenditure classes. Elasticities were calculated simply as the coefficient of the regression of the ln of consumption from the second lowest to the second highest categories against the ln of total expenditure defined at the mid-points of those categories.

places where only rich people shop – over the past ten years or so, they have spread from the wealthy suburbs of major cities to poorer areas and smaller towns. This has happened in response to a number of forces, many of them interconnected: rising incomes (also associated with higher ownership of consumer durables such as refrigerators and cars, which facilitate supermarket shopping); urbanization; greater female participation in the labour force (increased opportunity cost of time); and the desire to emulate Western culture, spurred on by the globalization of media and advertising (linked in turn to the globalization of food manufacturers and the promotion of their products as well as of fast foods and soft drinks). There has also been a movement in most developing countries towards liberalization of trade and investment, which has brought the global supermarket chains on to the scene, along with economies of scale, buying power in purchasing and supply chain management skills.

The process of "supermarketization" began in Latin America in the early 1990s, and by 2000 supermarkets were delivering 50 to 60 percent of retail food sales in countries in the region (Reardon, Timmer and Berdegué, 2004). The take-off in Southeast Asia began between five and seven years later and is registering faster growth. A third wave has taken place in Eastern and Central Europe, while Africa is rapidly following, led by South Africa, which has seen a "spectacular" rise since 1994 (Reardon, Timmer and Berdegué 2004: 171). The process is also taking place in low-income Mediterranean countries such as Morocco and Tunisia (Codron *et al.,* 2004). The implication is that this is an ongoing, even accelerating, process that will soon see supermarkets as the dominant food suppliers around the world. Projections to 2015 (see Traill, 2006) only partially support this view and suggest that, while income growth and urbanization will be contributing factors in the ongoing spread of supermarkets, the continued liberalization of foreign direct investment, resulting as it does in competition with and/or entry of multinational retailers, is likely to be the main driving force for the future spread of supermarkets in developing countries. However, even an open economy will not quickly bring high levels of market share to the low-income and highly rural economies of Southern Asia, and even in countries such as China the supermarket share of total food sales is not projected to rise above 30 percent by 2015 (although this is a substantial increase from the 2002 level of about 11 percent).[5]

Nevertheless, it is clear that supermarkets are a fact of life, at least in urban areas, which implies that they will contribute to the nutrition transition by making available time-saving foods at lower prices, and these foods tend to be energy dense.

Globalization of food and soft drink manufacturing and fast foods, and their impacts on consumption

The spread of multinational food and soft drink manufacturers and fast food franchises has been well charted (see e.g., Bruinsma, 2003), but their impacts on food consumption have not been analysed. Conceptually, to the extent that they also increase availability and lower prices, they would also be expected to increase consumption. Wilkinson (2004) claims that United States investments in Mexico have concentrated on convenience and highly processed foods, especially snacks, beverages, instant coffee, mayonnaise and breakfast cereals. While it does not automatically follow that consumption of these products is higher than it would have been in the absence of multinational enterprises (MNEs), the controversy that reaches back at least as far as the debate about the ethics of Nestlé's selling of powdered infant formula milk in developing countries from the 1960s is set to continue rumbling. Some figures in Annex 2 suggest that there

---

[5] For the other case study countries projections are as follows: Mexico 61 percent (from 45 percent); South Africa 80 percent (from 55 percent); India 9 percent (from 2 percent); Egypt 13 percent (from 10 percent). Data not available for the Philippines.

has certainly been a very sharp increase in imports (and therefore, presumably, availability) of processed food products in the case study countries.

Fast food chains such as McDonald's and Domino's and soft drink companies (Pepsi, Coke) have also been blamed for unhealthy eating in developing countries (and also of course in developed countries, e.g., the film *Super-Size Me*). Pingali (2004) charts the growth of McDonald's from 951 stores in Asia and the Pacific in 1987 to 7 135 in 2002, and in Latin America from 99 to 887 over the same period. Hawkes (2002) has undertaken an extensive review of the marketing activities of leading soft drink and fast food companies in developing countries, concluding that their numerous techniques to target children and adolescents indicate their intention of changing soft drink and fast food consumption trends over the long term. However, of potentially far greater importance for diets are the domestic companies that have sprung up to imitate global brands at much lower prices, which therefore have much higher sales (Vepa, 2004). There is no quantitative information on the impact of these changes on nutrient intakes.

Gehlhar and Regmi (2005) obtained data from Euromonitor that show how soft drink sales are growing particularly rapidly in Southeast Asian countries such as the Philippines (12 percent per annum) and Indonesia (22 percent). The data they present give Mexico a per capita annual soft drink consumption of 342 litres, higher than the United States (313 litres), the United Kingdom (170 litres), South Africa and the Philippines (about 65 litres), China (17 litres) and India (3 litres). That looks like a lot of sugar in Mexico!

Overall, it is virtually impossible to gather evidence to prove, one way or another, the impact that various changes in food supply chains are having on diets. The industry would certainly argue that it is simply satisfying latent demand – which is doubtless true to a point – but logic and circumstantial evidence suggest that this is contributing to trends in overweight. In any case, the supply chain changes are inevitably associated with economic development, and the solution must be to develop policies that counter any negative side-effects rather than to hold back development more generally.

Conclusions on the transition

This has not been intended as a comprehensive review of how diets have changed as countries have become richer – Schmidhuber and Shetty (2006), for example, have already done this thoroughly with respect to total energy, saturated fats and fruit and vegetables. The attempt here has been to focus on two causal issues of importance with respect to overweight: incomes and changes in the supply chain.

Of the many conclusions that might be taken from this review, one is that although growing quantities of data exist from household surveys, these have not been collected or analysed in a way that informs knowledge of what foods people actually eat and how this varies by population sub-group. For example, although it is informative to know whether people eat more or less dairy products or fruit in urban and rural environments, it would also be useful in the context of the obesity debate to know what types of processed foods they are eating, particularly snack foods. Greater knowledge about specific sub-groups of the population, for example the extent to which urban and rural consumption patterns can be explained by income and demographic differences between urban and rural populations, would allow a better assessment of the importance of any residual "urbanization effect" and of whether this is narrowing over time. In this way a country-specific evidence base for informed policy-making can be developed.

POLICY ALTERNATIVES: LESSONS FROM DEVELOPED COUNTRIES?

Overweight and obesity result from an imbalance between energy input and output, and in principle can be regulated by reducing input or increasing output. A public health policy must inevitably tackle both sides of this equation, but the following sections focus only on the input side, restricting discussion to interventions in food markets.

Virtually all of the literature and evidence on policy measures cited in this section relate to developed countries. It is assumed that the issues emerging in the middle-income and developing countries will mirror the developed countries, although it is recognized that the priorities for policy action will be different and the institutions for some policy interventions and enforcement may be absent in many less developed countries.

Economic justification for government intervention

A usual justification for governments to intervene in markets is the existence of some form of market failure; in the absence of market failure, it is argued, liberal democracies should allow their citizens to make their own choices about how best to lead their lives, even if the choices they make are risky ones such as mountaineering, riding a bicycle through city traffic or eating too much. Another common reason for intervention is the reduction of health inequalities among social groups.

In relation to overweight, three types of market failure have been discussed in the economic literature: the social costs of overweight may exceed the private costs; there may be uncertainty and/or asymmetry in the available information; and some individuals may not act rationally because they lack self-control.

In middle- and high-income countries, society has already decided that there should be some form of safety net so that individuals who become unwell do not have to pay the full cost of medical treatment – i.e., there is a national health service or State-paid compulsory health insurance for the poor. Similarly, days missed from work because of ill health are communally paid for (through social service systems or requirements on employers to comply with labour laws). Thus, when people take risks such as overeating, others in society bear at least some of the costs (social costs therefore exceed private costs), and society may feel that government, on its behalf, should take action to limit these costs. In circumstances similar to these, many countries have already acted with respect to smoking in public places[6] and wearing seat belts and crash helmets – actions that were controversial when introduced because they were seen as intrusions on liberty, but over time have come to be widely accepted.

Uncertainty exists if a consumer is unable to make informed dietary choices, which may be because of inadequate nutritional knowledge or because too little information is provided on the nutritional content of food. The former may suggest a lack of nutritional education, but could also reflect the complexity and speed of change of nutritional knowledge. In the absence of information, even educated consumers are unable to make fully informed choices. The nutritional value of processed food in particular cannot be known accurately by the vast majority of consumers, who therefore find it difficult to regulate their intake from energy-dense foods of fats, sugar and salt. This is important when, for example, 75 percent of salt intake in the United Kingdom is from processed foods (Wanless, 2004).

Asymmetric information is a similar problem, occurring when one party in the market – almost invariably the seller – is better informed than the other, who is unable to judge quality by appearance. In the absence of regulation, the better informed partner therefore has an incentive to pass off low-quality (unsafe or unhealthy) produce to the more poorly informed.

Lack of self-control has a specific and technical definition within the economics profession, but essentially it means that with respect to certain decisions (such as whether to have another drink or piece of chocolate), some people discount the future to such an

---

[6] Although the extra justification of the dangers of passive smoking do not exist with respect to food.

extent that they make choices that are inconsistent with their true time preferences; doing so reduces their overall welfare (O'Donohue and Rabin, 1999). It would be contentious to argue that governments should intervene because individuals lack self-control, but the principle is widely accepted that intervention is justified when someone could be made better-off without anyone else being made worse-off, which in theory is the case here.

Children

Children are often seen as a special case when the right of an individual to choose an unhealthy lifestyle is questioned. Children are deemed unready to make a whole range of personal choices, from marriage, to voting, to education, so it is not surprising that governments feel justified in acting to influence children's diets, even if interventions have so far been very limited. Apart from questioning whether children should be permitted to make unhealthy choices even if they are informed, children generally have less knowledge and self-control than adults, and those who influence their behaviour (in determining their social norms) may not always be considered ideal role models (by adults).

Intervention may be justified both as a means of reducing the incidence of childhood overweight and obesity itself, and also by the theory that habits developed in childhood are carried forward into adulthood – overweight children usually become overweight adults.

Types of policy intervention

If the sole purpose of policy intervention is to make those who impose costs on society pay for them ("internalize the externality" as economists would put it), the best policy option is theoretically straightforward – a tax should be imposed on overweight people, in proportion to their degree of overweight and their consequent likelihood of imposing medical and other costs on society (this is the equivalent of the "polluter pays" principle). Of course this is impractical and ethically unacceptable given that it would imply taxing people with a genetic disposition to obesity. The tax would also be regressive, both because it would represent a higher share of the incomes of poorer people and because a larger proportion of poor than rich people are overweight, at least in developed and middle-income countries. In addition, in rich countries and among wealthier groups in poorer countries, where food is a small proportion of total expenditure and consumption is fairly unresponsive to price, it is unlikely that the tax would have much impact on obesity.

If the policy objective is to reduce overweight and obesity for reasons other than social cost, there are many practical opportunities to influence what people eat. In Table 1 these have been grouped according to the main objective of the intervention.

TABLE 1
Nutrition policy instruments classified by type of intervention

Policy instrument	Objective
Measures to change consumer preferences	
Information campaigns	Increase consumer awareness
Advertising regulations	Limit/ban advertising of unhealthy foods (especially when directed to children)
Nutrition education programmes in schools	Increase awareness and knowledge of nutritional requirements and health consequences
Measures to allow better-informed choice	
Labelling rules	Promote informed choice by signposting healthy and unhealthy nutrient levels in foods
Nutrition information on menus	Promote informed choice in eating-out situations
Regulating health claims	Define rules and monitor the use of nutrition and health claims in the promotion and labelling of food products
Funding epidemiological, behavioural and clinical research	Improve knowledge, evaluate policy options
Market measures to change actual choices without changing preferences	
Taxes on foods high in fats, salt, sugar etc. (e.g., salted snacks)	Reduce consumption of unhealthy foods
Price subsidies for healthy foods (e.g., fruit and vegetables)	Increase consumption of healthy foods
Measures to affect availability	
Regulate liability of food companies	Monetize negative externalities of production/sale of unhealthy foods
Food standards	Set nutritional standards for processed products in order to limit access to unhealthy nutrients
Facilitate access to shopping areas for disadvantaged categories	Address the issue of store dispersion in low-income areas by facilitating access to supermarkets for disadvantaged categories
Regulate catering in schools, hospitals, etc.	Counter the tendency of allowing snack vending machines or fast foods in public places in exchange for private funding of activities

Source: Adapted from Mazzocchi and Traill, 2006.

Non-market interventions

Ideally people would choose to consume a healthy diet, and the first two and last sets of policy instruments in Table 1 have this goal in mind – make sure that foods are available that enable a healthy diet to be chosen, educate and inform people about what a healthy diet entails (at the same time countering unhealthy messages and claims from industrial advertisers), and provide sufficient information so that healthy options can be selected. When successful, these policies contribute to reducing the social costs of overweight and obesity, and when directed to disadvantaged groups they can reduce health inequalities and influence social norms in such a way as to make healthy eating accepted behaviour.

Informing consumers of the nutritional content of food (nutritional labelling) has been the least controversial policy measure in developed countries, although even this has not been easy to implement. In most countries, nutritional labelling of processed food is voluntary (the United States is an exception, and the European Union [EU] is planning to make nutritional labelling compulsory); where labelling is voluntary, regulation often specifies the form it should take when used. Unsurprisingly, this has resulted in multiple formats internationally, despite the best efforts of Codex (which has established guidelines). Nutritional labelling of processed foods imposes costs on businesses (administration, testing, design and print of labels), especially when exporting to a range of countries with different requirements, but Golan, Kuchler and Mitchell (2000) estimate that the social benefits outweigh the costs in the United States; their research concludes that consumers read labels and alter their purchase decisions. Producers also respond by introducing new healthier formulations such as low-fat foods. On the negative side, these authors calculate that nutritional labelling has had a minimal impact on obesity in the years since it was introduced (1991). Labelling of unprocessed foods and meals taken outside the home (including takeaways) has proved much more difficult, and it appears that no country has yet introduced such requirements. It is unlikely that such labelling would pass a cost–benefit test.

The other pillar supporting the informed choice edifice is nutritional knowledge. Nutritional education has re-emerged as a necessary part of the school curriculum, and information campaigns promoting a healthy eating message have been publicly funded in many countries, particularly those promoting fruit and vegetable consumption. Observers have noted that commercial advertising expenditure is concentrated on the "big five" of pre-sugared breakfast cereals, soft drinks, confectionery, savoury snacks and fast food (e.g., Miller, Skinner and Bryant, 2006), none of which would feature strongly in many healthy eating campaigns. Some have deduced that governments need to counter this flood of "harmful" information with more "good" information, but it does not necessarily follow that people's choices among food groups would be affected by more balanced information. As Kuchler *et al.* (2005) state, again in an American context, "the sheer volume of media coverage devoted to diet and weight makes it difficult to believe that Americans are unaware of the relationship between a healthful diet and obesity". They quote surveys that show most American consumers to be aware of health problems associated with certain nutrients and able to discriminate among foods on the basis of fat, fibre and cholesterol. Adults in most middle- and high-income countries are all likely to have the same knowledge, although a case could be made for public service broadcasting to promote new knowledge as it emerges. The case of children however is the one that concerns most professionals. A major systematic review undertaken for the United Kingdom Food Standards Agency (Hastings *et al.,* 2003) concludes that advertising to children affects the categories of food eaten as well as brand choice.[7] Some countries, such as Sweden, Denmark and Finland, have introduced controls on advertising to children, others are looking to manufacturers to introduce a voluntary code, and this seems to be an area where there is widespread agreement that some action is desirable.

There is also a potential role for government policy in taking measures that affect what food is available to consumers. This is accepted with respect to some forms of food fortification, as well as the establishment of food safety and quality regulations to ensure minimum standards for food consumed. So far, however, standards have not been used to control the macronutrient content of foods offered for sale to the general public. However, governments have intervened to affect food availability in other ways, such as offering milk and fruit to schoolchildren and, in some American states (e.g., Texas), controlling the sale of soft drinks to children through vending machines. Collins and McCarthy (2006) show that the ease with which schoolchildren can obtain soft drinks, confectionery and salted snacks in schools is a major factor determining their overall consumption levels. This is consistent with the analysis of Cutler, Glaeser and Shapiro (2003), which emphasizes ease of access (time saving) as a determinant in the increased consumption of snack foods.

Governments are also beginning to take seriously their ability to influence diets through controlling the composition of meals in schools and other government institutions such as hospitals, prisons and public sector cafeterias. They may also act to regulate the salt, sugar, saturated and trans fatty acid contents of processed food that consumers cannot tell from the food's appearance or taste – many consumers may be unprepared to read or unable to interpret labels. Rather that compulsory regulation, policy-makers in some countries such

---

[7] Watching television is not thought to consume many calories either.

as Finland have entered into dialogue with industry, which has voluntarily reduced the levels of "harmful" nutrients.

On the supply side there have also been calls in some quarters for more attention to be paid to access to healthy food (mainly fruit and vegetables) by disadvantaged groups who live in "food deserts" devoid of traditional local shops and who are unable to reach out-of-town supermarkets unless they own cars. The evidence that this is the case is far from compelling (White *et al.*, 2004). Concern is also often expressed that healthy food is too expensive for the poor and that fats and sugars are the cheapest source of calories, so poor people consume a lot of them (e.g., Kennedy, 2005). This is sometimes presented as an industry conspiracy, calling for government control. The notion that healthy food costs more is usually based on a direct comparison between the prices of a regular product (e.g., mayonnaise) and its healthier derivative (low-fat mayonnaise), or between the prices per calorie of, say, asparagus and butter. In fact, it is quite possible to eat a diet that meets all health recommendations at very low cost (Henson, 1991), but doing so is time-consuming as it requires preparation from raw ingredients rather than buying time-saving prepared food.

Market measures

There has been increasing discussion in developed countries about the desirability of taxing unhealthy foods and/or nutrients – often referred to as "fat taxes". The issues are similar for middle-income countries. The idea is to increase the price of unhealthy foods relative to healthy foods or ingredients, thereby encouraging consumers to switch to healthy alternatives. However the pitfalls are also well known: the tax would be ineffective because the demand for foods is price-inelastic – there would be limited response to anything other than a very high level of tax; it would be regressive, hitting the poorest consumers hardest; and it would be unfair because slim people would also have to pay it (see e.g., Schmidhuber, 2004, Kuchler, Tegene and Harris, 2004). The tax might be more effective in developing countries, where consumers are more responsive to price, but it would ethically be very difficult to recommend a policy that taxed the poor and undernourished at the same rate as it taxed the rich and overnourished. The obverse of a fat tax has been called a "thin subsidy" (e.g., Cash, Sunding and Zilberman, 2006), which is a subsidy to encourage the consumption of fruit and vegetables. The authors find that demand for fruit and vegetables in the United States is quite responsive to price and that the cost of a statistical life saved by such a subsidy would be in the order of US$1.3 million, well below the typical benchmark figure used in United States government programmes of about $10 million. Nevertheless, for a cash-strapped government the total cost would still be substantial and would be subject to the charge that wealthy consumers also were having their food subsidized. Although this is true, it is also the case that poorer consumers would be the major health beneficiaries because their consumption is more responsive to price and they have lower fruit and vegetable consumption to start with, at least in urban areas. It is not unreasonable to contemplate a package whereby the money raised by a fat tax (e.g., on salty snacks, soft drinks and confectionery) was used to finance a thin subsidy.

The middle-income and developing country context

As already indicated, this review of nutrition policies and assessment of their effectiveness has been based almost entirely on developed countries. To what extent is it relevant to developing or middle-income countries, and how high a priority should anti-obesity policies be? Obesity has already become a problem in many developing countries and is set to become a much larger problem (Schmidhuber and Shetty, 2006). The social–private cost divergence may be less of a justification for action because few developing countries operate a health care system based on free access, nor do they have employment law that protects employees who are absent because of ill health. This means that the costs of obesity are largely borne by the individuals concerned and their families. Imperfect and asymmetric information, lack of self-control, changing social norms and reducing health inequalities remain reasons for policy action, and in this context it can be argued that policy should be a priority long before a problem arises; for example, it would be much better to influence social norms so that being overweight was never viewed as something to aspire to, rather than waiting until it becomes a health problem – although in many cases this has already happened, particularly where AIDS is prominent.

Concerning specific policies, it is probable that levels of nutrition education are lower in developing countries and it would be relatively cheap to introduce nutrition education into school curricula, at least in middle-income countries.[8] The Republic of Korea and Malaysia have done this. Public information campaigns should be feasible, although they may not be seen as a first priority for the use of scarce public finances. Control of advertising to children would however be cheap and likely effective. Nutritional labelling is highly desirable in principle, but given that proportionately far fewer packaged groceries are sold in developing than in developed countries and that the enforcement of existing labelling legislation is often patchy, this may not be a priority. Measures to control the availability of snack foods and soft drinks for children in schools would be feasible and cheap, although some schools may be tempted to use vending machines as money raisers. Taxes and subsidies would be feasible in principle, but in practice are likely to be expensive to operate.

A package of measures

It is currently fashionable to state that policy-making should be "evidence-based", but with respect to diet and obesity, as indeed with respect to much policy-making in the area of public health, evidence is sadly lacking, even in the developed world. One reason for the difficulty in obtaining evidence is that changing diets is only one aspect of public health policy to reduce the incidence of non-communicable diseases (NCDs), alongside the promotion of exercise and reducing smoking and drinking. Advances in medicine may sometimes provide a substitute for dietary change (e.g., control of hypertension). A comprehensive, integrated and long-term package of policy measures may also work in synergy to provide benefits that cannot be identified with respect to individual policies in the short term. The famous Finnish North Karelia project adopted such an approach, and its achievements in terms of reduced coronary heart disease (CHD) deaths have been widely acclaimed. However, since the project was introduced and later extended countrywide, the incidence of overweight in Finland has steadily increased (Puska, 2002).

A report on encouraging behavioural change for sustainable development (United Kingdom Department of the Environment, Food and Rural Affairs, 2004) develops the "four Es of a new approach". Measures relating to *enabling change* include many of the educational and availability policies mentioned in Table 1. The object is to make it easy for people to change their behaviour, if they want to, by making sure that healthy foods are available and that people know what comprises a healthy diet. *Engagement* is about involving people in a policy so that they feel they own it and believe in its objectives; it is much more than telling people what they should do and needs to be long-term and consultative and to involve key nodes in social communication networks. *Encouragement* involves giving the right signals, which may include a combination of taxes and subsidies, as discussed earlier. *Exemplifying* means government leading by example, which may involve ensuring that its own mass catering provides healthy foods (and facilities for exercise), as well as taking care that its policies are consistent across the multitude of

---

[8] Capacity building may be required to train the trainers.

departments whose work impinges on obesity, as is increasingly recognized, for example by the World Health Programme (WHO) in its global strategy (WHO, 2004).

Conclusions on policy measures

Even for developed countries, there is an absence of strong evidence for what works and what does not at the individual policy instrument level, let alone for the effectiveness of a package of measures. For developing countries with limited resources for public health, it is especially important that: 1) interventions are directed to serious problems, which requires good data and proper analysis to assess where the problems lie; and 2) the effectiveness of any policy intervention is carefully monitored, ideally against realistic targets. Although there are lessons to be learned from experiences in other countries, many problems are country-specific and the way people react to policy measures is culture-specific. Once again this puts great emphasis on the collection of good data, and their careful analysis.

OVERALL SUMMARY AND CONCLUSIONS

Overweight and obesity are already common in middle-income countries and are becoming prevalent among some groups in less developed countries. Over the medium to long time horizon, the problems associated with overweight and obesity will become serious public health issues, and actions to tackle them should be taken sooner rather than later.

The reasons for overweight are many, not least economic development and the increasing availability of low-cost, time-saving alternatives to home food preparation. Although household surveys routinely collect information on the foods that people actually consume, these tend to be converted back into raw-product equivalents before analysis – dairy products, meat, cereals, etc., rather than cornflakes, carbonated soft drinks and potato chips. However, if these and other calorie-dense prepared foods are what people are increasingly eating and getting fat on, the existing data need to be analysed and new data collected with this in mind.

There are many possible policy interventions that might bring about dietary change, and a package of measures as part of an overall public health policy is most likely to be effective, especially when it comes to long-term change in social norms. Of course, policy-making should be evidence-based, but there is very little hard evidence on policy effectiveness, even in developed countries. At a minimum, well-targeted policy interventions require knowledge of which groups are most at risk. Children are one such group in all countries, but in many other respects problems are likely to depend on the stage of economic development and to be culture-specific. Identifying at-risk groups and their characteristics is another important task for data analysts. Which socio-economic groups are overweight? what are they eating? and how is this changing over time? are fundamental questions.

REFERENCES

Bruinsma, J., ed. 2003. *World agriculture: Towards 2015/30, an FAO perspective.* London, Earthscan and Rome, FAO.

Cash, S.B., Sunding, D.L. & Zilberman, D. 2006. Fat taxes and thin subsidies: prices, diet and health outcomes. *Food Economics,* (forthcoming).

Chopra, M. 2004. Globalization, urbanization and nutritional changes in South Africa. *In* FAO. *Globalization of food systems in developing countries: impact on food security and nutrition,* pp. 5–80 and 119–133. FAO Food and Nutrition Paper No. 83. Rome, FAO.

Codron, J.-M., Bouhsina, Z., Fort, F., Coudel, E. & Pueh, A. 2004. Supermarkets in low-income Mediterranean countries: impacts on horticultural systems. *Development Policy Review,* 22(5): 587–602.

Collins, A. & McCarthy, M. 2006. Adolescents' eating motives, constraints and behaviours during the school day. *Food Economics,* (forthcoming).

Cutler, D.M., Glaeser, E.L. & Shapiro, J.M. 2003. Why have Americans become more obese? *Journal of Economic Perspectives,* 17: 93–118.

Ezzati, M., Vander Hoorn, S., Lawes, C.M.M., Leach, R., James, W.P.T., Lopez, A.D., Rodgers, A. & Murray, C.J.L. 2005. Rethinking the diseases of affluence paradigm: global patterns of nutrition risks in relation to economic development. *PLoS Medicine,* 2(5).

Farina, E.M.M.Q. 2002. Consolidation, multinationalisation, and competition in Brazil: Impacts on horticulture and dairy products systems. *Development Policy Review,* 20(4): 441–457.

Gehlar, M. & Regmi, A. 2005. Factors shaping global food markets. *In New directions in global food markets.* AIB-794, 5-17. Washington, DC, USDA Economic Research Service.

Golan, E., Kuchler, F. & Mitchell, L. 2000. *Economics of food labeling.* Agricultural Economic Report No. 793. USDA Economic Research Service. 41 pp.

Hastings, G., Stead, M., McDermott, L., Forsyth, A., MacKintosh, A.M., Rayner, M., Godfrey, C., Caraher, M. & Angus, K. 2003. *Review of research on the effects of food promotion to children.* Report for the Food Standards Agency. London. 218 pp.

Hawkes, C. 2002. Marketing activities of global soft drink and fast food companies in emerging markets: a review. *In* WHO. *Globalization, diets and non-communicable diseases.* Geneva, WHO. 78 pp.

Henson, S. 1991. Linear programming analysis of constraints upon human diets. *Journal of Agricultural Economics,* 42(3): 380–393.

Hu, D., Reardon, T., Rozelle, S., Timmer, P. & Wong, H. 2004. The emergence of supermarkets with Chinese characteristics: challenges and opportunities for China's agricultural development. *Development Policy Review,* 22(5): 557–586.

Kennedy, E.T. 2005. The global face of nutrition: what can governments and industry do? *Journal of Nutrition,* 4: 913–915.

Kuchler, F., Tegene, A. & Harris, M. 2004. *Taxing snack foods: what to expect for diet and tax revenues.* AIB-747-08. Washington DC, USDA, Economic Research Service.

Kuchler, F., Golan, E., Variyam, J.N. & Crutchfield, S.R. 2005. Obesity policy and the law of unintended consequences. *Amber Waves (June).* Washington DC, USDA, Economic Research Service. 8 pp.

Lackdawalla, D. & Philipson, T. 2002. *The growth of obesity and technological change: a theoretical and empirical examination.* Working Paper No. 8946. Cambridge, Massachusetts, USA, National Bureau of Economic Research. 41 pp.

Mazzocchi, M., Lobb, A.E. & Traill, W.B. 2005. The Sparta model: an econometric analysis of consumer behaviour under risk. Paper presented at the European Association of Agricultural Economists Conference, 23 to 27 August, Copenhagen.

Mazzocchi, M. & Traill, W.B. 2006. Nutrition, health and economic policies in Europe. *Food Economics,* (forthcoming).

Mendez, M.A. & Popkin, B.M. 2004. Globalization, urbanization and nutritional change in the developing world. *In* FAO. *Globalization of food systems in developing countries: impact on food security and nutrition,* pp. 55–80. FAO Food and Nutrition Paper No. 83. Rome, FAO.

Miller, H., Skinner, T. & Bryant, C. 2006. The economics of obesity. *Food Economics,* (forthcoming).

O'Donoghue, T.O. & Rabin, M. 1999. Doing it now or later. *American Economic Review,* 89: 103–124.

Philipson, T.J. & Posner, R.A. 1999. *The long-run growth in obesity as a function of technological change.* Working Paper No. 7423. Cambridge, Massachusetts, USA, National Bureau of Economic Research. 35 pp.

Pingali, P. 2004. Westernization of Asian diets and the transformation of food systems: implications for research and policy. *ESA Working Paper 04-17.* Rome, FAO. 17 pp.

Puska, P. 2002. Successful prevention of non-communicable diseases: 25 year experiences with North Korelia Project in Finland. *Public Health Medicine,* 4(1): 5–7.

Reardon, T. & Berdegué, J.A. 2002. The rapid rise of supermarkets in Latin America: Challenges and opportunities for development. *Development Policy Review,* 20(4): 371–388.

Reardon, T. & Swinnen, J.F.M. 2004. Agrifood sector liberalisation and the rise of supermarkets in former state controlled economies: a competitive overview. *Development Policy Review,* 22(5): 515–523.

Reardon, T., Timmer, P. & Berdegue, J. 2004. The rapid rise in supermarkets in developing countries: induced organizational, institutional and technological change in agrifood systems. *Electronic Journal of Agricultural and Development Economics,* 1(2): 168–183.

Sawaya, A.L., Martins, P.A. & Martins, V.J.B. 2004. Impact of globalisation on food consumption, health and nutrition in urban areas: a case study of Brazil. *In* FAO. *Globalization of food systems in developing countries: impact on food security and nutrition,* pp. 253–274. FAO Food and Nutrition Paper No. 83. Rome, FAO.

Schmidhuber, J. 2004. The growing global obesity problem: some policy options to address it. *In* FAO. *Globalization of food systems in developing countries: impact on food security and nutrition,* pp. 81–99. FAO Food and Nutrition Paper No. 83. Rome, FAO.

Schmidhuber, J. & Shetty, P. 2006. The nutrition transition to 2030: why developing countries are likely to bear the major burden. *Food Economics,* (forthcoming).

Senauer, B. & Goetz, L. 2003. The growing middle class in developing countries and the market for high-value food products. Paper prepared for the Workshop on Global Markets for High-Valued Food, 14 February, Washington, DC, ERS, USDA.

Traill, W.B. 2006. The rapid rise of supermarkets? *Development Policy Review,* 24(2).

United Kingdom Department for the Environment, Food and Rural Affairs. 2004. *Changing behaviour through policy making.* London, Sustainable Development Unit. 5 pp.

Uustialo, U., Pietinen, P. & Puska, P. 2002. Dietary transition in developing countries: challenges for chronic disease prevention. *In* WHO. *Globalization, diets and non-communicable diseases.* Geneva, WHO. 25 pp.

Vepa, S.S. 2004. Impact of globalization on the food consumption of urban India. *In* FAO. *Globalization of food systems in developing countries: impact on food security and nutrition,* pp. 215–229. FAO Food and Nutrition Paper No. 83. Rome, FAO.

Vio, F. & Albala, C. 2004. Nutrition transition in Chile: a case study. *In* FAO. *Globalization of food systems in developing countries: impact on food security and nutrition,* pp. 275-284. FAO Food and Nutrition Paper No. 83. Rome, FAO.

Wanless, D. 2004. *Securing good health for the whole population.* Report to the Prime Minister, the Secretary of State for Health and the Chancellor of the Exchequer. London, HMSO. 204 pp.

Weatherspoon, D.D. & Reardon, T. 2003. The rise of supermarkets in Africa: implications for agrifood systems and the rural poor. *Development Policy Review,* 21(3): 333–355.

White, M., Bunting, J., Williams, E., Raybould, S., Adamson, A. & Mathers, J. 2004. *Do food deserts exist? A multi-level geographic analysis of the relationship between retail food access, socio-economic position and dietary intake.* London, Food Standards Agency. 261 pp.

Wilkinson, J. 2004. The food processing industry, globalization and developing countries. *eJADE,* 1(2): 184–201.

WHO. 2004. *Global strategy on diet, physical education and health.* WHA 57.17. Geneva 20 pp.

Zywicki, T.J., Holt, D. & Ohlhausen, M. 2004. Obesity and advertising policy. *George Mason Law & Economics Research Paper,* 04-45.

ANNEX 1: OVER- AND UNDERWEIGHT PROPORTIONS OF THE POPULATION BY COUNTRY

Country	Mendez and Popkin, 2004				IOTF		
	Overweight, women 20–49 years (%)		Underweight, women 20–49 years (%)		Category	Over-weight, men	Over-weight, women
	Urban	Rural	Urban	Rural	Age (years)		
Sub-Saharan Africa							
Benin (1996)	18.4	10.5	9.7	15.5	15–49 (2001)		16.0
Cameroon (1998)	36.7	19.5	5.2	5.9			
Kenya (1998)	27.9	15.3	7.0	12.1	15–49 (1998)		14.8
Madagascar (1997)	10.3	3.6	14.1	21.5	15–49 (1997)		3.7
Mali (1996)	21.6	6.1	13.5	14.6	15–49 (1996)		8.4
Niger (1998)	31.6	4.5	12.1	19.6	15–49 1998)		7.6
Nigeria (1999)	23.9	23.4	13.6	13.3			
South Africa (1998)	61.0	55.8	4.3	5.7	15+ (1998)	31.2	53.8
Tanzania, United Republic of (1996)	28.5	11.4	8.6	9.6			
Uganda (1995)	23.3	9.4	6.6	9.8	15–49 (2000/2001)		11.2
Zambia (1996)	25.9	11.5	5.9	9.9	15–49 (2001/2002)		10.3
Zimbabwe					15–49 (1999)		25.9
North Africa/West Asia/Europe							
Egypt (1995)	69.9	46.6	0.7	1.8	15–49 (2000)		71.2
Jordan (1997)	69.4	63.0	1.6	1.8			
Turkey (1998)	63.2	65.6	2.1	1.5	20+ urban (2001/2002)	63.0	58.0
South and Southeast Asia							
China (1997)	20.5	15.2	7.4	6.1	20–94 urban (1998–2000)	32.6	34.4
India (1999)	26.4	5.6	23.1	48.3	18+ (1998)	4.7	4.9
Korea, Republic of					15–79 (1998)	23.6	26.4
Philippines					20+ (1998)	17.0	23.3
Latin America and Caribbean							
Bolivia (1998)	57.9	47.1	7.4	6.1	15–49 (1998)		46.4
Brazil (1996)	42.8	33.0	5.2	9.3	20+ (1997)	37.9	39.0
Colombia (2000)	48.8	51.4	2.0	2.1	15–49 (2000)		40.8
Dominican Republic (1996)	50.2	40.2	4.5	6.2			
Guatemala (1998)	61.9	42.6	1.5	1.6	15–49 (1998/1999)		43.8
Mexico (1999)	65.4	58.6	1.5	2.2	20–69 (2000)	60.7	65.2
Peru (2000)	60.2	43.3	0.8	0.7	Adults (1996)	48.8	57.3
Transition economies							
Czech Republic					25+ (1997/1998)	73.2	57.6
Estonia					19–64 (1997)	41.9	29.9
Latvia					19–64 (1997)	50.5	40.4
Lithuania					19–64 (1997)	53.3	51.0
Kazakhstan (1999)	36.3	36.3	6.3	6.0			
Kyrgystan (1997)	34.7	34.5	4.9	4.4			
Developed countries							
Belgium					35–59 (1994–1997)	63	41
Finland					25–64 (1997)	67.8	52.4
Germany					25+ (2002)	75.4	58.9
Greece					19–64 (1994–1998)	78.6	76.7
Japan					20+ (2000)	26.8	20.7
Netherlands					20–59 (1998–2002)	53.9	38.6
United Kingdom					16+ (2003)	63.4	55.6

Overweight = BMI > 25
Underweight = BMI < 18.5.

ANNEX 2: PROCESSED FOOD IMPORTS: CASE STUDY COUNTRIES

The following figures support the view that dramatic increases have taken place in processed food imports in the case study countries; these changes will have led to large increases in availability. FAOSTAT trade data include a number of product categories that are candidates for having a high value-added content. The following products were selected from FAOSTAT as representing high added-value through further processing of agricultural raw material: pastry, breakfast cereals, beer, infant food, mixes and doughs, food preparations, flour and malt extract, frozen potatoes, sugar confectionery, olive oil, tomato juice (single strength), tomato paste, canned mushrooms, frozen vegetables, orange juice (single strength), wine, alcoholic distilled beverages, chocolate, fresh cream, butter, yoghurt, cheese, bacon, sausages, canned chicken, margarine, other prepared food. Although the presence of some items on this list may be disputed, it was applied uniformly across all countries. The figures show products that had the highest import levels *at the end* of the data period.

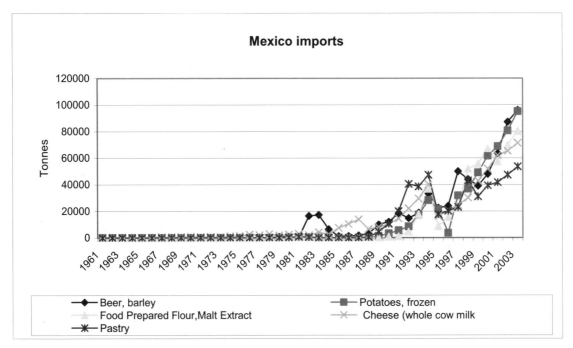

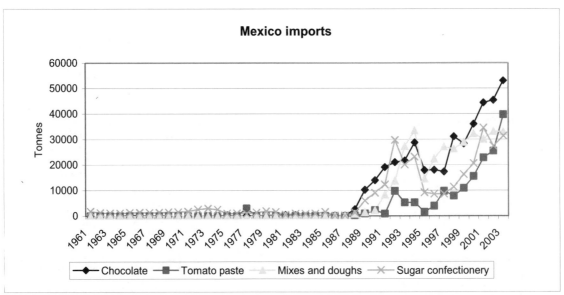

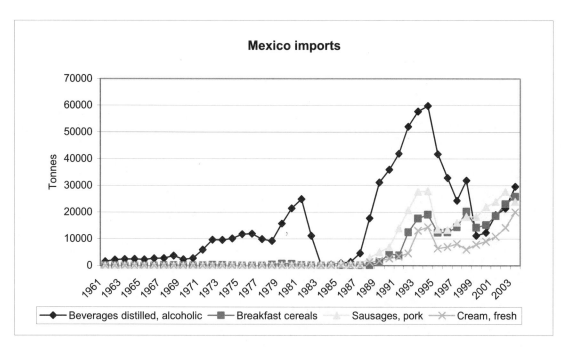

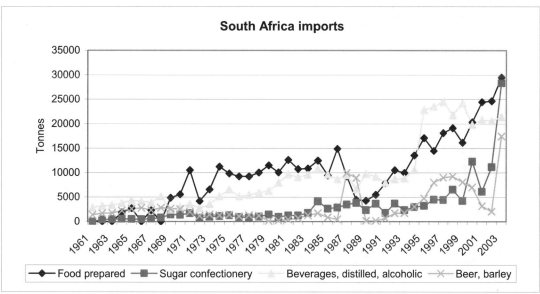

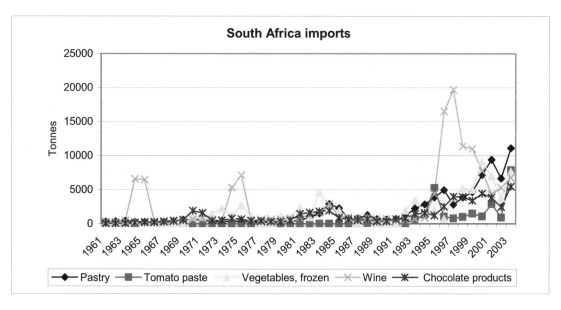

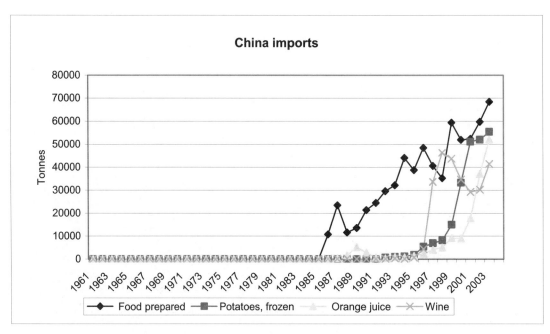

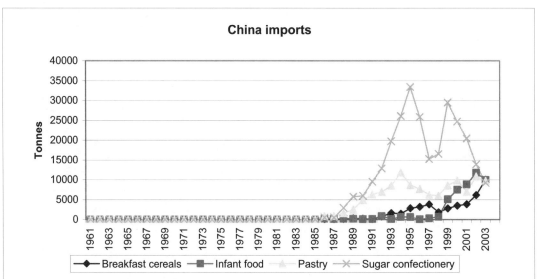

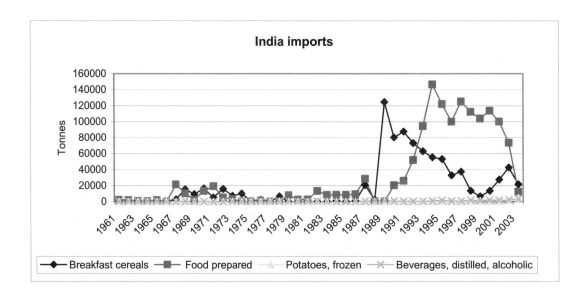

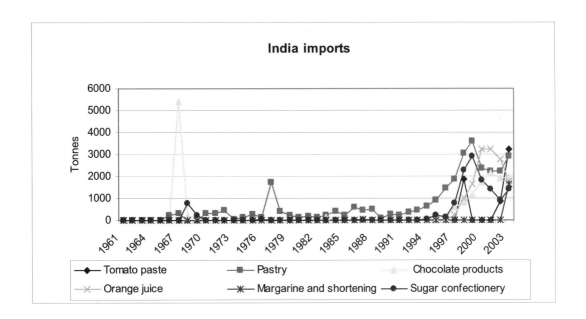

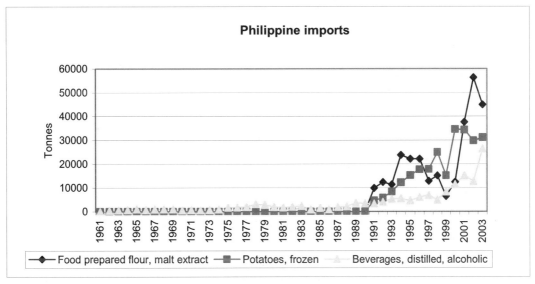

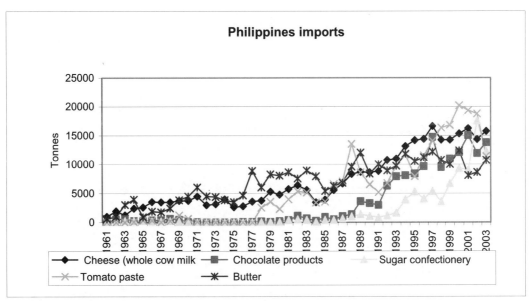

Workshop recommendations

A workshop including representatives from all of the case study countries was held in September 2005 to review the case study findings and draft a set of recommendations to address the double burden of malnutrition. The first set of recommendations relates to lessons learned during the process of compiling national-level time series data on the double burden of malnutrition. The second set of recommendations involves strategies at the individual and community levels to address the double burden. The third set of recommendations is aimed at identifying actions that can be taken at the national level. It is hoped that these recommendations will be useful for other countries interested in addressing the rising problem of the double burden of malnutrition.

LESSONS LEARNED AND CHALLENGES FACED DURING PRODUCTION OF THE COUNTRY REPORTS

The six case study countries faced certain common problems in the analysis of nationally representative time series data on the burden of malnutrition. A difficulty faced by many was the lack of systematically collected data on important dietary indicators, such as intakes of fruits and vegetables, saturated fats, processed food and food eaten outside the home. Only two countries (China and the Philippines) had nationally representative dietary intake data comparable over three or more time periods. Even in countries where repeated surveys had been conducted, there had often been an updating of methodology over time, for example updates to nutrient requirements or food composition tables, thus it was not always possible to compare directly older survey data with more recent data.

In terms of data on nutritional status and other risk factors for chronic disease, information on the spectrum of undernutrition was the most systematically and regularly collected. Time series data on other factors of interest, including physical activity, overnutrition in children and adults and risk factors for chronic diseases were lacking in most countries. In most countries, information on many risk factors of both under- and overnutrition was limited to data collected for specific small research projects. Typically these data were not nationally representative, and were collected for a very narrow research focus (e.g., vitamin A or iron deficiency). When another survey addressing the same or a similar nutritional problem was conducted, the data were often collected on different age or gender groups, thus restricting the potential to examine time series trends in indicators of nutritional status.

Another limitation noted was that of information management and related human resources. In some cases – particularly for older surveys – the raw data had been discarded and it was only possible to work with data from published reports. The presentation of data in published reports was not always compatible with more recent data structures; for example, changes were made to the ways in which foods were categorized. Computerized data storage systems in some countries did not exist or functioned poorly, and there was also a lack of trained personnel to help create appropriate data storage and management systems. Furthermore, some countries noted a lack of personnel skilled in higher-level data analysis.

RECOMMENDATIONS FOR ADDRESSING THE DOUBLE BURDEN OF MALNUTRITION AT THE INDIVIDUAL AND COMMUNITY LEVELS

Workshop participants listed underlying causes of the major malnutrition problems identified in the case study countries: overweight and obesity in adults, adolescents and children; undernutrition (stunting, wasting and underweight) in children; and micronutrient deficiencies, particularly iron but also other micronutrients, which are widespread in some countries. For each broad underlying cause, a matrix of determinants was elaborated and solutions were proposed. As part of this process, the solutions that were considered beneficial for reducing both under- and overnutrition were highlighted.

The following lists identify strategies that could be considered to address the spectrum of both under- and overnutrition. A more comprehensive list of the determinants and proposed strategies for each identified problem appears in Annex 1 at the end of this chapter.

Strategies to reduce the double burden of malnutrition in children

- Promote exclusive breastfeeding from birth to six months of age.
- Promote the introduction of complementary feeding at six months.
- Promote continued breastfeeding until two years of age or beyond.
- Promote age-appropriate complementary feeding.
- Promote eating a healthy breakfast at home.
- Promote the concept of bringing healthy meals and snacks prepared at home to school.
- Promote the consumption of home-prepared food at school.
- Make fruits and vegetables attractive and tasty.
- Promote the sale of healthy foods in the school environment (school shops, canteens and food vendors).
- Reduce children's exposure to the advertising and vending of unhealthy foods.
- Implement nutrition education for children, parents and child care givers using teacher–child–parent nutrition education.
- Promote community involvement in healthy eating at schools.
- Eliminate soda sales and marketing in school environments.
- Promote the consumption of dairy products (low-fat if appropriate).
- Promote eating of a variety of animal foods.
- Promote age-appropriate physical activity.

Strategies to reduce the double burden of malnutrition in adults

- Promote the concept of bringing healthy snacks and meals prepared at home to work.
- Implement nutrition education.
- Encourage decreased consumption of soda, and its substitution with water (encourage people to drink more water).
- Promote a diversity of animal source protein (for overweight the emphasis should be on reducing dependence on red meat only).
- Make fruits and vegetables available at the workplace.

Promoting awareness of the double burden of malnutrition

In addition, the working group recommended actions at the national level to promote greater awareness of the double burden of malnutrition.

The working group:

- recognizes that the double burden of malnutrition requires an intersectoral process for effective action;
- recommends the establishment of a permanent high-level intersectoral coordinating committee/council (ISCC) – which is independent of individual ministry authority and adequately resourced – to develop strategies and policy options that address the double burden of malnutrition;
- recommends that the ISCC includes representatives from all relevant stakeholders and sectors, coordinates the development and implementation of a plan of action, and coordinates the monitoring and reporting of progress;
- recommends that countries adopt nutrition goals specific to the analysis of their problems with the double burden of malnutrition and in keeping with Millennium Development Goals.

RECOMMENDATIONS TO IMPROVE NATIONAL DATA COLLECTION AND ANALYSIS OF THE DOUBLE BURDEN OF MALNUTRITION

The working group recognized that the following areas require improvement:

- Emphasize to the authorities the importance of collecting and making available nationally representative data from periodic surveys on nutritional status and physical activity in order to assess both under- and overnutrition.
- Coordinate and harmonize surveys to enable time series and trend analysis.
- Include variables that monitor both over- and undernutrition, and their health consequences.
- Establish a research agenda to be pursued nationally/internationally that deals with changes in cut-offs, interpretation and analysis of data; encourages presentation of data as frequency distributions; provides access to public sector data sources for analysis; and looks at regional and genetic/ethnic differences and the effect of infant undernutrition on adult disease (Barker hypothesis).
- Carry out capacity building in developing countries to collect, analyse and interpret data from relevant sectors.
- Highlight the importance of emerging overnutrition amid undernutrition, i.e., the rise of the double burden, and that the problem is not only one of affluence but also closely linked to poverty.

ANNEX 1: PROBLEM TREES ELABORATED DURING WORKING GROUP SESSIONS

The diagrams that follow represent the four main nutritional problems identified during working group sessions: overweight/obesity in children and adolescents; undernutrition in children and adolescents; overweight and obesity in adults; and iron-deficiency anaemia (IDA) and other micronutrient deficiencies in children, adolescents and adults. For each problem, a series of determinants were identified and a list of potential solutions suggested. Solutions that are shaded in grey were considered particularly appropriate for addressing problems of under- and overnutrition for the age group identified.

Problem tree for overweight/obesity in children and adolescents

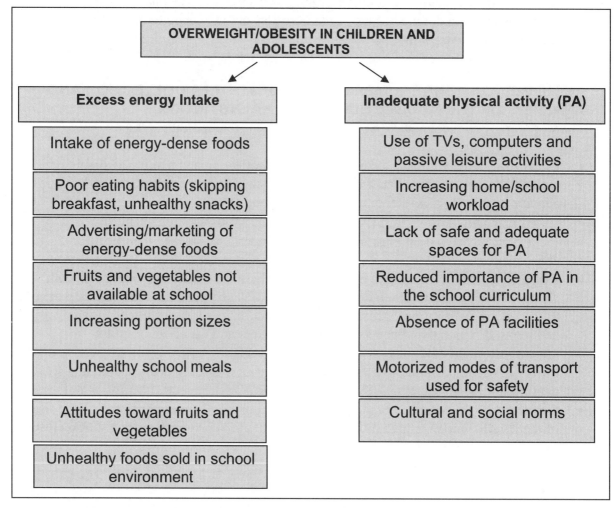

Strategies related to diet (high-energy density)

- Promote exclusive breastfeeding from birth to six months of age.
- Promote age-appropriate complementary feeding.
- Promote a diversity of animal source protein to reduce the dependence on red meat only.
- Make fruits and vegetables attractive and tasty.
- Promote the bringing to school of healthy meals and snacks prepared at home.
- Implement nutrition education for children, parents and child care givers.

- Promote healthy options in fast foods/encourage fast food outlets to reduce the energy density of their meals.
- Reduce (trans) fat in fast foods.
- Encourage consumption of water instead of soda and sugar-sweetened drinks.
- Promote low-fat dairy products.

Strategies related to diet (poor eating habits)

- Promote the eating of a healthy breakfast at home.
- Promote the sale of healthy foods in the school environment (school shops, canteens and food vendors).
- Reduce children's exposure to the advertising and vending of unhealthy foods.
- Implement nutrition education for children and their parents using teacher–child–parent nutrition education.
- Promote community involvement in healthy eating at schools.
- Eliminate the sale and marketing of soda in school environments.
- Promote dairy products.
- Promote the eating of a variety of animal foods.
- Make fruits and vegetables attractive and tasty.
- Reduce (trans) fat in fast foods.
- Encourage children to drink water.

Strategies related to physical activity

- Increase awareness of the importance of physical activity (PA) among teachers, parents and students.
- Increase time spent on PA in schools.
- Increase PA at home.
- At the local level, provide safe protected spaces for PA near the home.
- Promote sports days organized by schools/communities.
- Promote community exercise events.
- Increase awareness of the need for space for all children to do PA (young children, girls, etc.).
- Make PA an active part of school curricula (including homework).
- Provide incentives/awards for physical fitness in children.
- Increase awareness of the detrimental effects of TV viewing among teachers, parents and students.
- Encourage family exercise or participation in PA activities.

Problem tree for undernutrition in children and adolescente

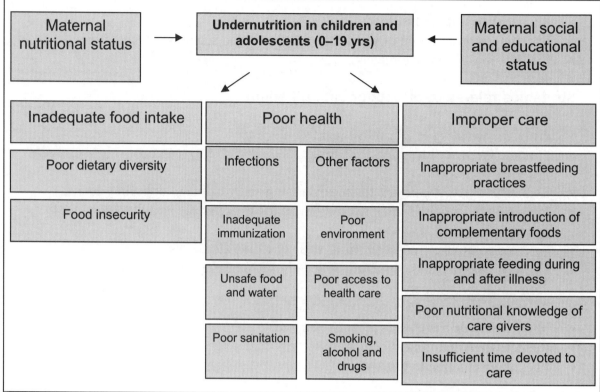

Strategies to improve undernutrition in children and adolescents

- Promote exclusive breastfeeding from birth to six months of age.
- Promote the introduction of complementary feeding at six months.
- Promote continued breastfeeding until two years of age or beyond.
- Promote age-appropriate complementary feeding.
- Promote the eating of a healthy breakfast at home.
- Promote the bringing to school of healthy meals and snacks prepared at home.
- Promote the sale of healthy foods in the school environment (school shops, canteens and food vendors).
- Promote age-appropriate physical activity.
- Reduce exposure to advertising.
- Implement nutrition education for children and their parents using teacher–child–parent nutrition education.
- Promote community involvement in healthy eating at schools.
- Promote dairy products.
- Promote the eating of a variety of animal foods.
- Make fruits and vegetables attractive and tasty.
- Improve reproductive-age and maternal health and nutrition status.
- Promote the prevention, detection and appropriate management of infections.
- Promote correct feeding practices during illness and recovery.
- Carry out timely immunization.
- Raise awareness of alcohol/tobacco/drugs risks.

Problem tree for overweight and obesity in adults

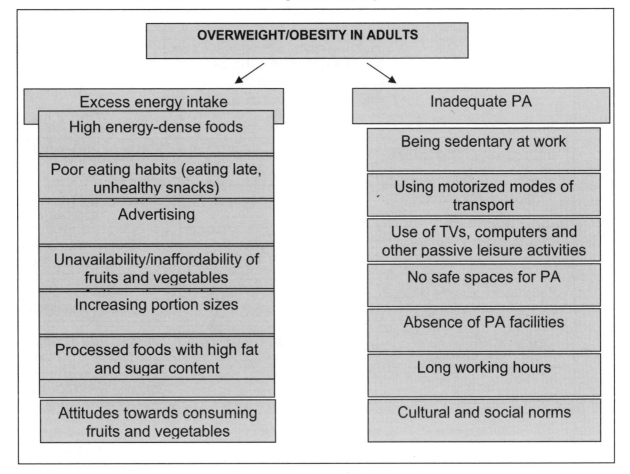

Strategies to decrease overweight in adults (reducing the energy density of the diet)

- Promote the bringing to work of healthy snacks and meals prepared at home.
- Implement nutrition education.
- Make fruits and vegetables available at the workplace.
- Promote healthy options in fast foods/encourage fast food outlets to reduce the energy density of their meals.
- Reduce (trans) fat in fast foods.
- Encourage decreased consumption of soda and its substitution with water (encourage people to drink more water).
- Promote low-fat dairy products.
- Promote a diversity of animal source protein to reduce the dependence on red meat only.

Problem tree for iron-deficiency anaemia and other micronutrient deficiencies

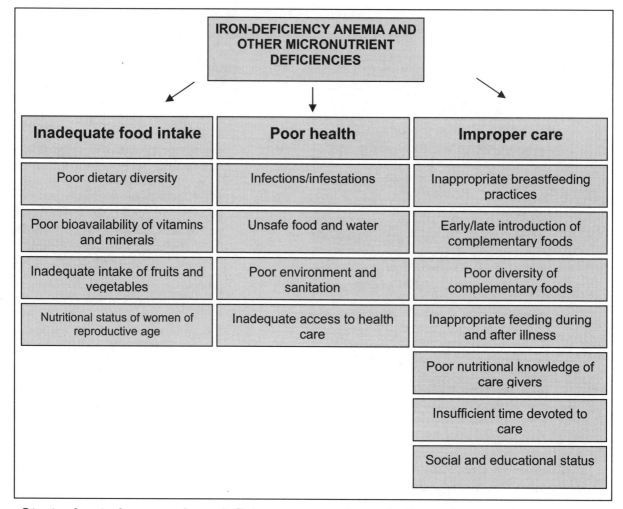

Strategies to improve iron-deficiency anaemia and other micronutrient deficiencies

- Promote dietary diversification.
- Increase intake of fruits and vegetables.
- Promote exclusive breastfeeding until six months of age.
- Promote the introduction of complementary feeding at six months.
- Promote continued breastfeeding until two years of age or beyond.
- Promote age-appropriate weaning practices.
- Promote the use of iodized salt and other fortified foods.
- Promote the prevention, detection and appropriate management of infections/infestations.
- Improve reproductive-age and maternal health and nutrition status.
- Promote micronutrient-rich food in school environments.
- Reduce children's exposure to the advertising and vending of unhealthy foods.
- Implement nutrition education for children and their parents using teacher–child–parent nutrition education.
- Promote community involvement in healthy eating at schools.

FAO TECHNICAL PAPERS

FAO FOOD AND NUTRITION PAPERS

1/1   Review of food consumption surveys 1977 – Vol. 1. Europe, North America, Oceania, 1977 (E)
1/2   Review of food consumption surveys 1977 – Vol. 2. Africa, Latin America, Near East, Far East, 1979 (E)
2   Report of the joint FAO/WHO/UNEP conference on mycotoxins, 1977 (E F S)
3   Report of a joint FAO/WHO expert consultation on dietary fats and oils in human nutrition, 1977 (E F S)
4   JECFA specifications for identity and purity of thickening agents, anticaking agents, antimicrobials, antioxidants and emulsifiers, 1978 (E)
5   JECFA – guide to specifications, 1978 (E F)
5 Rev. 1 JECFA – guide to specifications, 1983 (E F)
5 Rev. 2 JECFA – guide to specifications, 1991 (E)
6   The feeding of workers in developing countries, 1976 (E S)
7   JECFA specifications for identity and purity of food colours, enzyme preparations and other food additives, 1978 (E F)
8   Women in food production, food handling and nutrition, 1979 (E F S)
9   Arsenic and tin in foods: reviews of commonly used methods of analysis, 1979 (E)
10   Prevention of mycotoxins, 1979 (E F S)
11   The economic value of breast-feeding, 1979 (E F)
12   JECFA specifications for identity and purity of food colours, flavouring agents and other food additives, 1979 (E F)
13   Perspective on mycotoxins, 1979 (E F S)
14   Manuals of food quality control:
14/1   Food control laboratory, 1979 (Ar E)
14/1 Rev.1 The food control laboratory, 1986 (E)
14/2   Additives, contaminants, techniques, 1980 (E)
14/3   Commodities, 1979 (E)
14/4   Microbiological analysis, 1979 (E F S)
14/5   Food inspection, 1981 (Ar E) (Rev. 1984, E S)
14/6   Food for export, 1979 (E S)
14/6 Rev.1 Food for export, 1990 (E S)
14/7   Food analysis: general techniques, additives, contaminants and composition, 1986 (C E)
14/8   Food analysis: quality, adulteration and tests of identity, 1986 (E)
14/9   Introduction to food sampling, 1988 (Ar C E F S)
14/10 Training in mycotoxins analysis, 1990 (E S)
14/11 Management of food control programmes, 1991 (E)
14/12 Quality assurance in the food control microbiological laboratory, 1992 (E F S)
14/13 Pesticide residue analysis in the food control laboratory, 1993 (E F)
14/14 Quality assurance in the food control chemical laboratory, 1993 (E)
14/15 Imported food inspection, 1993 (E F)
14/16 Radionuclides in food, 1994 (E)

14/17 Unacceptable visible can defects – a pictorial manual, 1998 (E F S)
15   Carbohydrates in human nutrition, 1980 (E F S)
16   Analysis of food consumption survey data for developing countries, 1980 (E F S)
17   JECFA specifications for identity and purity of sweetening agents, emulsifying agents, flavouring agents and other food additives, 1980 (E F)
18   Bibliography of food consumption surveys, 1981 (E)
18 Rev. 1 Bibliography of food consumption surveys, 1984 (E)
18 Rev. 2 Bibliography of food consumption surveys, 1987 (E)
18 Rev. 3 Bibliography of food consumption surveys, 1990 (E)
19   JECFA specifications for identity and purity of carrier solvents, emulsifiers and stabilizers, enzyme preparations, flavouring agents, food colours, sweetening agents and other food additives, 1981 (E F)
20   Legumes in human nutrition, 1982 (E F S)
21   Mycotoxin surveillance – a guideline, 1982 (E)
22   Guidelines for agricultural training curricula in Africa, 1982 (E F)
23   Management of group feeding programmes, 1982 (E F P S)
23 Rev. 1 Food and nutrition in the management of group feeding programmes, 1993 (E F S)
24   Evaluation of nutrition interventions, 1982 (E)
25   JECFA specifications for identity and purity of buffering agents, salts; emulsifiers, thickening agents, stabilizers; flavouring agents, food colours, sweetening agents and miscellaneous food additives, 1982 (E F)
26   Food composition tables for the Near East, 1983 (E)
27   Review of food consumption surveys 1981, 1983 (E)
28   JECFA specifications for identity and purity of buffering agents, salts, emulsifiers, stabilizers, thickening agents, extraction solvents, flavouring agents, sweetening agents and miscellaneous food additives, 1983 (E F)
29   Post-harvest losses in quality of food grains, 1983 (E F)
30   FAO/WHO food additives data system, 1984 (E)
30 Rev. 1 FAO/WHO food additives data system, 1985 (E)
31/1   JECFA specifications for identity and purity of food colours, 1984 (E F)
31/2   JECFA specifications for identity and purity of food additives, 1984 (E F)
32   Residues of veterinary drugs in foods, 1985 (E/F/S)
33   Nutritional implications of food aid: an annotated bibliography, 1985 (E)
34   JECFA specifications for identity and purity of certain food additives, 1986 (E F)
35   Review of food consumption surveys 1985, 1986 (E)
36   Guidelines for can manufacturers and food canners, 1986 (E)
37   JECFA specifications for identity and purity of certain food additives, 1986 (E F)

38	JECFA specifications for identity and purity of certain food additives, 1988 (E)	47/1	Utilization of tropical foods: cereals, 1989 (E F S)
39	Quality control in fruit and vegetable processing, 1988 (E F S)	47/2	Utilization of tropical foods: roots and tubers, 1989 (E F S)
40	Directory of food and nutrition institutions in the Near East, 1987 (E)	47/3	Utilization of tropical foods: trees, 1989 (E F S)
41	Residues of some veterinary drugs in animals and foods, 1988 (E)	47/4	Utilization of tropical foods: tropical beans, 1989 (E F S)
41/2	Residues of some veterinary drugs in animals and foods. Thirty-fourth meeting of the joint FAO/WHO Expert Committee on Food Additives, 1990 (E)	47/5	Utilization of tropical foods: tropical oil seeds, 1989 (E F S)
41/3	Residues of some veterinary drugs in animals and foods. Thirty-sixth meeting of the joint FAO/WHO Expert Committee on Food Additives, 1991 (E)	47/6	Utilization of tropical foods: sugars, spices and stimulants, 1989 (E F S)
41/4	Residues of some veterinary drugs in animals and foods. Thirty-eighth meeting of the joint FAO/WHO Expert Committee on Food Additives, 1991 (E)	47/7	Utilization of tropical foods: fruits and leaves, 1990 (E F S)
		47/8	Utilization of tropical foods: animal products, 1990 (E F S)
41/5	Residues of some veterinary drugs in animals and foods. Fortieth meeting of the Joint FAO/WHO Expert Committee on Food Additives, 1993 (E)	48	Number not assigned
		49	JECFA specifications for identity and purity of certain food additives, 1990 (E)
41/6	Residues of some veterinary drugs in animals and foods. Forty-second meeting of the Joint FAO/WHO Expert Committee on Food Additives, 1994 (E)	50	Traditional foods in the Near East, 1991 (E)
		51	Protein quality evaluation. Report of the Joint FAO/WHO Expert Consultation, 1991 (E F)
41/7	Residues of some veterinary drugs in animals and foods. Forty-third meeting of the Joint FAO/WHO Expert Committee on Food Additives, 1994 (E)	52/1	Compendium of food additive specifications – Vol. 1, 1993 (E)
41/8	Residues of some veterinary drugs in animals and foods. Forty-fifth meeting of the Joint FAO/WHO Expert Committee on Food Additives, 1996 (E)	52/2	Compendium of food additive specifications – Vol. 2, 1993 (E)
		52 Add. 1	Compendium of food additive specifications – Addendum 1, 1992 (E)
41/9	Residues of some veterinary drugs in animals and foods. Forty-seventh meeting of the Joint FAO/ WHO Expert Committee on Food Additives, 1997 (E)	52 Add. 2	Compendium of food additive specifications – Addendum 2, 1993 (E)
		52 Add. 3	Compendium of food additive specifications – Addendum 3, 1995 (E)
41/10	Residues of some veterinary drugs in animals and foods. Forty-eighth meeting of the Joint FAO/WHO Expert Committee on Food Additives, 1998 (E)	52 Add. 4	Compendium of food additive specifications – Addendum 4, 1996 (E)
		52 Add. 5	Compendium of food additive specifications – Addendum 5, 1997 (E)
41/11	Residues of some veterinary drugs in animals and foods. Fiftieth meeting of the Joint FAO/WHO Expert Committee on Food Additives, 1999 (E)	52 Add. 6	Compendium of food additive specifications – Addendum 6, 1998 (E)
		52 Add. 7	Compendium of food additive specifications – Addendum 7, 1999 (E)
41/12	Residues of some veterinary drugs in animals and foods. Fifty-second meeting of the Joint FAO/WHO Expert Committee on Food Additives, 2000 (E)	52 Add. 8	Compendium of food additive specifications – Addendum 8, 2000 (E)
		52 Add. 9	Compendium of food additive specifications – Addendum 9, 2001 (E)
41/13	Residues of some veterinary drugs in animals and foods. Fifty-forth meeting of the Joint FAO/WHO Expert Committee on Food Additives, 2000 (E)	52 Add. 10	Compendium of food additive specifications – Addendum 10, 2002 (E)
		52 Add. 11	Compendium of food additive specifications – Addendum 11, 2003 (E)
41/14	Residues of some veterinary drugs in animals and foods. Fifty-eighth meeting of the Joint FAO/WHO Expert Committee on Food Additives, 2002 (E)	52 Add. 12	Compendium of food additive specifications – Addendum 12, 2004 (E)
		52 Add. 13	Compendium of food additive specifications – Addendum 13, 2005 (E)
41/15	Residues of some veterinary drugs in animals and foods. Sixtieth meeting of the Joint FAO/WHO Expert Committee on Food Additives, 2003 (E)	53	Meat and meat products in human nutrition in developing countries, 1992 (E)
		54	Number not assigned
41/16	Residues of some veterinary drugs in animals and foods. Monographs prepared by the sixty-second meeting of the Joint FAO/WHO Expert Committee on Food Additives, 2004 (E)	55	Sampling plans for aflatoxin analysis in peanuts and corn, 1993 (E)
		56	Body mass index – A measure of chronic energy deficiency in adults, 1994 (E F S)
42	Traditional food plants, 1988 (E)	57	Fats and oils in human nutrition, 1995 (Ar E F S)
42/1	Edible plants of Uganda. The value of wild and cultivated plants as food, 1989 (E)	58	The use of hazard analysis critical control point (HACCP) principles in food control, 1995 (E F S)
43	Guidelines for agricultural training curricula in Arab countries, 1988 (Ar)		
44	Review of food consumption surveys 1988, 1988 (E)		
45	Exposure of infants and children to lead, 1989 (E)		
46	Street foods, 1990 (E/F/S)		

59	Nutrition education for the public, 1995 (E F S)
60	Food fortification: technology and quality control, 1996 (E)
61	Biotechnology and food safety, 1996 (E)
62	Nutrition education for the public – Discussion papers of the FAO Expert Consultation, 1996 (E)
63	Street foods, 1997 (E/F/S)
64	Worldwide regulations for mycotoxins 1995 – A compendium, 1997 (E)
65	Risk management and food safety, 1997 (E)
66	Carbohydrates in human nutrition, 1998 (E S)
67	Les activités nutritionnelles au niveau communautaire – Expériences dans les pays du Sahel, 1998 (F)
68	Validation of analytical methods for food control, 1998 (E)
69	Animal feeding and food safety, 1998 (E)
70	The application of risk communication to food standards and safety matters, 1999 (Ar C E F S)
71	Joint FAO/WHO Expert Consultation on Risk Assessment of Microbiological Hazards in Foods, 2004 (E F S)
72	Joint FAO/WHO Expert Consultation on Risk Assessment of Microbiological Hazards in Foods – Risk characterization of *Salmonella* spp. in eggs and broiler chickens and *Listeria monocytogenes* in ready-to-eat foods, 2001 (E F S)
73	Manual on the application of the HACCP system in mycotoxin prevention and control, 2001 (E F S)
74	Safety evaluation of certain mycotoxins in food, 2001 (E)
75	Risk assessment of *Campylobacter* spp. in broiler chickens and *Vibrio* spp. in seafood, 2003 (E)
76	Assuring food safety and quality – Guidelines for strengthening national food control systems, 2003 (E F S)
77	Food energy – Methods of analysis and conversion factors, 2003 (E)
78	Energy in human nutrition. Report of a Joint FAO/WHO/UNU Expert Consultation, 2003 (E). Issued as No. 1 in the FAO Food and Nutrition Technical Report Series entitled Human energy requirements, Report of a Joint FAO/WHO/UNU Expert Consultation, 2004 (E)
79	Safety assessment of foods derived from genetically modified animals, including fish, 2004 (E)
80	Marine biotoxins, 2004 (E)
81	Worldwide regulations for mycotoxins in food and feed in 2003, 2004 (C E F S)
82	Safety evaluation of certain contaminants in food, 2005 (E)
83	Globalization of food systems in developing countries: impact on food security and nutrition, 2004 (E)
84	The double burden of malnutrition – Case studies from six developing countries, 2006 (E)

Availability: March 2006

Ar	–	Arabic	Multil	– Multilingual
C	–	Chinese	*	Out of print
E	–	English	**	In preparation
F	–	French		
P	–	Portuguese		
S	–	Spanish		

The FAO Technical Papers are available through the authorized FAO Sales Agents or directly from Sales and Marketing Group, FAO, Viale delle Terme di Caracalla, 00100 Rome, Italy.